Specialty Board Review

FAMILY PRACTICE

Sixth Edition

Specialty Board Review

FAMILY PRACTICE

Sixth Edition

Ernest Yuh-Ting Yen
Cerritos, California

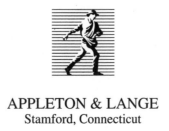

APPLETON & LANGE
Stamford, Connecticut

Copyright © 1999 by Appleton & Lange
A Simon & Schuster Company
Copyright © 1995, 1990 by Appleton & Lange
Copyright © 1985, 1980, 1975 by Prentice Hall, Inc.

www.appletonlange.com

99 00 01 02 03 / 10 9 8 7 6 5 4 3 2 1

Prentice Hall International (UK) Limited, *London*
Prentice Hall of Australia Pty. Limited, *Sydney*
Prentice Hall Canada, Inc., *Toronto*
Prentice Hall Hispanoamericana, S.A., *Mexico*
Prentice Hall of India Private Limited, *New Delhi*
Prentice Hall of Japan, Inc., *Tokyo*
Simon & Schuster Asia Pte. Ltd., *Singapore*
Editora Prentice Hall do Brasil Ltda., *Rio de Janeiro*
Prentice Hall, *Upper Saddle River, New Jersey*

Library of Congress Cataloging-in-Publication Data

Yen, Ernest Yuh-Ting, 1937–
    Specialty board review, family practice / Ernest Yuh-Ting Yen. —
6th ed.
      p.   cm.
    Includes bibliographical references.
    ISBN 0-8385-8739-9 (pbk : alk. paper)
    1. Family medicine—Examinations, questions, etc.   I. Title.
    [DNLM: 1. Family Practice examination questions.   WB 18.2 Y45s
1999]
    RC58.Y46   1999
    610'.76—dc21
    DNLM/DLC
    for Library of Congress   98-3615
                                                                CIP

Acquisitions Editor: Marinita Timban
Production Editor: Mary Ellen McCourt
Production Service: Rainbow Graphics, LLC
Cover Designer: Libby Schmitz

ISBN 0-8385-8739-9

90000

9 780838 7393

PRINTED IN THE UNITED STATES OF AMERICA

Contents

7. Internal Medicine

8. Pediatrics

Preface

The primary objective of a family practice residency training program is to produce family physicians who provide comprehensive and continuous total health care for the family in meeting community health needs. Accordingly, learning environments are organized for family practice residents to experience comprehensive and continuous total health care for their assigned panels of families. Although supervision is conducted by the attending physicians, the experiential learning is characterized by individual residents' self-assessment and self-growth. Didactic lectures, seminars, and conferences are offered to build a conceptual framework in facilitating residents' experiential learning. Computer-assisted learning, simulation instructions, and problem-solving techniques are used to enhance the residents' experiences. The present volume is designed to augment residents' experiential learning, reinforce their self-assessment and

self-growth, and better prepare them for the certification examination of the American Board of Family Practice.

There are many family medicine continuing medical education programs that prepare family physicians for the recertification examination. The present volume prepares many materials from subject areas of these programs and should be of interest to family physicians planning to take the recertification examination.

Many materials in the present volume were reviewed, updated, and prepared by faculty members and graduates of the Harbor–UCLA Family Practice Residency Training Program, Torrance, California. Their efforts are highly appreciated. Secretarial assistance from Ms. Rebecca Sun, Hui-Mei Huang, and Su-Yueh Yang of the Tainan Municipal Hospital, Tainan, Taiwan, was invaluable in the completion of the work.

Introduction

HELPFUL TIPS FOR EXAMINATION

Applications for Taking Examinations

A petition to take the examination should be made early to allow for a possible delay in application procedures. Complete and accurate applications should be submitted along with all required documents and correct fees.

Preparation Plans

1. In drafting a study schedule, remember that the date of the examination is the deadline date by which all preparations are to be completed. It is important to stick to the study schedule and complete it.
2. Start early and allocate ample time for preparation.
3. Review all subject areas; start with those subjects that are less familiar, and spend more time on those subjects that will probably constitute a large part of the examination.
4. Family practice cuts across all clinical disciplines; review first the more focused areas (such as urology and otorhinolaryngology) and then the broad disciplines (such as internal medicine and pediatrics).
5. Read familiar textbooks first; use question-and-answer books to assess the progress. Enhance weak areas through further readings of reference sources.
6. As the date of the examination approaches, the golden rule of contentment is essential.
7. On the day before the examination, keep a clear head, calm mind, and confident outlook. A good night's sleep before the examination is beneficial. Do not take any sedatives that are unfamiliar.

On the Day of the Examination

1. Be sure to wake up in time—an alarm clock may be needed.
2. Do not get hypoglycemic. Eat a good, light breakfast and bring candies, soda, or gum with you.
3. Dress comfortably and casually; bring along a working watch, two pencils, and necessary identifications.
4. Arrive at the examination site ahead of time; take into account a possible traffic jam.
5. If you must smoke, request special permission to leave the room for a break.
6. Ask permission for use of the toilet facilities.
7. Time yourself on the test. Reserve time for rechecking the answers. For multiple-choice answers, plan to spend no more than 40 seconds per item.
8. Follow directions printed at the beginning of each section of the test. Follow the directions given for each special group of questions. Be aware of the changes in examination format.
9. Make sure that the answer corresponds correctly to the question and that the correct answer is given on the answer sheet.
10. Answer all multiple-choice questions.

11. Try not to discuss the examination during the breaks; use the breaks to prepare for the next session.

COMMON TYPES OF MULTIPLE-CHOICE EXAMINATION QUESTIONS

One-Best-Response Type

The question contains the stem followed by five suggested lettered answers (A, B, C, D, E). Only one answer is correct. The examinee is instructed to select only the best or most appropriate answer among five alternative answers given. There is a 20% (one out of five) chance of choosing the correct answer just by random guessing. Through the process of elimination (discussed later in this introduction), the examinee can guess intelligently to select the correct answer.

Excluded-Term Type (Negative-Term Type)

The stem of the question is followed by five suggested lettered answers (A, B, C, D, E) of which all but one (ie, four answers) are applicable to the statement or situation described by the stem. The examinee is instructed to choose the one answer that is least applicable to the statement or situation of the stem. The commonly used negative words include EXCEPT, LEAST, and NOT. The examinee should remember that the "wrong" answer is the "correct" response.

Matching Type

A matching question consists of a list of lettered headings followed by a list of numbered words or phrases. The examinee is asked to select one or several headings most closely related to each of the numbered words or phrases. There are usually five lettered headings (A, B, C, D, E) and fewer than five numbered items (usually two or three). Only one lettered heading is matched with each numbered item, and each lettered heading can be used once, more than once, or not at all. To prepare for the matching questions, a familiarity with word association in medicine is useful.

Modified Matching Type

The list of numbered questions (often two or three) is preceded by four lettered answers (A, B, C, D). The examinee is instructed to answer:

A, if the numbered question is associated with A only.

B, if the numbered question is associated with B only.

C, if the numbered question is associated with both A and B.

D, if the numbered question is associated with neither A nor B.

Each lettered answer (A, B, C, D) can be used once, more than once, or not at all. This type of question is used to make the examinee identify the similarity (association) of and difference between A and B, and the questions usually concern the differential diagnosis of A and B.

Modified Multiple True–False Type

Each test item consists of an item followed by four or five lettered options (ie, options A, B, C, D, or options A, B, C, D, E). The examinee is asked to evaluate all options: if the option is true (or correct), answer the option with "T"; If the option is false (or incorrect), answer the option with "F."

In this type of question, all options are listed randomly and do not denote priority or sequential relationships among options. All options may be correct or all may be incorrect; there is no specific pattern that can be identified. Although all options are somehow related to each other (eg, describe the different aspects of the same illness), each option needs to be examined separately, independent of other options listed. This question type forms the basic unit of the clinical set problems.

Pictorial Quizzes

Pictorial quizzes may use all seven types of multiple-choice questions (one-best-response type, excluded-term type, matching type, modified matching type, standard and modified multiple true–false type, and situation type) in presenting the pictorial illustrations in the question either as numbered items or as lettered items. The pictorial illustration includes x-rays, ECGs, skin conditions, eye problems, eye grounds, blood smears, bone-marrow smears, urine sediments, audiograms, gross and microscopic specimens, experimental graphs, anatomic atlases, statistical charts, and summary tables. Pictures, graphs, tables, or x-rays that are used in the examination are usually typical cases, and the examinee should look for the central focus to select the correct responses. Whenever pictorial questions are accompanied by case histories, the examinee should review the case histories in detail *first,* then analyze the illustrations according to the characteristics expected from the case histories given in the question. The pictorial quizzes will be further discussed later in this introduction.

HELPFUL HINTS FOR GUESSING MULTIPLE-CHOICE QUESTIONS WHEN THE ANSWERS ARE NOT KNOWN

1. Use the process of elimination. Cross out wrong responses, and eliminate the unlikely responses; then select the most probable response among the remaining ones.
2. Look for verbal cues. A statement with "may" is often correct; a statement containing "always," "never," or "100% of the patients" may be incorrect.
3. The content of one item may indicate the answer to another item. Similar questions are often, repeated; often, the same questions appear.
4. Look for the design of the alternatives. A statement that does not grammatically follow the stem of the question may be incorrect. The shortest or the longest alternative may be the correct one.
5. In the best-response–type question, if two alternatives are similar, both may be incorrect. If they are contradictory, one may be correct.
6. A statement with unfamiliar technical terms may be an incorrect response.
7. "All of the above" or "none of the above" is usually the correct response.
8. In the situation-type question, the answer is often related to the correct response for a previous question.
9. Generally, true–false tests have a greater number of true answers.
10. Occasionally, rely on your intuition.

THE PICTORIAL QUIZ

The pictorial quiz is a form of the multiple-choice question. Each question concerning a pictorial illus-

tration may have to be answered within 30 to 45 seconds, as with other multiple-choice questions. Thus, the examinee should concentrate on the recognition of specific patterns in the pictorial illustration related to the disease or problem situation presented in the question, so as to answer the question correctly within an allowable span of time, rather than spending a great deal of time analyzing and interpreting the pictorial illustrations. To do this, the examinee is expected to become thoroughly familiar with the popular topics listed below.

Radiology

Chest x-ray
1. Miliary tuberculosis
2. Interstitial pneumonitis
3. Pulmonary infarction
4. Diaphragmatic hernia
5. Staphylococcal pneumonia
6. Hiatal hernia
7. Mitral stenosis
8. Transposition of the vessels
9. Tetralogy of Fallot
10. Retrosternal goiter
11. Posterior mediastinal tumor
12. Silicosis
13. Asbestosis
14. Hyaline membrane disease
15. Pneumothorax
16. Aspergilloma
17. Lobar pneumonia

Bones
1. Severe iron deficiency anemia—skull
2. Multiple myeloma
3. Paget's disease
4. Lead poisoning
5. Hyperparathyroidism
6. Rheumatoid arthritis
7. Gout
8. Psoriatic arthritis
9. Sarcoidosis
10. Osteoarthritis
11. Ankylosing spondylitis—spine
12. Osteoporosis
13. Osteomalacia
14. Congenital syphilis
15. Chronic osteomyelitis

16. Congenital dislocation of the hip
17. Tuberculosis of the spine
18. Femoral slipped epiphysis
19. Avascular necrosis of the femur head
20. Child abuse
21. Osteogenic sarcoma
22. Gaucher's disease
23. Osteogenesis imperfecta
24. Bursitis, muscle calcification
25. Fracture, radial styloid process
26. Fracture, femoral supracondyle

Gastrointestinal Tract
1. Carcinoma of the esophagus
2. Duodenal atresia
3. Chronic duodenal ulcer
4. Gastric carcinoma
5. Ulcerative colitis
6. Crohn's disease
7. Perforated bowel
8. Paralytic ileus
9. Volvulus
10. Intussusception
11. Intestinal mechanic obstruction
12. Diverticulosis
13. Polyposis coli
14. Chronic pancreatitis
15. Meconium ileus
16. Esophageal varices
17. Fecalith—appendix
18. Carcinoma of the cecum
19. Gallstones

Genitourinary Tract
1. Hydronephrosis
2. Wilms' tumor
3. Neuroblastoma
4. Vesicoureteric reflux
5. Renal stones

Skull and CT Scan
1. Subdural hematoma
2. Hydrocephalus
3. Brain tumor—astrocytoma
4. Meningioma
5. Intracranial calcification—toxoplasmosis, tuberous sclerosis, Sturge—Weber syndrome, cytomegalovirus
6. Craniopharyngioma
7. Brain abscess

Bone Scan
1. Osteomyelitis
2. Bone cysts

Thyroid Scan
1. Cold and hot nodules

Ophthalmology
1. Optic atrophy
2. Diabetic retinopathy
3. Hypertensive retinopathy
4. Central vein occlusion
5. Central artery occlusion
6. Choroiditis
7. Tay–Sachs' disease
8. Papilledema
9. Glaucoma
10. Kayser–Fleischer ring
11. Subconjunctival hemorrhage
12. Chalazion
13. Pterygium
14. External hordeolum

Audiogram
1. Serous otitis media
2. Congenital deafness (rubella)
3. Ménière's disease
4. Otosclerosis
5. Noise exposure
6. Presbycusis
7. Acoustic neuroma
8. Drug ototoxicity

Electrocardiogram
1. Mitral stenosis
2. Left ventricular enlargement
3. Heart block—1º, 2º, 3º, Wenckebach phenomenon
4. Atrial fibrillation
5. Atrial flutter
6. Digitalis poisoning
7. Hypokalemia
8. Hyperkalemia
9. Hypocalcemia
10. Hypercalcemia
11. Myxedema
12. Infarction—anterior, anterolateral, inferior
13. Pulmonary embolism
14. Pericarditis
15. Bundle branch blocks

Hematology

1. Iron deficiency
2. Hemolytic disease of the newborn
3. Lead poisoning
4. Infectious mononucleosis
5. Megaloblastic anemia—peripheral smear
6. Megaloblastic anemia—bone marrow
7. Acute leukemia—bone marrow
8. Lupus erythematosus cell
9. Sickle cell anemia
10. Thalassemia major
11. Spherocytosis
12. Idiopathic thrombocytopenic purpura (ITP)—bone marrow
13. Ovalocytosis
14. Bone marrow neuroblastoma
15. Reed–Sternberg cells (bone marrow)
16. Auer rod in acute myeloblastic leukemia
17. Pernicious anemia
18. Multiple myeloma

Dermatology and Photographs

1. Psoriasis
2. Primary and secondary syphilis
3. Rosacea
4. Measles
5. Rocky Mountain spotted fever
6. Chickenpox
7. Stevens–Johnson syndrome
8. Erythema nodosum
9. Lupus erythematosus
10. Scleroderma
11. Dermatomyositis
12. Von Recklinghausen's disease, neurofibromatosis
13. Adenoma sebaceum (tuberous sclerosis)
14. Sturge–Weber syndrome
15. Peutz–Jegher syndrome
16. Hereditary telangiectasia
17. Cellulitis
18. Pemphigus
19. Atopic dermatitis
20. Drug eruptions—fixed
21. Dermatitis herpetiformis
22. Melanoma
23. Poison ivy
24. Scabies
25. Tinea capitis, cruris
26. Acanthosis nigricans
27. Chancroid and chancre
28. Condyloma acuminatum and lata

29. Zoster
30. Impetigo
31. Pityriasis rosea
32. Seborrheic dermatitis
33. Herpes progenitalis and labialis
34. Gonococcal arthritis—dermatitis syndrome
35. Lymphogranuloma venereum
36. Congenital syphilis
37. Klinefelter syndrome
38. Turner syndrome
39. Down syndrome

Electroencephalogram

1. Petit mal
2. Brain tumor
3. Stroke—intracranial hemorrhage
4. Epilepsies
5. Head injury—hematomas

CLINICAL SET PROBLEMS

The clinical set problems are used to assess the examinee's clinical problem-solving ability. In clinical set problems, the modified multiple true–false-type question format is adopted.

The clinical set problem is constructed from simulated case studies, which often include the following patient management processes: history, physical, laboratory, diagnosis, treatment, and follow-up. Other relevant data of the clinical problems can also be included in the test items such as pathophysiology, high-risk factors, preventive measures, etiologic factors, cost consideration, facility, and staffing needs. In most clinical set problems, two or more clinical aspects of the simulated cases are selected to form a "clinical set."

At the beginning of each clinical set, initial information (eg, symptoms, signs, situation, laboratory and clinical findings) is provided to describe a clinical setting. Following this clinical framework, there are two or more (mostly three or four) test items presented. Each test item is constructed by the modified multiple true–false question format. Each test item consists of the lead-in stem and two or more (mostly five or six) numbered options. Each test item consists of a clinical aspect of the simulated case and often is represented by a question or an incomplete statement. With available information (often not complete) from the initial clinical presentations and the description in the stem, the examinee is asked to decide the truth or falsity of the numbered options listed following the stem. These options are listed randomly and are not listed according to priority or any orderly sequence. All options may be true or all options may be false. The examinee is asked to answer "T" if the option is essential and important in the total management of the patient or family; and to answer "F" if the option is irrelevant or inappropriate in the total management of the patient or family. To determine the truth of each option, the examinee should follow the basic principles of family medicine including comprehensive (eg, psycho-social and preventive care) and continuous (eg, follow-ups) total health care for the patient and family. Although rare and uncommon clinical problems in daily practice may appear in the clinical set problems, the examinee needs to be thoroughly familiar with common clinical problems seen in family practice. The updated information of the pathophysiology of these common problems is frequently requested.

The following clinical case studies are to be familiarized:

1. Migraine headache
2. Acute neurolabyrinthitis
3. Acute sinusitis
4. Acute otitis media
5. Depression
6. Anxiety
7. Alzheimer's disease
8. Streptococcal pharyngitis
9. Bronchial asthma
10. Pneumonia
11. Graves' disease
12. Angina pectoris
13. Hypertension
14. Congestive heart failure
15. Breast cancer
16. Peptic ulcer disease
17. Acute appendicitis
18. Irritable bowel syndrome
19. Acute gastroenteritis
20. Colorectal cancer
21. Urinary tract infection
22. Nephrolithiasis
23. Pelvic inflammatory disease
24. Endometriosis
25. Vaginitis
26. Ectopic pregnancy
27. Contraception counseling
28. Normal prenatal care
29. Newborn care
30. Well-child care
31. Genetic counseling
32. Lumbar disk disease
33. Parkinson's disease
34. Panic disorder
35. Drug abuse
36. Alcoholism
37. Smoking cessation
38. Pernicious anemia
39. HIV care
40. Constitutional growth delay
41. Somatization
42. Anterior cruciate ligament injury of the knee
43. Periodic health screening
44. Pinworm infestations
45. Clostridial myonecrosis
46. Psittacosis
47. Polymyalgia rheumatica
48. Kawasaki syndrome
49. Dysfunctional uterine bleeding
50. Pigmented lesions

References

1. Taylor R. *Family Medicine, Principles and Practice*, 4th ed. New York: Springer-Verlag, 1994

2. Rakel E. *Textbook of Family Practice*, 5th ed. Philadelphia, PA: W.B. Saunders, 1995

3. Sloane P. *Essentials of Family Medicine*, 2nd ed. Baltimore, MD: Williams & Wilkins, 1993

4. Rakel E. *Essentials of Family Practice*. Philadelphia, PA: W.B. Saunders, 1993

5. Birrer B. *Urban Family Medicine*. New York: Springer-Verlag, 1987

6. Albert DM, et al. *Principles and Practice of Ophthalmology Clinical Practice*. Philadelphia, PA: W.B. Saunders, 1994

7. Kaplan H. *Comprehensive Textbook of Psychiatry VI*. Baltimore, MD: Williams & Wilkins, 1995

8. Morrey BF. *The Elbow and Its Disorders*, 2nd ed. Philadelphia, PA: W.B. Saunders, 1993

9. Matzen RN, et al. *Clinical Preventive Medicine*. St. Louis, MO: Mosby-Year Book, 1993

10. Donald PJ, et al. *The Sinuses*. New York: Raven Press, 1995

11. Berek JS. *Novak's Gynecology*, 12th ed. Baltimore, MD: Williams & Wilkins, 1996

12. Avery M. *Pediatric Medicine*. Baltimore, MD: Williams & Wilkins, 1989

13. Cummings CW, et al. *Otolaryngology—Head and Neck Surgery*, 2nd ed. St. Louis, MO: Mosby-Year Book, 1993

14. Pernoll M. *Current Obstetric & Gynecologic Diagnosis & Treatment*. Norwalk, CT: Appleton & Lange, 1991

15. Krane RJ, et al. *Clinical Urology*. Philadelphia, PA: J.B. Lippincott, 1994

16. Wyngaarden J. *Cecil Textbook of Medicine*, 19th ed. Philadelphia, PA: W.B. Saunders, 1992

17. Taylor R. *Fundamentals of Family Medicine*. New York: Springer, 1996

18. Scott J. *Danforth's Obstetrics and Gynecology*, 6th ed. Philadelphia, PA: J.B. Lippincott, 1990

19. Cunningham FG, et al. *Williams Obstetrics*, 19th ed. Norwalk, CT: Appleton & Lange, 1993

20. Wilson R. *Obstetrics and Gynecology*, 9th ed. St. Louis, MO: Mosby-Year Book, 1991

21. Sabiston D. *Textbook of Surgery*, 14th ed. Philadelphia, PA: W.B. Saunders, 1991

22. Weatherall DJ, et al. *Oxford Textbook of Medicine*, 3rd ed. Oxford: Oxford Medical Publications, 1996

23. Barker R. *Principles of Ambulatory Medicine*, 3rd ed. Baltimore, MD: Williams & Wilkins, 1991

24. White GM. *Color Atlas of Regional Dermatology*. New York: Mosby-Wolfe, 1994

25. Apley AG, et al. *Apley's System of Orthopedics and Fractures*, 7th ed. Oxford: Butterworth Heinemann, 1993

26. Fitzpatrick T. *Color Atlas and Synopsis of Clinical Dermatology*, 2nd ed. New York: McGraw-Hill, 1992

27. Fitzpatrick T. *Dermatology in General Medicine*, 4th ed. New York: McGraw-Hill, 1993

28. Colman BH. *Disease of the Nose, Throat and Ear, and Head and Neck*, 14th ed. New York: Churchill Livingstone, 1992

29. Vaughan D. *General Ophthalmology*, 13th ed. Norwalk, CT: Appleton & Lange, 1992

30. Misbell DR Jr., et al. *Management of Common Problems in Obstetrics and Gynecology*, 3rd ed. Boston: Blackwell Scientific Pub., 1994

31. Carr PL, et al. *The Medical Care of Women*. Philadelphia, PA: W.B. Saunders, 1995

32. Moore TR, et al. *Gynecology & Obstetrics, a Longitudinal Approach.* New York: Churchill Livingstone, 1993

33. Isselbacher KJ, et al. *Harrison's Principles of Internal Medicine,* 13th ed. New York: McGraw-Hill, 1994

34. Copeland LJ. *Textbook of Gynecology.* Philadelphia, PA: W.B. Saunders, 1993

35. Tanagho E. *Smith's General Urology,* 14th ed. Norwalk, CT: Appleton & Lange, 1995

36. Lee K. *Essential Otolaryngology.* New York: Medical Examination Publishing Co., 1991

37. Harvey M. *The Principles and Practice of Medicine,* 22nd ed. Norwalk, CT: Appleton & Lange, 1988

38. Ballenger J. *Diseases of the Nose, Throat, Ear, Head and Neck,* 14th ed. Philadelphia, PA: Lea & Febiger, 1991

39. Wiesel S. *Essentials of Orthopedic Surgery.* Philadelphia, PA: W.B. Saunders, 1993

40. McCarty D. *Arthritis and Allied Condition,* 12th ed. Philadelphia, PA: Lea & Febiger, 1993

41. Schrier R. *Diseases of the Kidney,* 5th ed. Boston: Little, Brown & Co., 1993

42. Oski F. *Principles and Practice of Pediatrics.* Philadelphia, PA: J.B. Lippincott, 1990

43. Hardman JG, et al. *Goodman & Gilman's The Pharmacological Basis of Therapeutics,* 9th ed. New York: McGraw-Hill, 1996

44. Hazzard W. *Principles of Geriatric Medicine and Gerontology,* 3rd ed. New York: McGraw-Hill, 1994

45. Williams JL, et al. *Rowe and Williams' Maxillofacial Injuries,* 2nd ed. Edinburgh: Churchill Livingstone, 1994

46. Spiro H. *Clinical Gastroenterology,* 4th ed. New York: McGraw-Hill, 1993

47. Ham R. *Primary Care Geriatrics,* 2nd ed. St. Louis, MO: Mosby-Year Book, 1992

48. Massry SG, et al. *Massry & Glassock's Textbook of Nephrology,* 3rd ed. Baltimore, MD: Williams & Wilkins, 1995

49. Hulley S. *Designing Clinical Research.* Baltimore, MD: Williams & Wilkins, 1988

50. Shott S. *Statistics for Health Professionals.* Philadelphia, PA: W.B. Saunders, 1990

51. Barker D. *Epidemiology in Medical Practice,* 4th ed. Edinburgh: Churchill Livingstone, 1988

52. Hennekens C. *Epidemiology in Medicine.* Boston: Little, Brown & Co., 1987

53. Hudson W. *Clinical Preventive Medicine.* Boston: Little, Brown & Co., 1988

54. Last J. *Maxy-Rosenau-Last Public Health and Preventive Medicine,* 13th ed. Stamford, CT: Appleton & Lange, 1992

55. Habif TP. *Clinical Dermatology: A Color Guide to Diagnosis and Therapy,* 3rd ed. St. Louis, MO: Mosby-Year Book, 1996

56. Kanski JJ. *Clinical Ophthalmology a Systematic Approach,* 3rd ed. Oxford: Butterworth Heinemann, 1994

57. Kaplan HI, et al. *Pocket Handbook of Psychiatric Drug Treatment.* Baltimore, MD: Williams & Wilkins, 1993

58. La Dou J. *Occupational Medicine.* Norwalk, CT: Appleton & Lange, 1990

59. Glass RH. *Office Gynecology,* 4th ed. Baltimore, MD: Williams & Wilkins, 1993

60. Woodley M. *Manual of Medical Therapeutics,* 27th ed. Boston: Little, Brown & Co., 1992

61. Kendell RE, et al. *Companion to Psychiatric Studies,* 5th ed. New York: Churchill Livingstone, 1993

62. Schwartz SI, et al. *Principles of Surgery,* 6th ed. New York: McGraw-Hill, 1994

63. Kelly W. *Textbook of Rheumatology,* 4th ed. Philadelphia, PA: W.B. Saunders, 1993

64. Cassidy J. *Textbook of Pediatric Rheumatology,* 2nd ed. New York: Churchill Livingstone, 1990

65. Tierney L. *Current Medical Diagnosis & Treatment,* 33rd ed. Norwalk, CT: Appleton & Lange, 1994

66. Behrman R. *Nelson Textbook of Pediatrics,* 15th ed. Philadelphia, PA: W.B. Saunders, 1996

67. Yao F, et al. *Anesthesiology: Problem-Oriented Patient Management,* 3rd ed. Philadelphia, PA: J.B. Lippincott, 1993

68. Rudolph A. *Rudolph's Pediatrics,* 19th ed. Norwalk, CT: Appleton & Lange, 1991

69. McAnarny E. *Textbook of Adolescent Medicine.* Philadelphia, PA: W.B. Saunders, 1992

70. Strosburger V. *Adolescent Medicine.* Boston: Little, Brown, & Co., 1991

71. Hoffman A. *Adolescent Medicine,* 2nd ed. Norwalk, CT: Appleton & Lange, 1989

72. Hanbrich WS, et al. *Bockus Gastroenterology,* 5th ed. Philadelphia, PA: W.B. Saunders, 1995

73. Lee GR, et al. *Wintrobe's Clinical Hematology,* 9th ed. Philadelphia, PA: Lea & Febiger, 1993

74. Mandell GL, et al. *Mandell, Douglas and Bennett's Principles and Practice of Infectious Disease,* 4th ed. New York: Churchill Livingstone, 1995

75. Stein JH, et al. *Internal Medicine,* 4th ed. St. Louis, MO: Mosby-Year Book, 1994

76. Pope AM, et al. *Environmental Medicine Integrating a Missing Element into Medical Education.* Washington, DC: National Academy Press, 1995

77. O'Donoghue GM, et al. *Clinical ENT: An Illustrated Textbook.* Oxford: Oxford University Press, 1992

78. Williamson RCN, et al. *Scott: An Aid to Clinical Surgery,* 5th ed. Edinburgh: Churchill Livingstone, 1994

79. Greenfield LJ, et al. *Surgery: Scientific Principles and Practice.* Philadelphia, PA: J.B. Lippincott, 1993

80. Balderston RA, et al. *The Hip.* Philadelphia, PA: Lea & Febiger, 1992

81. Brown JS. *Minor Surgery: A Text and Atlas,* 2nd ed. London: Chapman & Hall Medical, 1992

82. Driscoll CE, et al. *Procedures for Your Practice,* 2nd ed. Los Angeles: Practice Management Information Corporation, 1991

83. Strange GR. *Pediatric Emergency Medicine: A Comprehensive Study Guide.* New York: McGraw-Hill, 1996

84. Jahss MH. *Disorders of the Foot & Ankle: Medical and Surgical Management,* 2nd ed. Philadelphia, PA: W.B. Saunders, 1992

85. Lin CC, et al. *The High-Risk Fetus: Pathophysiology, Diagnosis, and Management.* New York: Springer-Verlag, 1993

CHAPTER 1

Psychiatry
Questions

DIRECTIONS (Questions 1 through 142): Each of the numbered items or incomplete statements in this section is followed by answers or by completions of the statement. Select the ONE lettered answer or completion that is BEST in each case.

1. Which of the following descriptions on medical ethics is correct?

    (A) Medical ethics attempts to motivate physicians to act more morally.
    (B) Medical ethics applies ethical principles in medical practice.
    (C) Medical ethics is a full-fledged subspecialty in medicine.
    (D) Medical ethics accounts for 75% of curricular time in urban family-practice residency programs.
    (E) Medical ethics is a new religion in the United States. *(Ref. 5)*

2. Which groups of women are most likely to divorce?

    (A) women who marry in their 30s
    (B) women who marry in their teens
    (C) women who marry in their 20s
    (D) women who marry late
    (E) women who are Catholic *(Ref. 5)*

3. The highest incidence of divorce comes at which stage of the family life cycle?

    (A) independent adulthood
    (B) early partnership
    (C) child rearing
    (D) late independent adulthood
    (E) middle and late partnership *(Ref. 5)*

4. Both biological parents are in the household of

    (A) single-parent families
    (B) adoptive families
    (C) step-families
    (D) nuclear families
    (E) foster families *(Ref. 5)*

5. In single-parent families

    (A) 20% are headed by women
    (B) 5% are due to the couple's separation or divorce
    (C) 80% of the parents are never married
    (D) the average income is much lower than the two-parent families
    (E) their number accounts for less than 1% of all families *(Ref. 5)*

6. Three times in the past month, a 32-year-old married white woman has arrived unexpectedly for consultation after hours at her family physician's office. She has complained of chest pain, but no specific physical findings can be discovered. She has also complained about the arrogance of the receptionist. The next time she arrives to see the doctor when he is working alone in the evening, he should

   (A) tell her firmly that there is nothing wrong with her and that she should see a psychiatrist
   (B) point out that she needs careful, thorough evaluation and give her the next available appointment during scheduled office hours
   (C) ask her to call the office next morning
   (D) sit down and have a good, long, heart-to-heart talk with her
   (E) drive her out of the office   (Ref. 7)

7. The first phase of the family life cycle is the

   (A) child-centered phase
   (B) contraction phase
   (C) adult-centered phase
   (D) expansion phase
   (E) grandparent-centered phase   (Ref. 5)

8. To make a legally acceptable will, the person making the will must fulfill all of the following criteria EXCEPT that he need not

   (A) know that he is making a will
   (B) know the nature and extent of his property
   (C) know the natural objects of his bounty
   (D) know what he is doing when he signs it
   (E) be able to read and write   (Ref. 2)

9. Three weeks after her 3-year-old son was killed in an auto accident, a previously well 28-year-old mother is suffering from waves of somatic distress, is irritable and unfriendly toward her husband, accuses herself unjustly of negligence, is unable to attend to her housework, and is preoccupied with visual images of her son in which she sees him calling her. The situation is probably

   (A) a normal grief reaction
   (B) acute psychotic depression
   (C) psychoneurosis
   (D) a paranoid state
   (E) toxic psychosis   (Ref. 7)

10. As part of the adjustment reaction of adolescence, all of the following symptoms may be present EXCEPT

   (A) school failure
   (B) delinquency
   (C) depression
   (D) sexual impulse
   (E) paranoid delusions   (Ref. 2)

11. A 35-year-old housewife is very anxious about being at home alone when her husband is away. She states that she is afraid someone may break into the house at night and says, "I don't see anything wrong with that. None of the women I know like to be alone at night." To facilitate her statement, you should say

   (A) "Well, it is reassuring to know you have the same anxieties that other housewives have."
   (B) "First, let us try to understand your feelings and what these feelings do to you."
   (C) "You are right, nothing is wrong with that."
   (D) "You mean that most of your friends like to be alone in the daytime."
   (E) "When you say 'alone' perhaps you are worried about sexual attack."   (Ref. 2)

12. When a patient encourages a physician to assume a directive position and then procrastinates in following the physician's suggestions, he is most likely to be

   (A) displaying a weak ego
   (B) trying to compensate for low self-esteem
   (C) malingering

(D) expressing hostility with passive rebellion

(E) afraid of the physician   *(Ref. 2)*

13. Separation anxiety in early childhood may be associated with

    (A) hospitalization
    (B) school phobia
    (C) maternal deprivation
    (D) transient normal reaction
    (E) all of the above   *(Ref. 2)*

14. A child with school phobia

    (A) requires tranquilizers
    (B) should be hospitalized to observe how he or she functions when separated from his or her family
    (C) should remain at home until he or she gets over it
    (D) should be sent back to school immediately, and then the underlying problem worked out
    (E) should go to school part-time   *(Ref. 2)*

15. Adjustment reactions are characterized by

    (A) transient reactions
    (B) symptomatic reaction to the current situation
    (C) symptomatic reaction to emotional conflict
    (D) relief when the situation is corrected
    (E) all of the above   *(Ref. 2)*

16. Alcoholism is often suspected by the following unexplained laboratory result

    (A) decreased hemoglobin
    (B) increased hemoglobin
    (C) decreased serum amylase level
    (D) increased mean corpuscular volume (MCV)
    (E) decreased MCV   *(Ref. 3)*

17. A young female patient gives a history of aching anterior chest pain interspersed with sharp stabs. She also complains of palpitations, difficulty in breathing, lightheaded-

ness, tingling of the extremities, and exhaustion, and you note that she sighs frequently. Physical examination is negative. The most likely diagnosis is

    (A) hyperventilation syndrome
    (B) metabolic alkalosis
    (C) respiratory acidosis
    (D) asthma
    (E) anemia   *(Ref. 7)*

18. Among the following, the most common reason to see a physician is

    (A) for health maintenance
    (B) for an annual physical examination
    (C) for discussing family problems
    (D) reaching tolerance threshold of a symptom
    (E) consultation on sexual dysfunctions   *(Ref. 5)*

19. Which of the following attitudes may enhance patient rapport?

    (A) nonjudgmental
    (B) prejudiced
    (C) hostile
    (D) businesslike
    (E) arrogant   *(Ref. 7)*

20. Common fantasies preceding suicidal acts include

    (A) fantasies of identification
    (B) fantasies of a reunion
    (C) fantasies of destroying a "bad" part
    (D) fantasies of rebirth
    (E) all of the above   *(Ref. 7)*

21. Active listening is most useful in

    (A) understanding patients' health-seeking behaviors
    (B) reconciling perception distance between the physician and the patient
    (C) obtaining information on family trees
    (D) assessing mental status
    (E) completing a review of systems   *(Ref. 5)*

22. To stabilize a conflicting dyad system, the couple will most likely

    (A) join another dyad
    (B) seek a third person to form a triangle
    (C) recruit two additional individuals to form a rectangle
    (D) resolve the original dyad and each person form a new dyad
    (E) invite three additional individuals to form a polygon   *(Ref. 5)*

23. In the management of somatization, it is best to educate the patient, shifting somatic preoccupation to productive life endeavors through an appointment schedule that is

    (A) spare
    (B) frequent
    (C) frequent and long
    (D) frequent and brief
    (E) spare and brief   *(Ref. 3)*

24. An ethical decision is made by

    (A) gut feelings
    (B) considering only information that you like
    (C) personal preferences
    (D) universal principles
    (E) an instant burst of emotions   *(Ref. 5)*

25. Trichotillomania is characterized by

    (A) manic–depressive behaviors
    (B) alopecia areata
    (C) broken hairs of varying length
    (D) silver, scaling plaques
    (E) vellus hairs in the genitalia   *(Ref. 27)*

26. Good results in achieving abstinence with alcoholics are obtained by

    (A) phenothiazine medication
    (B) vitamin B injections
    (C) membership in Alcoholics Anonymous
    (D) long-term hospitalization at mental hospitals
    (E) imprisonment   *(Ref. 7)*

27. Methadone is an opiate that

    (A) does not produce habituation
    (B) blocks the euphoric effects of other opiates
    (C) causes no withdrawal symptoms when stopped
    (D) is a morphine antagonist
    (E) has no analgesic effect   *(Ref. 7)*

28. During an interview, stroking the chin is most likely to be interpreted as

    (A) impatience
    (B) tension
    (C) interest
    (D) contemplation
    (E) relaxation   *(Ref. 5)*

29. A consequence-oriented approach is most likely to be used for

    (A) teleological ethics
    (B) deontologic ethics
    (C) descriptive ethics
    (D) normative ethics
    (E) golden ethics   *(Ref. 5)*

30. Professional autonomy is most highly regarded in which of the following practice options?

    (A) health maintenance organizations
    (B) family-practice residency teachings
    (C) multispecialty groups
    (D) solo practice
    (E) public health institutions   *(Ref. 5)*

31. A 74-year-old depressed female has improved by drug therapy. However, she now complains of weight gain. She probably is taking a

    (A) monoamine oxidase inhibitor (MAOI)
    (B) selective serotonin reuptake inhibitor (SSRI)
    (C) tricyclic antidepressant (TCA)
    (D) benzodiazepine
    (E) thyroid hormone   *(Ref. 7)*

32. What type of psychiatric disorder is frequently associated with carcinoma of the pancreas or large bowel?

(A) paranoid reaction
(B) phobic state
(C) depressive reaction
(D) schizophrenia
(E) antisocial personality   *(Ref. 7)*

33. Illness is

(A) an anomaly in the body structure
(B) cultural reactions to discomfort
(C) dysfunction of the cardiovascular system
(D) something an organ has
(E) laboratory abnormalities   *(Ref. 5)*

34. A 17-year-old white male was seen by you for a laceration wound in his hand. He told you that "bad guys" wanted him and injured his hand because he was an important person in the school. He also told you about his homosexual desires and that he planned to leave his girlfriend because of her promiscuity. You are possibly dealing with a case of

(A) depression
(B) juvenile delinquency
(C) adjustment reaction
(D) delusional disorder
(E) schizophrenia   *(Ref. 7)*

35. A response to the proverb "Two heads are better than one," or "A person with two heads could think better" is characteristic of

(A) a hysterical disorder
(B) good abstraction
(C) a schizophrenic reaction
(D) severe mental retardation
(E) an organic psychotic reaction   *(Ref. 7)*

36. Alcoholism is often associated with all of the following syndromes EXCEPT

(A) cirrhosis
(B) microcytic anemia
(C) gastritis
(D) encephalopathy
(E) labile hypertension   *(Ref. 3)*

37. A patient exhibits stiffness, tremor, and an expressionless face. The medication he has been taking is most likely

(A) barbiturates
(B) Tofranil (imipramine)
(C) Thorazine (chlorpromazine)
(D) Valium (diazepam)
(E) Miltown (meprobamate)   *(Ref. 7)*

38. Which of the following statements does not jeopardize confidentiality of the doctor–patient relationship?

(A) Suspected child abuse information should not be reported to protect the child.
(B) Reporting requirements for tuberculosis should be ignored for patients for whom you have cared for many years.
(C) Information on drug abuse by teenagers should be shared with their teachers.
(D) Information on contraceptive use by adolescents should be revealed to their mothers to institute corrective moral sanction.
(E) Positive gonococcal culture should be reported to the public health agency.

(Ref. 5)

39. To depict the significant life events of the family history, which of the following presentations is most commonly used?

(A) family life line
(B) family genogram
(C) family life cycle
(D) family system map
(E) family structure graph   *(Ref. 5)*

40. Pick's disease

(A) typically shows symptoms of apathy
(B) is more common in men than in women
(C) is more common than Alzheimer's disease
(D) typically affects the occipital lobe
(E) is characterized by senile plaques   *(Ref. 7)*

41. A patient with acute myocardial infarction is admitted to the coronary care unit (CCU). He is extremely anxious. You would

    (A) prescribe benzodiazepines
    (B) start corticosteroid continuous infusion
    (C) tell the patient that he will die soon
    (D) reassure the patient that he has no illness
    (E) promise the patient that you will discharge him in the morning   (Ref. 7)

42. Thomas is a frequent visitor to the family practice center, where he presents himself as a helpless person who feels he is not being adequately taken care of by the staff there. He is probably

    (A) passive–aggressive
    (B) a schizophrenic, hebephrenic type
    (C) an obsessive–compulsive neurotic
    (D) a drug addict
    (E) a phobic neurotic   (Ref. 7)

43. A 35-year-old housewife has had three episodes of chest pain during the past two weeks. Each time she has visited the emergency room, with normal electrocardiogram (ECG) and isoenzymes. Today she visited your office complaining of chest pain of one hour's duration. Results of physical examination and ECG are essentially normal. You would now

    (A) prescribe digitalis
    (B) prescribe dobutamine
    (C) prescribe hydralazine
    (D) provide psychotherapy
    (E) give IV morphine   (Ref. 7)

44. A 30-year-old housewife has been afraid of snakes and heights since childhood. During the past six months, she has experienced repeated panic attacks whenever she has driven an automobile across the downtown area. The treatment of choice is

    (A) benzodiazepines (Valium)
    (B) phenothiazines (Thorazine)
    (C) alprazolam (Xanax)
    (D) phenobarbital
    (E) propranolol (Inderal)   (Ref. 7)

45. The most dramatic responses to treatment with neuroleptics are generally seen in

    (A) severely depressed individuals
    (B) withdrawn and apathetic schizophrenics
    (C) manic and hypomanic individuals
    (D) agitated paranoid schizophrenics
    (E) chronic organic brain syndromes   (Ref. 7)

46. The pleasure principle is utilized by the

    (A) id
    (B) ego
    (C) ego ideal
    (D) superego
    (E) libido   (Ref. 7)

47. The most commonly abused drug in the United States is

    (A) diazepam
    (B) alcohol
    (C) heroin
    (D) cocaine
    (E) marijuana   (Ref. 5)

48. Lithium may cause

    (A) central diabetes mellitus
    (B) central diabetes insipidus
    (C) nephrogenic diabetes insipidus
    (D) peripheral diabetes insipidus
    (E) nephrogenic diabetes mellitus   (Ref. 7)

49. Steepling is most commonly indicative of

    (A) sadness
    (B) contemplation
    (C) defensiveness
    (D) suspicion
    (E) confidence   (Ref. 2)

50. Olfactory hallucinations most often occur in

    (A) amphetamine abuse
    (B) a tumor at the frontal lobe
    (C) depressive illnesses
    (D) a patient with phobic state
    (E) chiasma lesions   (Ref. 7)

51. A patient tells you that her husband wants her to engage in "unnatural sexual activity." She feels it is wrong but doesn't know what to do and asks your help. You can

   (A) call in the husband and tell him to respect his wife's sensitivities
   (B) tell the wife that she should try to satisfy her husband's sexual needs; otherwise, he might look for gratification elsewhere
   (C) suggest she come in with the husband and try to refer them for sex counseling
   (D) attempt to clarify the wife's sexual attitudes and her reasons for feeling the activity is wrong, and give her some preliminary guidance
   (E) tell her that sex is dirty and not in the realm of family practice   (Ref. 7)

52. A husband complains of his wife's being overweight, her sloppiness, and her improper training of the children. He is embarrassed to be seen with her and mentions a miserable childhood with an obese mother he was ashamed of. His wife was thin prior to marriage, but gradually gained considerable weight during the childbearing and child-rearing years. The wife, although wishing she were thin, dismisses her husband's concern about the problem and feels it indicates his lack of understanding of the pressures she is under. You should now

   (A) point out to the husband that he is overreacting to the wife's appearance because of his experience with his mother
   (B) point out to the wife the fact that she may be jeopardizing the marital relationship and offer help with dieting
   (C) discuss with both the apparent seeds of a serious problem in the marriage, pointing out that this could lead to more serious difficulty which might eventually jeopardize the marriage, and say that professional help should be seriously considered
   (D) tell the couple that their problems are not in the realm of family practice
   (E) refer the couple to a psychiatrist immediately since this is a psychiatric emergency   (Ref. 7)

53. The prime responsibility for providing emotional support for the terminally ill patient rests with the

   (A) head nurse on the ward
   (B) social worker
   (C) patient's friends
   (D) oncologist
   (E) attending family physician   (Ref. 7)

54. You are called by the police to examine a patient for alcoholism after an accident. The patient refuses to be examined. You then proceed to

   (A) examine the patient
   (B) draw blood from the patient for determination of alcohol concentration
   (C) call for physician assistants to restrain the patient
   (D) refuse to examine the patient
   (E) inject diazepam intravenously to calm the patient, then examine the patient at your ease   (Ref. 7)

55. In the absence of a special contract, the family physician

   (A) may guarantee a cure
   (B) should guarantee that the treatment will benefit his patient
   (C) is under obligation to exercise ordinary degrees of skill, care, and judgment, as exercised by members of his profession practicing in the same or a similar locality in the light of the present state of medical and surgical science
   (D) who is practicing in sparsely settled areas must have the same degree of skill and judgment as a physician practicing in urban areas
   (E) is required by law to exercise an extraordinary degree of special care for his own patients to show physicians' benevolence   (Ref. 7)

56. Mr. A. has been your patient for a number of years, and you know he has a serious cardiac condition. He is married, has seven children, and drives a school bus for a living. You have pleaded with him to quit driving the bus, but he has adamantly and consistently refused to do so. His reason for refusing is that he knows he will be unable to find another job, and without work his family will undergo severe economic hardship. His employer, the school board, does not require a physical examination for the job; consequently, there is no method by which they can find out about Mr. A.'s condition independently. Which of the following statements is true?

    (A) As his physician, you are legally bound to inform the school board of Mr. A.'s condition.
    (B) As his physician, you are bound by your professional code of ethics to keep the information in confidence.
    (C) As his physician, you are bound by your professional code of ethics to inform the school board of his condition.
    (D) You should gossip with the mother of a school child who boards your patient's bus.
    (E) none of the above   (Ref. 7)

57. The percentage of Americans affected by alcohol abuse is approximately

    (A) 0%
    (B) 5%
    (C) 50%
    (D) 75%
    (E) 100%   (Ref. 5)

58. Full recovery in anorexia nervosa can be expected in

    (A) 0% of patients
    (B) 5% of patients
    (C) 10% of patients
    (D) 25% of patients
    (E) 85% of patients   (Ref. 7)

59. The treatment of posttraumatic stress disorder includes

    (A) amitriptyline
    (B) chlorpromazine
    (C) cyclosporine
    (D) all of the above
    (E) none of the above   (Ref. 7)

60. Which of the following drugs is most useful in the treatment of Parkinson's disease?

    (A) acyclovir
    (B) verapamil
    (C) propranolol
    (D) haloperidol
    (E) amantadine   (Ref. 57)

61. Which of the following medications should be avoided by a patient taking an MAOI?

    (A) salicylic acid
    (B) phenylpropanolamine
    (C) thiamine
    (D) ascorbic acid
    (E) amoxicillin   (Ref. 57)

62. Which of the following antidepressants is most potent in sedative effect?

    (A) desipramine (Norpramin)
    (B) doxepin (Sinequan)
    (C) nortriptyline (Aventyl)
    (D) amoxapine (Asendin)
    (E) protriptyline (Vivactil)   (Ref. 57)

63. A patient taking MAOIs should be advised to avoid food that contains a high concentration of

    (A) riboflavin
    (B) thiamine
    (C) iron
    (D) tyramine
    (E) copper   (Ref. 57)

64. A patient with closed-angle glaucoma develops depression. The LEAST desirable medication is

(A) MAOIs
(B) SSRIs
(C) carbonic anhydrase inhibitors
(D) parasympathomimetic agents
(E) TCAs   (Ref. 57)

65. The side effects of phenothiazines include

(A) blurred vision
(B) loss of ejaculation
(C) fainting
(D) jaundice
(E) all of the above   (Ref. 57)

66. Paranoid behaviors may be described as

(A) delusions of grandeur
(B) litigiousness
(C) delusions of persecution
(D) violence
(E) all of the above   (Ref. 7)

67. The common side reactions of SSRIs include all of the following EXCEPT

(A) agitation
(B) tremor
(C) anorexia
(D) increased libido
(E) nausea   (Ref. 7)

68. TCAs are the drug of choice for depressive patients with the following associated illness:

(A) acute myocardial infarction
(B) acute congestive heart failure
(C) bulimia
(D) bundle-branch block
(E) narrow-angle glaucoma   (Ref. 57)

69. Which of the following antidepressants is associated with most anticholinergic effects?

(A) doxepin
(B) imipramine
(C) desipramine
(D) amitriptyline
(E) trazodone   (Ref. 57)

70. A patient complains of excessive and vivid dreaming following the discontinuance of a drug; the drug is most likely to be

(A) amitriptyline
(B) verapamil
(C) hydralazine
(D) enalapril
(E) streptokinase   (Ref. 57)

71. The most useful working definition of family in the urban setting is

(A) intimate reciprocal, and continuous relationships between two or more persons
(B) two married persons
(C) two married persons with two children
(D) legal marriage between husband and wife
(E) legal marriage between husband and wife with two children, one boy and one girl   (Ref. 5)

72. Opiate ingestion is frequently suggested by

(A) needle marks
(B) miosis
(C) urine test
(D) abstinence syndrome
(E) all of the above   (Ref. 57)

73. Youths who abuse and become dependent on amphetamines are likely to have a history of

(A) school failure
(B) treated hyperkinesis
(C) alienation from society
(D) gang behavior
(E) all of the above   (Ref. 57)

74. Which of the following statements is incorrect with regard to anorexia nervosa?

    (A) Patients see themselves as obese.
    (B) Patients desire to lose weight.
    (C) There is a 100% cure rate.
    (D) Behavior therapy is useful.
    (E) Patients may often perform self-induced vomiting.   (Ref. 75)

75. Mary and John have heard about a sensitivity training group (T-group) that is sponsoring a marathon group therapy session. They come to you for advice about such groups and are curious about the possibility of attending. In offering such advice, you would want to determine which of the following?

    (A) the emotional integrity of the couple
    (B) the mental illnesses suffered by the couple, if any
    (C) the qualification and the training of the sponsoring group staff
    (D) the reasons for attending
    (E) all of the above   (Ref. 7)

76. The characteristics of a healthy urban family include

    (A) family members are cohesive
    (B) family maintains a clear boundary within the community
    (C) family members are proud of historic and cultural heritage
    (D) family's internal structure is adaptive to its developmental stages
    (E) all of the above   (Ref. 5)

77. The family structure of urban psychosomatogenic families is most likely to be characterized by

    (A) predictable hierarchy
    (B) flexibility
    (C) overprotectiveness
    (D) ready resolution of conflicts
    (E) clear boundaries with family's subsystems   (Ref. 5)

78. Compared to rural families, urban families are more likely to be

    (A) diversified in family types and relationships
    (B) heterogeneous in class, race, and ethnicity
    (C) adaptive to changing environment, including influences from social and employment agencies
    (D) multicultured and economically interdependent
    (E) all of the above   (Ref. 5)

79. Poor families in urban areas are more likely to be

    (A) maintaining a strict boundary with the community
    (B) dependent on public social welfare programs
    (C) well organized in the family structure
    (D) very much integrated in family memberships
    (E) two-parent families   (Ref. 5)

80. The incidence of suicide is higher in

    (A) advanced age
    (B) males than females
    (C) peacetime than in wartime
    (D) physicians
    (E) all of the above   (Ref. 7)

81. Motives for suicide include

    (A) a need for self-punishment
    (B) a wish to join a dead parent
    (C) revenge
    (D) psychosis
    (E) all of the above   (Ref. 7)

82. Adaptation stages of a dying patient usually include

    (A) denial
    (B) anger
    (C) depression
    (D) acceptance
    (E) all of the above   (Ref. 7)

83. The best evidence that informed consent was given is

   (A) the nurse's words
   (B) a laboratory technician's witness
   (C) the physician's statement
   (D) documentation
   (E) the receptionist's impression   *(Ref. 7)*

84. There is a need to bring new family physicians into inner-city communities to practice; the most ideal characteristic of these family physicians is

   (A) missionary zeal
   (B) belief only in biomedical models
   (C) intention to conduct molecular research in the most advanced technologic medical center
   (D) training in the biopsychosocial model of health care
   (E) a dislike of government intervention in health-care delivery   *(Ref. 5)*

85. Which of the following statements is correct?

   (A) Spanish-origin households account for 11% of total American households.
   (B) Most Haitians reside in urban areas.
   (C) 90% of Native American Indians reside in urban areas.
   (D) 10% of black households are located in the center of cities.
   (E) 84% of Spanish-origin families are settled in the suburbs.   *(Ref. 5)*

86. Which of the following urban families need immediate family therapy?

   (A) parentified child
   (B) children reared by the grandmother
   (C) adolescent parenting
   (D) peripheral male
   (E) none of the above   *(Ref. 5)*

87. In response to which of the following signs should the family physician suggest immediate family therapy to restructure a well-functioning urban family?

   (A) when the family puts immediate survival issues ahead of health-care issues
   (B) when the family has a strong gender-role separation
   (C) when the mother uses an extensive female network from her family of origin to help with child care
   (D) when the sibling subsystem plays an important role
   (E) none of the above   *(Ref. 5)*

88. Depression may occur with which of the following medications?

   (A) alpha-methyldopa
   (B) propranolol
   (C) alcohol
   (D) oral contraceptives
   (E) all of the above   *(Ref. 7)*

89. During adolescence, an individual's most important developmental task is to develop

   (A) identity
   (B) trust
   (C) industry
   (D) generativity
   (E) initiative   *(Ref. 3)*

90. Psychotic symptoms can be caused by

   (A) alcohol withdrawal
   (B) cocaine abuse
   (C) psychomotor epilepsy
   (D) all of the above
   (E) none of the above   *(Ref. 7)*

91. Which of the following methods is most helpful for the urban immigrant family to protect against stress and illness?

    (A) social networking
    (B) scapegoating of a family member
    (C) power realignment of family members serving those who speak English
    (D) cutting relationships with the family of origin in the homeland
    (E) parent–child coalition   *(Ref. 5)*

92. In urban single-parent families

    (A) divorce is the cause of all single-parent situations
    (B) all heads of the family were once married
    (C) all are headed by a male
    (D) all of the above
    (E) none of the above   *(Ref. 5)*

93. In urban psychosomatic families, which of the following conditions is most likely to occur?

    (A) The parents are united to focus on their executive functioning.
    (B) There is a clear boundary between the parental and sibling subsystems.
    (C) The ill child forms a stable coalition with one parent and rejects the other parent.
    (D) Family structure is flexible to accommodate developmental tasks of the ill child.
    (E) The family has an adequate social network to support the ill child's exploration of the extrafamilial world.   *(Ref. 5)*

94. Your 68-year-old female patient complains of insomnia for 2 months. Physical examinations are unremarkable. You will suggest

    (A) a glass of red wine before bedtime
    (B) two cups of freshly brewed coffee at bedtime
    (C) one pack of cigarettes prior to retiring
    (D) elimination of exercises altogether
    (E) establishment of a bedtime routine
                                       (Ref. 2)

95. The most common mental illness in the urban setting is

    (A) schizophrenia
    (B) functional psychoses
    (C) substance abuse
    (D) manic–depressive illnesses
    (E) sexual dysfunction   *(Ref. 5)*

96. In the urban family practice, the family circle is often used for family mapping. The family circle is the patient's

    (A) biological family
    (B) spiritual family
    (C) adoptive family
    (D) emotional family
    (E) legal family   *(Ref. 5)*

97. A 42-year-old female complains of diffuse hair shedding for the past 3 months following abrupt termination of her job due to a budget crisis. She noticed a loss of 150 hairs a day and is very anxious. You will

    (A) prescribe Premarin 0.625 mg PO per day for 3 months
    (B) offer reassurance
    (C) order 5-—reductase serum level
    (D) start 2% topical minoxidil (Rogaine) solution
    (E) use intralesional bismuth injection
                                       (Ref. 27)

98. Recent immigrants in the urban areas are at higher health risk due to

    (A) cultural discontinuity
    (B) disruption of social supports
    (C) residential mobility
    (D) unavailability of family members who may remain in the motherland
    (E) all of the above   *(Ref. 5)*

99. Urban patients with chronic stable schizophrenia are best managed by

    (A) family physicians
    (B) internists
    (C) social workers

(D) mental health agencies

(E) alcohol counselors   *(Ref. 5)*

100. Today, an 18-year-old man appearing somewhat more disheveled than his current peers states that he does not know the date. He is concerned that some friends have misplaced objects in his apartment to trick him and are now laughing at his plight. The most likely diagnosis is

(A) depression

(B) manic–depressive

(C) organic brain syndrome (presenile or senile dementia)

(D) schizophrenia

(E) toxic psychosis   *(Ref. 7)*

101. In the underserved urban setting, the primary care team is usually composed of multiprofessional and multiethnic team members. Due to their different backgrounds and diversified training, there may often be conflicts between the primary-care team members. These conflicts are best resolved by

(A) team development programs

(B) eliminating the fighting team members

(C) dissolving the team entirely

(D) replacing team members by computers

(E) establishing a new team   *(Ref. 5)*

102. Violent crime is more prevalent in the urban setting, which is most likely related to

(A) spacious dwelling place

(B) abundance of housing

(C) high rate of unemployment

(D) highly educated dwellers

(E) high-income population   *(Ref. 5)*

103. Compared to rural patients, urban patients with mental illnesses are more likely to be

(A) similar in social status to their family physicians

(B) homogeneous in their social backgrounds

(C) in crisis

(D) maintaining long-lasting professional relationships with their family physicians

(E) employing the same linguistic speech with the same cultural explanations

          (Ref. 5)

104. The primary prevention in the urban setting includes

(A) treatment of hypertension

(B) screening for glaucoma

(C) detection of asymptomatic gonorrhea

(D) removal of lead-based paints from inner-city tenements

(E) liver transplantation for cirrhotic patients   *(Ref. 5)*

105. In an urban clinical setting, a medical ethicist

(A) determines the absolute truths of a clinical situation

(B) dictates definitive answers to complex clinical issues

(C) offers patient counseling as a clinical psychologist

(D) assists physicians in medical decision making

(E) educates health-care providers in analysis of concepts   *(Ref. 5)*

106. Which of the following guidelines is most useful for family physicians practicing cross-cultural medicine in the urban setting?

(A) Report local curanderos to the police authority.

(B) Establish residence away from the practice neighborhood.

(C) Convert patients to the same religion if their religions are different from yours.

(D) Insist on speaking only English (the official language) at the office.

(E) Acknowledge and discuss situations and differences about the perception of the problem.   *(Ref. 5)*

107. Acculturation of new immigrants is most likely to be helped by

(A) social isolation
(B) fluent English
(C) low socioeconomic status
(D) unemployment
(E) congregation with own ethnic group

(Ref. 5)

108. With "AIDS stigma," when you encounter a Haitian patient at your urban family practice office, you will

(A) immediately refer the patient to an AIDS clinic
(B) send the patient to a hospital emergency room
(C) provide concerned comprehensive and continuous care for the patient and the families
(D) politely ask the patient to see another family physician located on the next street
(E) politely refuse to see the patient   *(Ref. 5)*

109. Which of the following statements is true in the urban family practice setting?

(A) A competent patient has the right to refuse treatment.
(B) The family physician can withhold any information to the patient.
(C) The family physician can only withhold the information when it is for the good of the patient.
(D) The family physician should only tell the family the unfavorable prognosis.
(E) The family physician should not tell the patient the risks of the treatment regimen.   *(Ref. 5)*

110. Good health habits include

(A) excessive alcohol consumption
(B) 7 to 8 hours of sleep every night
(C) moderate cigarette smoking
(D) sedentary lifestyle
(E) steady weight gains   *(Ref. 5)*

111. Which of the following complications may be seen in bulimia?

(A) benign parotid and submandibular gland swelling
(B) erosion of dental enamel
(C) mild elevation of serum amylase
(D) hypokalemia
(E) all of the above   *(Ref. 7)*

112. Etiologic hypothesis of schizophrenia includes which of the following?

(A) The disease is partly genetically determined.
(B) A hyperdopaminergic state may produce symptoms.
(C) Information overload is a high risk factor.
(D) Enlarged ventricles indicate a poor treatment response.
(E) all of the above   *(Ref. 7)*

113. The lowest blood alcohol concentration that most states recognize as showing that persons are legally intoxicated is (in mg/100 mL)

(A) 600
(B) 300
(C) 150
(D) 80
(E) 5   *(Ref. 7)*

114. An adolescent athlete complains of depression, school failure, nasal congestion, and a period of feeling high. He is tremulous, and there is tachycardia and nasal mucosal irritation. The clinical picture may suggest

(A) infectious mononucleosis
(B) paranoid personality
(C) steroid abuse
(D) cocaine abuse
(E) manic–depressive phychosis   *(Ref. 3)*

115. Common untoward effects of anorectic drugs include

(A) palmar sweating
(B) blurred vision

(C) insomnia

(D) dry mouth

(E) all of the above   *(Ref. 7)*

116. Children with runaway reactions

(A) often feel that they are rejected at home

(B) are mostly teenagers (average age being 15 years)

(C) often steal

(D) may not return home at all

(E) all of the above   *(Ref. 7)*

117. "Rewards for desired behavior" is the application of the basic principle of

(A) free association

(B) psychoanalysis

(C) family life cycle

(D) operant conditioning

(E) social punishment   *(Ref. 7)*

118. Coping behavior may

(A) diminish the pathology of the illness

(B) keep the level of distress manageable

(C) enhance the risk of divorce

(D) increase social isolation

(E) lessen the effectiveness of minor tranquilizers   *(Ref. 7)*

119. An effective primary-care team requires all of the following characteristics EXCEPT

(A) explicit goal setting

(B) fair allocation of responsibility

(C) close affectionate intimacy between members

(D) flexible and adaptable members

(E) professional competency   *(Ref. 5)*

120. Static and kinetic tremor is most likely indicative of

(A) parkinsonism

(B) hyperthyroidism

(C) tardive dyskinesia

(D) cerebellar disease

(E) hepatic coma   *(Ref. 7)*

121. Flight of ideas is characteristic of

(A) schizophrenia

(B) manic state

(C) Korsakoff's psychosis

(D) depression

(E) somatization   *(Ref. 7)*

122. When a patient indicates: "I know I shouldn't feel this way, but . . ." she probably possesses a(n)

(A) obsessive–compulsive personality

(B) hysterical personality

(C) phobic personality

(D) depressed personality

(E) paranoid personality   *(Ref. 7)*

123. Which of the following defense mechanisms is the separation of an unacceptable impulse from the memory origin?

(A) repression

(B) isolation

(C) denial

(D) suppression

(E) sublimation   *(Ref. 7)*

124. Which of the following is an intelligence test?

(A) WAIS

(B) TAT

(C) Bender–Gestalt

(D) MMPI

(E) house drawing   *(Ref. 7)*

125. Understanding of right and wrong is the basis of

(A) M'Naghten rule

(B) irresistible impulse

(C) AMA ethical codes

(D) clinical policy guidelines

(E) managed competition   *(Ref. 7)*

126. When an individual understands that the number of objects in a set does not change with spatial arrangement, he is in the

    (A) Piaget's sensorimotor period
    (B) Piaget's period of concrete operations
    (C) Piaget's period of formal operations
    (D) Freud's latency period
    (E) Erikson's latency period   (Ref. 7)

127. The reproduction function of the family

    (A) is no longer existent
    (B) is not viable in the childless couple
    (C) has never been seen as a source of stress in the marital relationship
    (D) should not be discussed by the couple premaritally
    (E) is not existent in the single-parent family
                                          (Ref. 7)

128. Which of the following is true regarding conversion reaction?

    (A) persistent intrusion of unwanted thoughts, urges, or actions that the patient cannot control
    (B) usually involves sensory or motor system dysfunction with no organic dysfunction
    (C) intense fear of object or situation with no actual danger
    (D) diffuse anxiety not restricted to specific situations or objects
    (E) alteration in patient's state of consciousness or identity, including amnesia, somnambulism, and multiple personality
                                          (Ref. 7)

129. A normal grief reaction may cause

    (A) feelings of sadness
    (B) loss of appetite
    (C) insomnia
    (D) hostility to the primary-care practitioner
    (E) all of the above   (Ref. 7)

130. Erik Erikson's formulation of the adolescent stage of psychosocial development gives central importance to the development of a sense of

    (A) trust
    (B) generativity
    (C) efficacy
    (D) identity
    (E) stagnation   (Ref. 7)

131. The Eriksonian stage in which the individual becomes somewhat less involved with his or her own needs and more concerned with providing life and sustenance to a new generation is termed

    (A) intimacy vs. isolation
    (B) generativity vs. stagnation
    (C) mutuality vs. egocentrism
    (D) integrity vs. despair
    (E) industry vs. inferiority   (Ref. 7)

132. A family may be in trouble when

    (A) the wage earner suddenly loses his or her job
    (B) the parents are talking about divorce
    (C) the adolescent boy is dropping out of school
    (D) the father has had acute myocardial infarction
    (E) all of the above   (Ref. 7)

133. Confabulation is characteristic of

    (A) acute organic brain syndrome
    (B) Korsakoff's psychosis
    (C) hepatic encephalopathy
    (D) amphetamine psychosis
    (E) schizophrenia   (Ref. 7)

134. Paranoid psychotic reactions can be produced by

    (A) MAOIs
    (B) barbiturates

(C) amphetamines

(D) doxepin (Sinequan)

(E) chlordiazepoxide (Librium)   *(Ref. 7)*

135. Gender identity is formed

(A) in utero

(B) at birth

(C) during early childhood (1–3 years)

(D) in school age (7–12 years)

(E) at adolescence (12–18 years)   *(Ref. 7)*

136. A recent immigrant from Southeast Asia visited your office for the first time. In reviewing his history, you found that he spent 8 months in a concentration camp. He is at an increased risk to develop

(A) pancreatic cancer

(B) cholelithiasis

(C) Alzheimer's disease

(D) prostatic cancer

(E) complex posttraumatic stress disorder   *(Ref. 7)*

137. The most common clinical feature of a patient with borderline personality disorder is

(A) stable interpersonal relationship

(B) appropriate anger for the circumstance

(C) high sense of self-identity

(D) chronic boredom

(E) consistent mood   *(Ref. 7)*

138. If you encountered an angry patient at your office, you would

(A) call the police

(B) refer the patient to a psychiatrist

(C) call a clinical psychologist to deal with the patient

(D) continue to provide needed care for the patient

(E) terminate the care of the patient   *(Ref. 61)*

139. An overly dependent patient should be treated by

(A) antidepressants

(B) minor tranquilizers

(C) conforming to the patient's demands

(D) setting limits on appointment time

(E) terminating the professional relationship with him   *(Ref. 61)*

140. When you are rejected by a patient, you may

(A) feel inadequate

(B) avoid that patient thereafter

(C) terminate the professional relationship with that patient

(D) tell all your colleagues about that patient's rejection

(E) continue to provide needed care through genuine concerns   *(Ref. 61)*

141. When you encounter a malingering patient, you

(A) reward the patient with his demands (such as a disability certificate)

(B) continue to provide needed care to foster appropriate health-care behavior

(C) refer the patient to another family physician

(D) "damp" the patient to the nearest family practice center or a family practice residency training program

(E) refuse the patient's demands and terminate the professional relationship   *(Ref. 7)*

142. When you suspect a patient is somatizing, you

(A) say to the patient that there is nothing physically wrong

(B) tell the patient that he is a hypochondriac

(C) repeat again and again the same negative test in search of obscure organic disease

(D) provide continuity of care with short regular appointment time

(E) offer premature and definite reassurance   *(Ref. 7)*

DIRECTIONS (Questions 143 through 179): Each question consists of an introduction followed by some statements. Mark T (true) or F (false) after each statement.

143. In tricyclic antidepressants

(A) if the patient does not respond to the first dose, he or she should be changed to an MAOI

(B) sudden withdrawal of the medication may result in sleep disturbance with vivid dreams

(C) the first therapeutic effect is the resolution of sexual dysfunction

(D) urinary retention may occur in the elderly with prostatic hypertrophy

(E) may produce ECG nonspecific ST changes and cardiac arrhythmias

(Ref. 57)

144. Sexual dysfunction is commonly seen in patients who have

(A) chronic renal failure

(B) diabetes mellitus

(C) hypertension

(D) hypothyroidism

(E) anemia   (Ref. 7)

145. Managements of anorexia nervosa include

(A) hospitalization

(B) amitriptyline

(C) cyproheptadine

(D) chlorpropamide

(E) family to force food intake and to punish the patient if the patient does not finish the meal   (Ref. 7)

146. In the elderly, which of the following common medications may cause depression?

(A) doxepin

(B) clonidine

(C) estrogen

(D) cimetidine

(E) theophylline   (Ref. 7)

147. Reversible causes of dementia are

(A) congestive heart failure

(B) subdural hematoma

(C) hypocalcemia

(D) chronic use of antacids

(E) hyperthyroidism   (Ref. 7)

148. Clinical presentations of anorexia nervosa include

(A) hyperglycemia

(B) hypermenorrhea

(C) relative monocytosis

(D) 20% weight loss

(E) hypothermia of 90°F to 95°F   (Ref. 7)

149. Clinical manifestations of depression include

(A) eosinophilia

(B) serum cortisol level of 2 ng/dL

(C) thyroid-stimulating hormone (TSH) rises 15 ng/mL following thyrotropin-releasing hormone administration

(D) hypomagnesemia

(E) slow velocity in nerve conduction study

(Ref. 7)

150. A housewife confides in you that her husband is putting pressure on her to consider "switching" or even the possibility of a group marriage. You would now

(A) advise the patient that the marriage has no chance for survival

(B) advise the patient to conform to her husband's suggestions

(C) advise her to seek care elsewhere

(D) offer family counseling to explore the situation

(E) indicate your strong opinion against switching   (Ref. 7)

151. A husband and wife complain bitterly of each other's lack of consideration or concern for the other. They are engaged in active feuding, including withholding of money by the husband and refusal to prepare meals by the wife. Each one's complaints center on the

refusal of the other to behave in a fashion that would convey caring and consideration about the other. The husband is very worried about money and is enraged that his wife won't economize. The wife states that her husband's worries are exaggerated, that he has always been a miser, and that she can't live as if the wolf were constantly at the door. You would

(A) side with the husband in demanding that the wife prepare meals for him

(B) provide family counseling to help them work together in less destructive ways

(C) provide reassurance for the wife that this quarrel is commonplace in marriage

(D) help both parties to clarify expectations

(E) suggest divorce   (Ref. 7)

152. Common effects of marijuana are

(A) euphoria

(B) dreamy fantasy state

(C) improved memory

(D) improved motor coordination and skillfulness

(E) time–space distortions   (Ref. 7)

153. The following statements are concerned with family problems:

(A) 20 to 50% of all murders in the United States are committed by a family member.

(B) Violence occurs more frequently between family members than between other individuals.

(C) Spouse abuse occurs in 16% of American homes.

(D) 35% of sons and 20% of daughters of parents with an abusive relationship had behavioral problems and retarded social skills.

(E) 20 to 26% of battered women attempt suicide.   (Ref. 7)

154. An initial management of spouse abuse involves

(A) prescription for narcotics

(B) tranquilizers

(C) nonjudgmental direct inquiry about the possibility of abuse

(D) providing information about available shelters and community resources for help

(E) taking the abused spouse into custody against her will in a continuing abusive relationship   (Ref. 5)

155. Barriers to effective communication include

(A) aphasia in the patient

(B) presbycusis in the physician

(C) cultural differences between the physician and the patient

(D) language differences between the physician and the patient

(E) religious differences between the patient and the physician   (Ref. 5)

156. Obstacles to blood pressure control in hypertensive patients include

(A) poor physician–patient communication

(B) inadequate patient education

(C) costly antihypertensive drugs

(D) side effects of antihypertensive medications

(E) use of drugs that interfere with antihypertensive agents   (Ref. 5)

157. Neuroleptic malignant syndrome is characterized by

(A) hypothermia

(B) muscular hypotonicity

(C) tachycardia

(D) dazed mutism

(E) profuse diaphoresis   (Ref. 7)

158. The laboratory pictures of the neuroleptic malignant syndrome include

(A) marked leukopenia

(B) elevated serum creatine kinase

(C) elevated serum alkaline phosphatase

(D) elevation of serum aminotransferases

(E) diffuse spikes on the electroencephalogram (EEG)   (Ref. 7)

159. Management of the neuroleptic malignant syndrome includes

    (A) dantrolene (Dantrium)
    (B) bromocriptine (Parlodel)
    (C) phenelzine (Nardil)
    (D) amitriptyline (Elavil)
    (E) discontinuing the neuroleptics   (Ref. 7)

160. Rigid routines, impersonal approaches, and lack of resident involvement in the nursing home may contribute to residents' problems, such as

    (A) wandering
    (B) incontinence
    (C) anger
    (D) agitation
    (E) depression   (Ref. 7)

161. Tourette syndrome is often associated with

    (A) obsessive–compulsive behavior
    (B) attention deficit–hyperactivity disorder (ADHD)
    (C) somnambulism
    (D) learning disabilities
    (E) mental retardation   (Ref. 7)

162. Features of Tourette syndrome include

    (A) coprolalia
    (B) inability to suppress tics voluntarily
    (C) echolalia
    (D) involuntary obscene gesturing
    (E) increased incidence of left-handedness   (Ref. 7)

163. Pharmacotherapy of Tourette syndrome involves

    (A) haloperidol (Haldol)
    (B) clonidine (Catapres)
    (C) pimozide (Orap)
    (D) benztropine mesylate (Cogentin)
    (E) diphenhydramine (Benadryl)   (Ref. 7)

164. Mescaline effects include

    (A) hallucinations
    (B) miosis

    (C) bradycardia
    (D) dry mouth
    (E) nausea   (Ref. 7)

165. Stress is often associated with

    (A) decreased cortisol levels
    (B) increased glucose intolerance
    (C) decreased cholesterol levels
    (D) increased platelet adhesion
    (E) impaired lipoprotein ratios   (Ref. 7)

166. Akathisia is frequently associated with

    (A) diphenhydramine (Benadryl)
    (B) haloperidol (Haldol)
    (C) prochlorperazine (Compazine)
    (D) propranolol (Inderal)
    (E) fluphenazine (Prolixin)   (Ref. 7)

167. The following behaviors will improve physician–patient relationships:

    (A) business dealings through undue influence
    (B) bartering goods for office visit
    (C) volunteering patients' domestic services at office for the fees charged
    (D) exchanging patients' professional services for the medical services rendered
    (E) engagement in sexual relations with the patient   (Ref. 7)

168. A patient consults you because he says that he does not know what to do—his wife has expressed much dissatisfaction with him and is currently engaged in an extramarital affair, which she makes little attempt to hide from him. The patient says everyone is telling him to leave her. Your contact with the wife reveals her to be unconcerned about her husband's feelings, and she openly states that if she could find someone else, she would leave him. They have one 13-year-old child. You should

    (A) tell the husband that the wife doesn't seem to care much about him and that he should seriously consider separation
    (B) talk with the wife about the advantages of trying to keep the family together and the destructive effect of her behavior on her husband and son

(C) suggest to the husband that perhaps if he stands by, his wife will realize that any relationship has its disappointments and she will then be ready to work on the marriage

(D) tell the husband that while you do not object to giving advice, it is obvious that he is deeply unhappy over his wife's behavior and yet he is neither capable nor desirous of leaving her (otherwise he would). Suggest that it would be helpful for him to talk to someone who may be able to help him find a less taxing way of dealing with the situation (whether he stays or goes)   *(Ref. 7)*

169. Which of the following statements is/are true for the relationship between the physician and patient?

(A) It is consensual.

(B) The physician is bound to render professional service to every patient who applies.

(C) It may be contractual.

(D) When a physician obtains a state license to practice medicine, he has to practice medicine immediately.   *(Ref. 7)*

170. Conditions that do not constitute abandonment are those in which the

(A) physician's answering service refuses to call the physician

(B) physician and patient mutually agree to terminate the relationship

(C) physician accuses the patient of ignorance and then suddenly refuses to see him

(D) patient terminates the relationship   *(Ref. 7)*

171. Which of the following statements is/are true concerning the physician's liability for negligence of third person?

(A) A family physician who is practicing in a three-man partnership is liable for the actions of the partners.

(B) A physician is not responsible for the negligence of a substitute if he uses reasonable care in his selection, and the substitute is not in his employment or associated with him as a partner.

(C) A surgeon who operates at a hospital not owned or controlled by him and who is assisted in an operation by nurses provided by the hospital is not responsible for the mistakes or negligence of such nurses.

(D) A physician is not responsible for the carelessness of a nurse who gives an erroneous sponge count during a hysterectomy so that a sponge is left inside the abdomen.   *(Ref. 7)*

172. Which of the following statements is/are true about informed consent?

(A) The physician's duty is fulfilled when the disclosure is sufficient to enable the patient to make an intelligent choice as to whether or not he desires to have the procedure performed.

(B) In a medical emergency in which the patient is in no condition to make an intelligent determination for himself, disclosure of collateral risks may not be required.

(C) When an explanation of every attendant risk may result in unnecessarily alarming the apprehensive patient, the disclosure can be limited to relevant facts.

(D) The physician has no duty to make a full disclosure to the patient of collateral risks and dangers inherent in the suggested treatment or procedure.   *(Ref. 7)*

173. A mother complains that her 3-year-old is shy with strangers, tends to cling to her, and does not respond positively to other children. In giving a history, the mother described the child as always having been a "difficult" child—her schedule was never regular, every new situation was met with resistance, she cried easily, and was irritable. The mother is wondering whether her own anxiety—this is her first child—and the negative feelings she sometimes experiences played a role in the child's difficulties, and whether she should get treatment for herself, the child, or both. You will tell the mother that

(A) it is very commendable that she is willing to look at her own reactions; it is possible that her negative feelings have perhaps caused her to be overprotective and to interfere with the child's separation from her, and treatment for her might be an excellent idea

(B) she should get treatment for the child since she is bound to have difficulties when she starts school

(C) the child will get through the difficulty eventually so there is no reason for her to worry, and that neither she nor her child needs counseling or guidance

(D) some children are from birth much more "difficult" than others, may require special handling, and are bound to heighten any mother's anxiety; and that it might be worthwhile for her to get some help in dealing with the issues that arise, or you could try to help her with it   *(Ref. 7)*

174. A family has a child with cystic fibrosis (CF). The parents seek your guidance concerning the possibility of other children being born with the disease and whether they should have other children. You should now

(A) reassure them that the chances are only one in four that the next child will be born with the illness

(B) tell them they owe it to the unborn children not to bring them into the world if there is a chance they will have this disease, because the chances of unhappiness for them and an affected child are over-

whelming; suggest adoption if they want more children

(C) tell them that much has been done to prolong life expectancy in CF, and perhaps by the time their children reach adolescence, a cure will have been found

(D) help them think through how much they want children and consider the risks—what it would mean for a child and for them   *(Ref. 7)*

175. You are called in because a 15-year-old has made a suicide attempt. She claims that her parents don't love her and are too restrictive, but her parents claim that her behavior shows poor judgment and could get her into serious trouble. You will now

(A) discuss with both the girl and the parents the fact that they have not found a way of living together that meets all their needs, and that they should seek professional help to see if matters could be made more comfortable for all of them

(B) suggest that the youngster receive treatment since she needs help both in relation to the behavior and because of the possibility of another suicide attempt

(C) suggest that they let her do what she wants so she will learn from the consequences of her behavior

(D) suggest that since the parents are having a difficult time controlling their daughter, they request a PINS petition (Persons In Need of Supervision) from the family court, which will put the power of the court behind them without giving the youngster a record   *(Ref. 7)*

176. A mother complains bitterly that her teenage daughter is secretive, consorts with kids who drink, is irresponsible about household chores, and is sullen when she tries to talk to her about it. She asks whether you could talk to the daughter and get her to behave differently. You do talk to both of them and find that a vicious cycle has been escalating between them in which the parents are more and more restrictive in relation to the girl's social life while the youngster is exhibiting anger and resentment toward her parents. You also find that the parents are right in some of their complaints. You will now

(A) reassure the mother that you have known the girl since she was a baby and you are sure that she can't be doing anything wrong, and that many teenagers go through periods like this

(B) refer both of them for intensive psychotherapy

(C) help the mother (parents) become less restrictive so that a break is made in the cycle of punishment and further defiance

(D) tell the daughter how much her mother has done for her and that she should show appreciation by being more cooperative   *(Ref. 7)*

177. Somatizing patients may be suspected from the following characteristics:

(A) specific single complaint

(B) fever of 102°F or above

(C) polypharmacy

(D) physician shopping

(E) hostile attitudes toward health care staff members   *(Ref. 7)*

178. Hysterical characters include the following:

(A) excitability

(B) hallucinations

(C) somatization

(D) self-dramatization

(E) overreactivity   *(Ref. 7)*

179. A high index of suspicion of malingering should be maintained when the patient has

(A) a medicolegal context in the presentation

(B) consistency of physical findings with claimed disability

(C) cooperation to suggestive diagnostic procedures

(D) identifiable secondary gains (such as disability incomes)

(E) a preexisting antisocial personality disorder   *(Ref. 7)*

DIRECTIONS (Questions 180 through 186): The following clinical set problems consist of clinical information presented in the format of questions or incomplete statements followed by a group of numbered options.

Indicate T if the option is true;
Indicate F if the option is false.

John, a 5-year-old boy, is referred by his kindergarten teacher for aggressive and destructive behavior in the classroom. He has had a severe behavior problem since birth, showing aggressiveness toward his older sister and older brother. His sleeping and eating patterns are erratic. He is described by his mother as always being excitable, overreactive with poor attention, and accident prone, and he "refuses to listen or learn." Based upon the history, the diagnosis is most likely

180. autism

181. childhood schizophrenia

182. ADHD

The major treatment approaches for John will most likely be

183. parental counseling for the management of the behavioral difficulties

184. special education

185. medication

186. child guidance and follow-up   *(Ref. 7)*

Answers and Explanations

1. **(B)** Medical ethics is the study of the application of the principles of ethics to the practice of medicine and the biological sciences.

2. **(B)** The divorce rate of women who married in their teens is double that of women who married in their 20s. The divorce rate of women who married in their 20s is double that of women married in their 30s.

3. **(C)** The highest incidence of divorce comes at the stage of childbearing and child rearing.

4. **(D)** In step-families only one biological parent is in the household; in foster families neither biological parent is present.

5. **(D)** Single-parent families account for 15% of families with children: 80% are headed by women; 44% resulted from divorce or separation; 35% resulted from the husband's death; 13% of single mothers were never married; 4% have institutionalized or geographically remote husbands. The average income is half that of the two-parent family.

6. **(B)** The therapeutic distance can be maintained by seeing the patient during office hours with attendance of the nurse. To have a long talk with the patient after office hours will increase intimacy and may hamper the doctor–patient relationship. A seductive patient needs comprehensive medical and emotional care in a professional milieu by a family physician before calling for psychiatric consultation.

7. **(D)** The first phase of the family life cycle is the expansion phase, followed by the child-centered phase, then the contraction phase.

8. **(E)** A person's competency to make a will is known as testamentary capacity. The person signing a will must know clearly what he is doing when he signs it. This means that he knows that he is making a will, and he knows the nature and extent of his property and the natural objects of his bounty (ie, the members of his family, his warm friends, the institutions he is interested in).

9. **(A)** Grief reactions in mothers who lose small children are commonly severe, with a duration of four to six weeks.

10. **(E)** Adjustment reaction is a temporary, transitional period of maladaptation in response to unusual stresses. Adjustment disturbance in adolescence is usually the rule rather than the exception. An adolescent with paranoid delusions should be suspected as psychotic until proved to be otherwise.

11. **(B)** In order to secure the optimum rapport and maximum information, the physician must be flexible and the interview must be characterized by spontaneity. The patient usually feels that she is understood and her point of view appreciated if the physician permits her to tell her own story. To facilitate further communication, physicians should be nonjudgmental, with no presuppositions.

12. **(D)** This patient is passive–aggressive in personality. He expresses hostile wishes through covert and passive means. Subtle resistances

are likely to be masked under a facade of conformity to the therapeutic ritual, and the physician is frequently blamed for changes in the patient's life situation. In the face of overt acting-out behavior, realistic limit-setting by the physician may become necessary.

13. **(E)** The separation anxiety in early childhood is the child's fear and apprehension upon being removed from the parent or parent figure. This also happens in children who change foster homes too frequently. To avoid separation anxiety, the mother's overnight stay with her preschool child in the hospital is a valuable supportive measure.

14. **(D)** The child should be engineered back to school as quickly as possible. The parents may accompany the child to school but should not remain. The teacher must cooperate to keep the child in the classroom. The parents must avoid interest in the child's physical complaints and be firm in preparing the child for school attendance. Family therapy has been tried for severe cases.

15. **(E)** Adjustment reactions in infancy are symptomatic responses of the infant to separation from the mother and include developmental delay. Adjustment reactions of childhood are usually manifested in simple repetitive activities, such as nailbiting, thumbsucking, enuresis, masturbation, and temper tantrums. Adjustment reactions of adolescence are largely indicative of the youth's struggle for identity.

16. **(D)** Common laboratory abnormalities associated with alcoholism include elevated MCV, elevated serum gamma-glutamyl transpeptidase (GGT), elevated serum uric acid, elevated serum triglycerides, elevated serum amylase, elevated serum glutamic oxaloacetic transaminase (SGoT) and serum glutamic pyruvic transaminase (SGPT) (SGOT higher than SGPT).

17. **(A)** One of the most common complaints of anxious patients is difficulty in breathing. Patients often demonstrate this by deep sighs. They frequently complain of fainting, lightheadedness, or tingling of the extremities, which are due primarily to a decrease in blood carbonate (a respiratory alkalosis). The diagnosis is often confirmed by asking the patient to hyperventilate, which reproduces the lightheadedness, tingling, and faintness. This will also reassure the patient.

18. **(D)** The most common reason to see a physician is (1) the symptom's reaching the anxiety limit, followed by (2) a symptom's reaching the tolerance limit, (3) a hidden agenda, (4) an administrative problem, and (5) using an opportunity.

19. **(A)** A nonjudgmental attitude usually invites patients' and families' trust, which puts them at ease to provide the family physician the personal and intimate information that is important in making diagnostic and therapeutic plans.

20. **(E)** Fantasies precede suicidal acts. Family physicians who encounter patients with any of the fantasies mentioned should ask patients about thoughts of suicide. The suicide threat from a patient should call for immediate management.

21. **(A)** Active listening is most useful in a nondirective (patient-controlled) process: (a) medical concerns of patients (symptoms); and (b) emotional, spiritual, and environmental concerns of patient. A directed (doctor-controlled) process is useful in: (a) review of systems and emergent medical history; (b) social history, family tree, and mental status assessment.

22. **(B)** As a general principle of human behavior, the dyad (couple) seeks a third person to stabilize the relationship, especially in the face of conflicts between the original two.

23. **(D)** The usual treatment approach is to schedule frequent, brief office visits. Appointments should be regularly scheduled so that the patient does not need to develop a symptom to justify a visit to see the family physician. It is best for the session to be brief, around 10 to 20 minutes in length. The family physician and the patient need to focus on

one or two major issues. Over time, the family physician gradually shifts the conversation from somatic concerns toward productive life endeavors.

24. **(D)**   An ethical decision is made by (1) rational reasons, (2) objective consideration of all relevant data, (3) universally applicable principles, and (4) coherent and consistent moral beliefs.

25. **(C)**   Trichotillomania is a behavioral disorder resulting from repetitive pulling of own hair. The broken hairs are of unequal length. Trichotillomania is more likely in females; however, in preschoolers, it is more common in boys than in girls. The patient is associated with adjustment disorder, borderline personality, obsessive–compulsive disorder, ADHD, major depression, anxiety, mental retardation, severe medical illness, school conflict, and previous scalp injury. Behavioral modification and psychotherapy may be helpful.

26. **(C)**   Alcoholics Anonymous (AA) is a loosely organized voluntary fellowship of alcoholic persons. The largest identifiable group of abstinent former alcoholics are current or former AA members.

27. **(B)**   Although methadone is used for morphine addiction, it is a morphine substitute rather than an antagonist. Methadone will produce the same therapeutic effect (ie, analgesia) as other opiates, but not the euphoria of other similar substances. It will produce habituation and similar withdrawal symptoms which are milder and more prolonged than those of heroin.

28. **(D)**   Stroking the chin during an interview can be interpreted as contemplative thinking. Leaning forward means interest. Arms and legs tightly crossed and jaw set mean tension; and arms in lap, muscle groups relaxed indicate relaxation.

29. **(A)**   A consequence-oriented approach is most likely to be used for teleological ethics.

30. **(D)**   Solo practice usually produces a strong doctor–patient relationship and presents practice autonomy.

31. **(C)**   Weight gain is a common effect of cyclic antidepressants and may limit their use for obese patients or patients who desire weight reduction.

32. **(C)**   Depressive reactions are frequently encountered in carcinoma of the pancreas or large bowel. Symptoms of depression, anxiety, and premonition of serious illness are among the most common presenting complaints of patients with carcinoma of the pancreas.

33. **(B)**   Illness is personal, interpersonal, and cultural reactions to the disease or discomfort. Disease is an abnormality in the structure and function of body organs and systems.

34. **(D)**   The characteristics of the delusional disorder are hyperalertness; oversuspiciousness; reality distortion; and jealous, erotic, grandiose, persecutory, and litigious delusions. The paranoid psychotic often engages in homosexuality and is overly jealous toward the partner. The stress is often aggravated by injury.

35. **(C)**   One of the characteristics of schizophrenia is the disturbance of thinking. Patients with organic brain lesions will tend to omit important items, but schizophrenics think and reason in their own autistic terms, according to their own intricate private rules of logic.

36. **(B)**   Alcoholism is often associated with pancreatitis, hepatitis, peptic ulcer disease, cirrhosis, encephalopathy, macrocytic anemia, cardiomyopathy, labile hypertension, depression, and pneumonitis. The serum cholesterol level is usually normal or decreased.

37. **(C)**   The neuroleptic triad of parkinsonism, dystonia, and akathisia may occur with phenothiazine therapy. If symptoms are distressing or disabling, a reduction in dose or an antiparkinsonian medication may be indicated.

38. **(E)** Mandatory reporting includes child abuse and communicable diseases such as venereal disease and tuberculosis.

39. **(A)** The family life line is a chronologic sequence of events that have taken place in a family's history. It offers insight into family trends and the family's coping strategies during past significant events.

40. **(A)** Pick's disease is an uncommon chronic brain syndrome. It occurs much less frequently than does Alzheimer's. This affliction occurs twice as frequently in women as in men. Typically, the patient shows apathy, loss of memory, and inability to deal with new situations. Aphasia gradually develops, along with the established dementia. The brain areas involved are mainly the frontal and temporal lobes. Senile plaques, frequently found in senile dementia, are rarely found in Pick's disease.

41. **(A)** Patients admitted to the CCU may frequently show profound anxiety and deep depression due to pain, fear of death, uncertainty, confinement, cerebral hypoxia, sleep disturbances, and the frightening features of the environment. The defense mechanism of denial is commonly seen and may be beneficial for the patient. The family physician should deal with the patient with honesty and compassion.

42. **(A)** People with passive–aggressive personality show both passivity and aggressivity. The aggressiveness is usually expressed in such passive ways as obstructionism, pouting, procrastination, clinging, indecisiveness, and helplessness. These patients are often manipulative and are sometimes very annoying to the medical staff. A progressively wider spacing of appointments is frequently employed.

43. **(D)** Psychological factors appear to be significant determinants of chest pain severity in patients with coronary heart diseases. Moreover, chest pain may be the presentation of somatization and the patient requires comprehensive and continuous total health care from the family physician.

44. **(C)** Agoraphobia is characterized by fear of going out into the open, into closed spaces, or into streets and crowds. A spontaneous panic attack will develop with extreme fearfulness, feelings of impending doom, and cardiorespiratory symptoms (pounding heart and dyspnea). Confrontation with the avoided object or activity is needed to eliminate the patient's anxiety. Benzodiazepines and SSRIs are used.

45. **(D)** Common neuroleptics include chlorpromazine (Thorazine), trifluoperazine (Stelazine), thioridazine (Mellaril), thiothixene (Navane), and haloperidol (Haldol). The best response to neuroleptics is seen in acute schizophrenia, when agitation, paranoid delusions, and hallucinations are present. Response in withdrawn, apathetic, or chronic schizophrenics is less favorable.

46. **(A)** Libido is the sexual instinctual forces and drives. The id is composed of all the instinctual drives, including sexual (libido) and nonsexual, and is bound by the pleasure principle. The ego is motivated primarily by logical secondary process thinking, which makes possible the delay of gratification through the reality principle. Ego-ideal is the idealized self-image, the private personal optimal goal. Superego is the conscience part of the personality, derived largely from significant relationships in which standards and models, good and bad, have been set.

47. **(B)** Fifty percent of American adults drink little or no alcohol; 50% drink moderately or heavily; and 15% are seriously and adversely affected.

48. **(C)** Lithium is used for mania and depression in manic–depressive illness. Its side effects include nausea, vomiting, diarrhea, tremor, hypothyroidism, and nephrogenic diabetes insipidus (polyuria, polydipsia, and concentration defects).

49. **(E)** In steepling, the patient joins his hands with his fingers extended and his fingertips touched. This often indicates confidence and assurance. When the patient is sad, the hands are droopy and flaccid and the feet move in a slow, circular pattern. In contemplation, the hand is at the chin, stroking the chin or beard. In the defensive position, the arms are crossed, the legs are crossed, and the head is drawn back. A suspicious person often puts his hands in his pockets or behind his back and does not show open palms.

50. **(C)** Olfactory hallucinations are often central in origin, usually caused by lesions on the inferior and medial surface of one temporal lobe in or near the uncus; the seizure it produces is therefore called uncinate. Olfactory hallucination is commonly caused by patients with depressive illness or schizophrenia. In these patients, olfactory sensations are intact and the disagreeable-smelling odors are delusions.

51. **(D)** There is much the family physician can do before deciding that the sexual difficulty is serious enough to warrant referral for sex therapy. The patient's raising this question with the physician indicates that she trusts him or her enough to be receptive to his or her gradual suggestion that sexual satisfaction is "a continuum of experience with each position on the continuum equally important in and of itself," as opposed to the notion that only orgasm achieved through vaginal penetration is normal. The patient's reactions to sexuality can be briefly explored, with emphasis on helping her think of what would make the sexual experience more pleasurable for her. The couple can then be helped to communicate more effectively concerning each other's needs. The husband can be asked to come in, but at a time and in a way so that he will not perceive it as an occasion for chastisement.

52. **(C)** The problem presented by this couple contains the seeds of serious marital difficulty. The husband seems to be a compulsive character who cannot tolerate the disorganization that is attendant on family living. He sees raising the children as the wife's responsibility rather than a shared one, and is asking for something that may be quite impossible to achieve in this family: a wife and children who are compulsive in the same areas he is. The wife is rebelling against the husband's putting all responsibility on her, and her overweight may be a way of getting back at him. This only widens the gulf between them. It is important to help this couple get counseling, since otherwise they will either remain together with more and more friction and conflict or the marriage might break up.

53. **(E)** The dying patient arouses very uncomfortable feelings in the physician; death reminds him of his own mortality. All too often, the dying patient for whom nothing else can be done is neglected by the attending physician and the nursing staff. This should never be allowed to happen, as terminally ill patients suffer from extreme loneliness and hopelessness and must receive emotional support from the attending family physician.

54. **(D)** If a physician is called upon to examine the individual as a patient who is in need of treatment, he can proceed with all the freedom granted by the rules of his profession, provided that the patient does not object to the examination. If the patient objects, the physician should make a note that medical attention was refused and should not examine the patient; treatment without consent can become assault and battery.

55. **(C)** The liability of a physician's cure is compared with the careful and skillful physicians practicing in a similar community or in accordance with his school of medicine.

56. **(E)** Principles of medical ethics provide that a family physician may not reveal the confidences entrusted to him in the course of medical attendance, or the deficiencies he may observe in the character of patients, unless he is required to do so by law or unless it becomes necessary to do so to protect the welfare of the individual or of the community. The family physician is the judge of the

need for disclosure, except when commanded to speak by a court.

57. **(B)** Eleven million Americans are alcoholics, and another 33 million family members and significant others are affected by the disease.

58. **(E)** The prevalence of anorexia nervosa among adolescent girls from upper-middle-class backgrounds has been estimated to be one in 200. Full recovery is expected in the majority of patients, with improvements in an additional 25% of patients. Mortality is estimated at 5%.

59. **(A)** The treatments of the posttraumatic stress disorder include individual psychotherapy, family therapy, hypnosis, relaxation and desensitization therapy, and antidepressants (TCAs, SSRIs), axiolytics and anticonvulsants are used.

60. **(E)** Parkinson's disease is usually treated with amantadine (Symmetrel), benztropine (Cogentin), trihexyphenidyl (Artane), levodopa (Larodopa), and bromocriptine (Parlodel).

61. **(B)** The following drugs are to be avoided in a patient taking MAOIs: indirect-acting sympathomimetics (ephedrine, phenylephrine, phenylpropanolamine), antihypertensives (methyldopa, propranolol, reserpine), amphetamines, levodopa, meperidine, methylphenidate, cocaine, and imipramine.

62. **(B)** Many antidepressants have significant antihistaminic properties, which include sedation, drowsiness, weight gain, and hypotension. Doxepin and trimipramine have strong sedative effect; desipramine and protriptyline have little sedative effect.

63. **(D)** MAOIs may produce hypertensive crisis if consumed with drugs or food that contains tyramine. Aged cheese, red wine, fava beans, and broad bean pods should be avoided.

64. **(E)** Common side reactions of TCAs include fatigue, insomnia, arrhythmia, seizures, jaundice, and amenorrhea. It produces anticholinergic effects including urinary retention, and aggravation of the narrow-angle glaucoma. In patients with glaucoma, pilocarpine eye drops must be administered concurrently.

65. **(E)** The side reactions of phenothiazines include pseudoparkinsonism, blurred vision, inhibition of ejaculation, postural hypotension, and jaundice.

66. **(E)** The characteristic paranoid behaviors are jealousy, eroticism, grandiosity, litigiousness, and persecution. The most frequent and the most important behavior is the delusion of persecution, which often leads the patient to believe that he is threatened, causing him to take violent action in self-defense.

67. **(D)** The common side effects of SSRIs include nervousness, agitation, sleep disturbance, nausea, diarrhea, anorgasmia, and weight loss.

68. **(C)** TCAs are not recommended for patients with bundle-branch block, acute myocardial infarction, acute congestive heart failure, narrow-angle glaucoma, urinary retention, prostatic hypertrophy, and leukopenia.

69. **(D)** Anticholinergic side reactions include dry mouth, constipation, impotence, arrhythmia, restlessness, tachycardia, and paralytic ileus.

70. **(A)** The withdrawal symptoms of antidepressants includes malaise, anxiety, excessive and vivid dreaming, bradykinesia, akathisia, and mania.

71. **(A)** A working definition of family in an urban setting is a unit that comprises some kind of special relationship between any two or more persons that implies intimacy, reciprocity, and continuity.

72. **(E)** Bluish phlebitic scars and needle marks may indicate that the patient has used opioids in the past. The presence of miosis and some degree of drowsiness would suggest that the patient is under the influence of opioids at the time of examination. A characteristic abstinence syndrome (yawning, pupillary dilatation, muscle twitching, abdominal cramps, vomiting, hypertension, and sweating) can be elicited by withdrawal of the opioids. If the patient has used opioids in the previous 24 hours, their presence in the urine can be demonstrated by chemical or chromatographic tests.

73. **(E)** Drug-dependent youths have used drugs in an attempt to solve their maladaptive behavior problems, such as school failure and alienation from society. The use of amphetamines may also lead to dependence on the drugs without careful monitoring. Some youths become addicted to earn respect from peers.

74. **(C)** Anorexia nervosa is commonly seen in adolescents because of their interest in losing weight. It is characterized by intense fear of gaining weight, and altered body image (the patient believes that he or she is obese). It carries an increased risk of death but can be treated by behavioral therapy.

75. **(E)** A sensitivity training group seeks to develop self-awareness and an understanding of group processes rather than to gain relief from emotional disturbances. The emotionally disturbed person should not be referred to the T-group with the expectation that he will thereby achieve relief of his illness. Mentally ill individuals should not be referred to the T-group, which will only increase the psychiatric casualties. The staff members of the encounter group have to be trained to deal with difficult complications of group encounters and to select the members carefully to be useful in the group dynamic process. The motives of the couple are also important considerations.

76. **(E)** Characteristics of a healthy urban family include: (1) rules that maintain boundaries within the community and within the family's subsystems that are clear and not mystified; (2) boundaries and hierarchy that are predictable and yet adaptive to changing circumstances; (3) permeable boundaries; and (4) power and internal structure that are appropriate for the family's development level.

77. **(C)** The family structure of the urban psychosomatogenic family is characterized by (1) physiologic vulnerability; (2) child involved in parental conflicts; and (3) family structure of enmeshment, overprotectiveness, rigidity, and lack of conflict resolution.

78. **(E)** Compared to rural families, urban families are more likely to possess the following characterictics: (1) responsive to a heterogeneous, diverse, and complicated environment; (2) economically interdependent; (3) the homeless, homosexuals, and runaways gather in cities—different kinds of family relationships; (4) two breadwinners in nuclear families, female-headed families (Aid to Families with Dependent Children [AFDC]), delayed to create family of procreation; (5) mobile and to change the structure rapidly; and (6) recent immigrant families with diversified culture and ethnicity.

79. **(B)** Poor families in urban areas are often limited in resources to meet the demands of adequate housing, clothing, food, and even heat in the winter; thus, many poor families may have to depend on public social welfare programs. As such, they often cannot maintain boundaries, and the family may exhibit fragmentation and disorganization. This is simply their response to the contradictory demands of employers, social agencies, clinics, schools, foster care agencies, and public assistance.

80. **(E)** Suicide is the tenth most prevalent cause of death in the United States. The suicide rate is higher in peacetime than in wartime, and it is four times higher for men than for women. The incidence of suicide increases with increasing age. Physicians have a higher suicide risk than the general popu-

lace. The suicide rate is also higher for single, divorced, and widowed adults.

81. **(E)** Suicide frequently occurs in psychotics, associated with delusions or hallucinations; it is also common in depressed patients. Some patients commit suicide out of revenge against a loved person. The act of dying by suicide is often perceived by the patient as a pleasurable reunion with a dead person, frequently the parental figure. A need for self-punishment in patients is usually associated with failure at work.

82. **(E)** Kübler-Ross has postulated five stages of dying: denial, anger, bargaining, depression, and acceptance. The family physician providing care for dying patients needs to offer support and to radiate realistic hope for the patient. The dying patient is badly in need of comprehensive and continuous care.

83. **(D)** Informed consent consists of consent, competence, and information. The best evidence of informed consent is documentation that includes the decision-making process, the clinician's rationale for treatment, and evaluation of costs and benefits in establishing clinical judgment.

84. **(D)** There is a need in the inner city to have family physicians who are trained in the biopsychosocial model of health care. However, the stress on the physician caring for people in often desperate circumstances may lead to burnout. To practice in the inner city, the family physician needs to recognize the realities of the setting without romanticization. Professional and social supports are imperative.

85. **(B)** Spanish-origin households account for 5% of total American households, and 84% are settled in large metropolitan areas. Black households comprise almost 11% of all households in the United States, but almost 60% are located in the central cities. Most Native American Indians reside in the rural reservations. There are over a half million Haitians in the United States, the majority of whom are concentrated in urban areas.

86. **(E)** Many characteristics of urban families may be different from those of the family physician's family of origin; however, if the family is well functioning, the family physician does not need to impose his own ideal of "normalcy" and does not have to regard "different" as pathologic.

87. **(E)** When a family physician finds that his or her own family differs from an urban patient's family with respect to the performance of tasks (survival, nurturance, and guidance) yet the patient's family is functioning well, the family physician can just respect the family's operation without imposing his or her own concepts or beliefs of model families.

88. **(E)** Reserpine gives the classic example of drug-induced depression. Many other drugs may also induce depression, and this should be detected early. These medications include corticosteroids, oral contraceptives, antihypertensives (alpha-methyldopa, guanethidine, clonidine, propranolol), alcohol, opiates, benzodiazepines, disulfiram, and digitalis.

89. **(A)** According to Erickson, during adolescence, an individual should develop identity to resolve role confusion; otherwise, the individual may develop an identity crisis.

90. **(D)** Psychotic symptoms can be the manifestations of organic diseases or can be drug induced. The following drugs and conditions commonly cause psychotic symptoms: intoxication, amphetamines and cocaine, hallucinogens, phencyclidine, anticholinergic drugs, withdrawal reactions, alcohol, barbiturates, systemic infections, metabolic and endocrine disorders, hypoxia or hypercapnia, hypoglycemia, ionic imbalances, hepatic or renal disease, thyroid disease, central nervous system disorders, encephalitis (especially due to herpes simplex), epilepsy (especially psychomotor epilepsy), Huntington's chorea, multiple sclerosis, cerebrovascular disease, and space-occupying lesions.

91. **(A)** Many immigrant families in urban centers have lost contact with people in their

homelands and are alone and isolated, in addition to being cut off from people who speak their primary language. Introducing the family to a social network that brings resources (material, emotional, and informational) can be a safeguard against stress and illness.

92. **(E)** Urban single-parent families are derived from separation, divorce, the husband's death, an institutionalized husband, or a husband away from home. Most single-parent families are headed by women; in many cases, the women were never married.

93. **(C)** In urban psychosomatic families, the following are most likely to occur: (1) triangulation (the child openly allied with one parent against another—the child always takes sides); (2) parent–child coalitions against the other parent; (3) detouring (parental conflict is submerged beneath protective or accusatory attentions for the sick child).

94. **(E)** Many elderly persons sleep less than 5 hours a day, decrease REM and deep sleep, and increase nocturnal awakening. A trial of good sleep hygiene (establishing a bedtime routine; elimination of alcohol, caffeine, and nicotine; increased daytime exercise; and a comfortable and quiet environment) is usually helpful.

95. **(C)** Substance abuse includes illegal use of opiates, alcoholism, and prescription drugs.

96. **(D)** The family circle is a person's "emotional family" (ie, the subjective perception of the person's family). A person can include any member of the biological and legal family, pets, institutions, and concerns or illness in the family circle. The data may shed light on the cause of the illness and the support and assistance available for the treatment plan.

97. **(B)** Telogen defluvium (or effluvium) is a temporary diffuse hair loss, resulting most likely from stressful life events, including the postpartum state, life-threatening injuries, severe illnesses, fever, surgical shock, crash diets, and psychological stresses. The adult scalp contains 90% anagen (growing phase) hairs, 10% telogen (resting phase) hairs and 0 to 1% catagen (transitional phase). The patient increases the telogen hairs to 25% or more. Spontaneous resolution is generally the case.

98. **(E)** Although not all immigrant groups suffer social and family disintegration, realignment of family social structure always takes place upon immigration. This discontinuity takes its toll. For reasons of economics, social contacts, and historic precedent, many immigrants settle first in the large cities, and the immigration-related stress becomes an urban health risk.

99. **(A)** Urban patients with chronic stable schizophrenia require comprehensive and continuous total care, and a family physician is certainly the best provider for them.

100. **(D)** Toxic psychosis can be caused by the use of hallucinogens (LSD), amphetamines, or alcohol. Hallucinogens often distort perceptions and may also cause hallucinations with vivid color images. The manic–depressive person is characterized by a recent high and current depression; during the manic cycle he may overspend, while in the depression cycle he may feel impending bankruptcy. Schizophrenics are so preoccupied with paranoid delusions that the date is unimportant to them anyway.

101. **(A)** A primary-care team development program consists of in-service training as well as continuing medical education. The curriculum includes group skills (role clarification, preparation of role changes, sense of belonging, cooperation, and problem-solving ability), leadership skills, and primary-care skills.

102. **(C)** Urban areas often have higher rates of unemployment, crowding, and inadequate housing. These conditions have been associated with higher crime rates. High crime rates increase the stress for people living in these areas, and fear of crime may inhibit people from meeting health and education needs.

103. **(C)** Compared to rural patients, urban patients with mental illness are more likely to be in crisis for the following reasons: (1) In urban family practice, the physician is less likely to be familiar with the patient and the family. (2) The family physicians are often different from the patients/families in cultural concepts, linguistic competence, and ethnic and social backgrounds. (3) Many urban patients/families are often overtaxed with many economic and social problems (overcrowding, broken families, and child abuse). They are often different in ethnic and social backgrounds themselves. Many urban families receive public assistance, including help from social work agencies experienced in the care of "multiproblem" families. (4) Many patients are apt to be in crisis, and they may be reluctant to continue care once symptoms are relieved.

104. **(D)** The primary prevention in the urban setting is preventing the onset of a disease by eliminating the risk or predisposing cause. A secondary prevention is preventing the progress of a disease by early detection and treatment. The tertiary prevention is preventing chronic disability by rehabilitation and restoration of normal roles.

105. **(E)** In an urban clinical setting, a medical ethicist is (1) a consultant who makes recommendations on "difficult" cases for actions to take in patient care; (2) an educator who analyzes concepts and illuminates issues for health-care providers; (3) a counselor who allows health-care providers to ventilate and unburden themselves; and (4) a patient advocate who educates physicians about patient rights and the physician's responsibility to protect those rights.

106. **(E)** Family physicians practicing cross-cultural medicine in an urban setting should (1) listen with sympathy and understanding to the patient's perception of the problem; (2) explain the perception of the problem to the patient; (3) acknowledge and discuss the differences and similarities; (4) recommend treatment; and (5) negotiate agreement.

107. **(B)** Acculturation is the process of change that occurs when two culture groups are in contact over a sustained period of time. The rate of acculturation is dependent on the length of time immigrants reside in this country, language dominance, race, socioeconomic and educational consonance, urban or rural background, migration pattern, immigration status, developmental stage of the family, and the structural characteristics of the family (permeability of boundaries and the level of cultural evolution).

108. **(C)** The average Haitian is very friendly, polite, appreciative, hospitable, compassionate, and cheerful. The physician should be polite, friendly, and concerned when interacting with Haitian patients.

109. **(A)** The legal rule is that competent adult patients have the right to consent to or to refuse treatment. There is, moreover, a right to refuse treatment even if the result of that refusal is foolish, harmful, or leads to death.

110. **(B)** Good health habits include (1) no smoking, (2) limited alcohol, (3) appropriate weight for height, (4) 7 to 8 hours of sleep per night, and (5) physical activities.

111. **(E)** Bulimia is treated with behavioral (diary keeping, assertion training, group meals, positive and negative contingency planning) and psychodynamic (insight and support, imagery) therapy, along with medications which include MAOIs, TCAs, and SSRIs.

112. **(E)** Schizophrenia has significant genetic basis. Information overload is a high-risk factor; a hyperdopaminergic state and enlarged ventricles may be related.

113. **(D)** Approximately one half of crashes fatal to vehicle occupants and one fifth of crashes in which vehicle occupants were injured result at least in part from alcohol use. The increased risk begins with blood alcohol concentrations of 30 mg/100 mL (0.03% by weight), commonly reached with one or two drinks in most individuals. All individuals

are affected at or below 100 mg/100 mL. Concentrations of 80 to 100 mg/100 mL are usually regarded as evidence of alcohol influence in most states.

114. **(D)**   Adolescent athletes are at an increased risk for drug abuse, including alcohol, marijuana, cocaine, amphetamines, sedatives, steroids, hallucinogens, and heroin.

115. **(E)**   Common untoward effects of anorectic drugs include stimulation of the sympathetic and central nervous systems, palmar sweating, dry mouth, pupillary dilatation, blurred vision, dizziness, palpitations, nervousness, irritability, insomnia, hyperkinesis, and decreased sense of fatigue.

116. **(E)**   Consistent disciplines, cohesive family environment, avoidance of mass media programs on violence and gangs, stimulating educational outlet programs, adequate housing and a supportive neighborhood, and steady school and vocational activities may decrease the risk of delinquency, including runaways.

117. **(D)**   When the child performs desirable behavior, reward him immediately and consistently with reinforcers (such as money, attention, praise, physical contact, or privileges). Tell him that you like what he is doing. Record the behavior on a chart and encourage him to keep up the good behavior.

118. **(B)**   Physical illness is a special life crisis; to cope effectively with physical illness, the patient requires general adaptive tasks and specific illness-related ones.
   1. General adaptive tasks:
      (a) Preserving a reasonable emotional balance—Upsetting feelings (guilt, a sense of failure, apprehension, a sense of inadequacy) associated with illness must be managed and a sense of hope installed.
      (b) Preserving a satisfactory self-image— A sense of competency and mastery must be maintained. The patient should be able to accept the necessary help comfortably and participate in the decision and direction of his activities.

(c) Preserving relationships with family and friends—The patient needs to keep communication channels open with his significant others to alleviate the sense of isolation and alienation.
      (d) Preparing for an uncertain future— With preparation, the uncertain future can be coped with effectively.
   2. Illness-related adaptive tasks:
      (a) Dealing with discomfort and incapacitation.
      (b) Managing the stresses of diagnostic or treatment procedures.
      (c) Developing adequate relationships with the family physician.

119. **(C)**   In response to the increased patient and family load, even the solo primary-care practitioner employs a supporting staff (ie, the primary-care team) or joins with other primary-care practitioners (ie, the interprofessional team) to provide needed primary-care for growing patients and families. Thus, the proper functioning of the health-care team is essential for delivering efficient and quality primary care. The following approaches may be found to be useful in effecting the functions of the primary-care team.
   1. Clarify roles for each team member—The primary-care practitioner serves as the team leader who is ultimately responsible for the care of the patient and the family. Other team members participate in the patient management process, according to the direction and supervision of the primary-care practitioner.
   2. The extent of the authority delegated must be clearly defined to maintain quality of health care provided—In order to delegate patient care responsibility to the office personnel, the task of the patient-care process is broken down into component parts which are performed by the office personnel under the training and supervision of the primary-care practitioner. The use of automated equipment also facilitates the ancillary personnel's participation in the patient-management process. These tasks should be clearly stated to maintain the standard of patient care.

3. Adaptable and flexible role changes through training and development—Responding to the increase of patient and family load, the expansion of service scopes, the change of patient population (eg, the increase of the elderly population due to the extension of the practice to the nursing home), and the acquisition of new equipment (eg, the arrival of spirometry), the team members may have to change their roles and perform new tasks. Without the ability to be flexible and adaptable, the team will find it difficult to respond to changes.

4. Well-defined specific objectives and evaluation criteria must be established—All team members should understand the goals and objectives of the team that preferably are congruent with their own personal goals in life. Evaluation should be conducted periodically to reinforce the team members in sticking to the performance of the objectives. Apparent deviations from the expected norms are identified for developmental remedy through further education and training.

5. Generating respect and trust between team members—A sense of belonging should be established between the team members; motivate the team members by common aspirations (eg, providing comprehensive and continuous total health care for the patient and the family) to facilitate their self-actualization needs.

120. **(B)** Parkinsonism is characteristic for resting tremor (pill-rolling tremor), bradykinesia, mask face, loss of associated movements, and decreased range of movement and can be treated by giving L-dopa. Tardive dyskinesia is caused by phenothiazine administration; athetosis is the predominant characteristic of tremor. "Flapping tremor" (asterixis) is a nonrhythmic, asymmetric lapse involuntary, sustained posture of the extremities; this is seen in hepatic encephalopathy but not in hepatic coma. The tremor of hyperthyroidism is best seen with the arms extended and the fingers spread apart. It represents an abnormal accentuation of physiologic static–kinetic tremor and therefore predominantly involves the flexion–extension movements, is small in amplitude, and occurs at a rate of about 10 to 12 Hz. A terminal crescendo tremor is a hallmark of disorders of the outflow pathway of the cerebellum (from the dentate nucleus) and its connections in the midbrain and thalamus.

121. **(B)** Flight of ideas is a nearly continuous high-speed flow of speech. The patient leaps rapidly from one topic to another, with each topic being more or less related to the preceding topic or to environmental stimuli, but progression of thought is illogical and the goal is never reached. This is characteristic of an acute manic state.

122. **(A)** Hysterical patients are usually egocentric, helpless, attention seeking, and manipulative. Phobic patients usually express a magical wish along with fear that the wish may not be granted. Obsessive–compulsive patients will often use the defense of intellectualization. The depressed patient is preoccupied with worries. Paranoid patients frequently show suspiciousness and mistrust.

123. **(A)** Denial is an unconscious mechanism wherein one behaves as if the problem does not exist, but lying is a conscious process. Denial is the simplest form of ego defense and is closely related to rationalization. Repression, the motivated unconscious forgetting, is the earliest and one of the most commonly employed defense mechanisms; it is the cornerstone of psychodynamics. Suppression is conscious forgetting, is not a true defense, and is a commonly employed coping mechanism of normal personalities. Isolation can remove the emotional charge associated with the original memory. This mechanism is commonly used by obsessive–compulsive persons.

124. **(A)** The TAT (Thematic Apperception Test) is a semistructured projective test consisting of 20 drawings of persons engaged in various activities. The patient is asked to make up a story for each drawing. The Bender–Gestalt test is a test of organic involvement which measures an individual's ability to remember and reproduce complex geometric designs.

The WAIS (Wechsler Adult Intelligence Scale) is an individual test to measure intelligence by means of verbal and performance tests. The MMPI (Minnesota Multiphasic Personality Inventory) consists of 550 questions designed to construct the personality profile of the subject.

125. **(A)** The M'Naghten rule defines criminal responsibility, which concerns the ability of the defendant to know he was doing wrong. It is not a test of sanity and is not formulated as such; rather, it is a test of legal responsibility for acts. The M'Naghten rule is supplemented by the irresistible impulse rule, which states that the accused cannot be held responsible for his behavior if he was unable to resist acting as he did.

126. **(B)** In concrete operations (6 to 12 years), the child gains the conservation ability and is aware that he has one point of view and that there are other points of view held by his peers. Thus, he can cooperate with others and share a modified point of view. The child is able to show experience—independent thoughts such as reversibility. In the process of reversibility, the child understands that his position is not immutable and that the risk of trying a new idea will produce nothing worse than a return to the starting point of the operation. The child also can arrange objects on one dimension such as weight or size (the process of serialization).

127. **(B)** The primary care practitioner can offer family planning services to help the couple to arrive at an ideal family size through reproduction. The reproduction function can be seen in the single-person family, in communal families, and in unmarried adults living together. Infertile women can fulfill the reproduction function by adopting children; however, if the infertile couple decides not to adopt any children, reproduction will not be an important function in that family.

128. **(B)** In conversion reaction, the patient converts his unconscious psychic conflict into somatic dysfunction. These patients are often emotionally labile and excitable, overly dramatic, dependent and demanding, and highly suggestible. They yearn for affection, often establish superficial and sexualized relationships with others, and frequently use denial and repression for defense. The somatized conversion symptoms include the following characteristics: (1) involuntary disorder; (2) frequently precipitated by sudden environmental (interpersonal) stress; (3) symptoms are useful in avoiding anxiety; (4) usually involves the sensory or motor system rather than the autonomic system; (5) symptoms rarely make anatomical sense; (6) symptoms are frequently inconsistent in presentation; (7) symptoms may disappear with sleep, hypnosis, or situations that threaten self-preservation; (8) the presence of secondary gain—social or other benefits of the symptom or disorder; (9) La belle indifference may be found—a small proportion show indifference or lack of concern; most common when the symptom involves no perception of pain.

129. **(E)** Following a major loss in life (such as the loss of a loved one, the loss of a job, the loss of property or possession, the loss of status, or the loss of body functioning), the patient usually goes through a grief (mourning) reaction which includes somatic distress (nausea, choking, shortness of breath), guilt, sadness, hostile feelings, preoccupation with the lost person or object, irritability, or withdrawal activities. This grief reaction is normal if it lasts no more than 6 to 12 months. The primary-care practitioner should facilitate the patient's grief process by encouragement and support. Let the patient understand that the mourning is necessary and not embarrassing; provide an opportunity for the patient to express his feelings of sadness, anger, and guilt; assist the patient in reviewing the circumstances of the loss to enhance his understanding that the loss is inevitable and may even be beneficial to all concerned; mobilize the family and significant others to assist or to participate in the grief process; and arrange the patient's returning to normal social activities gradually. Do not intend to abort the grief; hypnotics may be needed if the patient complains of insomnia. Frequent follow-ups are arranged to support the progress, to evaluate possible depressive episodes, and to identify

patients with abnormal grief reactions. Patients who are inhibited, socially isolated, and who have had multiple losses are at high risk to develop abnormal grief reactions or depressions.

130. **(D)** Responding to rapid body growth and societal demand, the adolescent searches for the answer to the question "Who am I?." When the adolescent shows his fidelity toward an ideology and establishes a solid sexual role, he will be able to define himself and achieve a sense of identity. If the adolescent cannot find a role in society, he will be unable to resolve the identity crisis and will feel a sense of role confusion or identity diffusion. There is a danger that he may achieve negative identity formation by clinging with gangs, thus engaging in antisocial behavior.

131. **(B)**

Psychosocial Stage	Developmental Tasks to Be Resolved
1. Sensory–oral	Trust/mistrust
2. Muscular–anal	Autonomy/shame and doubt
3. Locomotor–genital	Initiative/guilt
4. Latency	Industry/inferiority
5. Puberty and adolescence	Identity/role confusion
6. Young adulthood	Intimacy/isolation
7. Adulthood	Generativity/stagnation
8. Maturity	Integrity/despair

132. **(E)** Family crises are acute, stressful situations that the family finds difficult to cope with due to inadequate resources and inadequate coping mechanisms. The most common episodes include:

1. Developmental or normal crisis—A period of change, upset, and uneasiness occurs in the family system at several predictable times. Since these are predictable, they are considered "normal" and because they occur simply due to the normal course of development, they are often called "developmental." Families must redefine themselves and adapt their methods of interaction, power, support, and communication at these times. Common developmental crises include:
   (a) The addition of a new member—birth, adoption, grandparent.
   (b) The departure of a member—death, divorce, children leaving home.
   (c) The development of a new identity for one member—going from infant to toddler, midlife crisis, retirement.
2. Internal crisis—This is an event in the family that is viewed as demoralizing to the group. In this type of crisis, one or more of the family members have done something that disrupts the equilibrium of the system by violating the expectations and acceptable behaviors family members have for one another. This may involve a premarital pregnancy, illegitimacy, drug abuse, and extramarital affairs.
3. External or situational crisis—This is the crisis that is imposed on the family from the outside. This includes severe illness, tornadoes, fires, accidents, loss of status (change of jobs), or sudden impoverishment (unemployment).
4. Piling up—It often seems that once a crisis occurs, others follow quickly and pile up on a person or family. This is due to:
   (a) Greater vulnerability to perceive common events as crises—A person having a minor traffic accident after finding her husband is divorcing her feels that is a crisis, whereas two weeks earlier it would have been an inconvenience.
   (b) Unresolved nature of initial crisis—If a person has not worked through the initial crisis event, he or she tends to stockpile new upsets and put them on hold. Eventually, this pile-up of little events becomes unbearable.
   (c) Inadequate coping strategies—Families sometimes respond to a crisis in ways that further their feelings of anxiety or hopelessness. By doing this, they pile further crises and crisis reactions on themselves. An example is the woman with an unwanted premarital pregnancy whose family arranges an abortion for her only to discover later that she has a great deal of difficulty in handling the guilt, she really wanted to parent the child, or she cannot have children later for some reason. The impulsive handling of the

event was well-intentioned but may compound the impact of the event. Piling up may be a series of very minor events that, when fully developed, lead to divorce or feelings of alienation from one another.

133. (B) Confabulation is an unconscious filling in of gaps in memory by imagined experiences. These recollections change from moment to moment and are easily induced by suggestion. It is characteristic in Korsakoff's psychosis.

134. (C) Amphetamine psychosis is characterized by vivid visual hallucination and paranoid reaction (persecutory delusions and ideas of reference). Foodstuffs containing tyramine (eg, cheese, beer, wines, chicken liver, and pickled herring) used concurrently with MAOIs will cause severe hypertensive crisis. Barbiturates are contraindicated in patients with acute intermittent porphyria, as they can precipitate an acute attack.

135. (C) Gender identity is the feeling of the gender (whether male or female) the person belongs to. As early as 18 months a child is aware of his or her own gender, and by age 2 or 3 the child is able to answer whether he or she is a boy or a girl. This is the private experience of sex role. In homosexuality one may dislike the opposite sex, while in transsexuality the gender identity is that of the opposite biologic sex.

136. (E) Patients with complex posttraumatic stress disorder often exhibit a sense of hopelessness and despair, isolation and withdrawal, shame, guilt, and self-blame, derealization/depersonalization, persistent dysphoria, and chronic suicidal preoccupation. Individuals at risk include hostages, prisoners of war, concentration camp survivors, and survivors of domestic battering or sexual abuse.

137. (D) A family physician may often develop a "sinking feeling" for patients with borderline personality disorder, which is characterized by unstable mood, shifting behaviors from anxiety to depression, intense but volatile interpersonal relationships, excessive uncontrollable constant anger, a poor sense of self-identity, and impulsiveness. Supportive and continuous care from the family physician may establish satisfactory relationships with these patients.

138. (D) When anger is expressed by the patient, the family physician should not be provoked by his own angry feelings and should not generate avoidance behavior to neglect his patient's needs. The family physician should recognize that the patient's expression of anger may not be directly related to his diagnostic and therapeutic plans; rather, the anger represents the patient's cry for assistance for his helplessness resulting from his illness. The family physician should be calm, confident, and empathetic to provide needed care for the patient.

A patient feels anger for many reasons. It may be a response to a current situation of interpersonal transaction. Discomfort in the office temperature, long waiting hours, delayed appointment time, or missed laboratory results will provoke his anger easily. The family physician needs to evaluate the situation to institute remedial action. A patient's anger may be displaced from other life situations or events to the family physician who just happened to be convenient as the focus of the angry feelings. When the patient attacks with anger without any appreciable reasons from the current interaction, the family physician should let the patient fully express his feelings of anger to determine the causes of displacement. When the opportunities are provided, the patient will be able to calm down and get himself together again. Anger is also generated in patients when they are grieving or coping with a loss of control and competency. The aggressive patient may be dealing with anxiety about helplessness and be especially uncomfortable with the "sick" role. The feeling of being "out of control" stimulated the denial of symptoms, an attempt to take charge, or the appearance of super-normal recovery or vigor. Refrain from giving the patient premature and unnecessary reassurance to abort his anger; rather, his anger needs to be recognized and acknowledged with understanding and empathy to assist him through the adaptation stages. The patient should be treated with candor and his feelings of competency encouraged by actively participating in his own care. At times, anger may reflect a characteristic response pattern of the patient used to control and intimidate. Dealing with these angry patients requires a quiet, consistent, and assured posture. Openness and candor are beneficial. These patients are suspicious of unfamiliar helping procedures and they require direct, consistent, and unambiguous instructions from the family physician. The patient is best managed by actively engaging him in the treatment plan through explaining treatment and diagnostic procedures and encouraging his collaboration through questions and participation in his own care.

139. **(D)** The patient needs to be assured the availability and frequent but short appointments are set. During the appointment, the primary-care practitioner should keep up the time, listen attentively to the patient's complaints, evaluate his problems, and pay full attention to him. However, when the appointment time is up, the patient is asked to leave with the next appointment scheduled. Set firm limits; avoid spending inappropriate extra time with the patient. The patient is educated to be able to express his feelings without resorting to somatic complaints. Keep professional distance with the patient; refrain from divulging personal information to the patient, avoiding the establishment of inappropriate social or intimate relationships with the patient. Arrange to see the patient and his spouse or his intimate others together. Mobilize ancillary health professionals in the helping relationships.

140. **(E)** Do not become irritated or frustrated and ignore the patient. Be comfortable in accepting the patient's refusal of diagnostic work-up, treatment plans, or surgical procedures. Be sure that these procedures are absolutely necessary; take time to explain to the patient the necessity and benefits of these procedures. Be nonjudgmental; do not interpret or criticize his behavior. Show genuine interest in his welfare to cultivate a trustworthy relationship. Involve him in the care of his illness; let him exercise choices of diagnostic and therapeutic paths. Elicit assistance from his family and significant others in persuading his cooperation. Watch for depression, psychosis, or organic brain syndrome.

141. **(B)** Malingering is the simulation of symptoms or injury with intent to deceive. Some patients may go to extremes to "con" the family physician for the purpose of gain, such as being relieved of responsibility, avoiding an unpleasant situation, or obtaining compensation. The malingering patient is usually pleasant, flattering, and very conformative. The family physician should not fall into his traps easily by rewarding him with labeled "illness," which will reinforce his motivation to remain "ill" or to repeat "illness" in achieving a beneficial advantage. Repeated detailed questioning over a period of time, with accurate and complete recordkeeping of the answers (best done with witness or audiotape), will often yield inconsistencies and contradictions. The malingerer, fearing detection of his malingering, is often unwilling to undergo medical reexamination and is not willing to undergo any exploratory surgery or painful procedures. He has no pain or disability to respond to treatment. The malingerer is often associated with antisocial personality. The definite diagnosis is often difficult and may require psychiatric evaluation.

142. **(D)** Listen openly to the patient's complaints, allowing for their full expression. In doing so, the patient may realize the imaginary or unfounded nature of his complaints, or he may identify the solution to the problems he has encountered. There is no need to argue or quarrel with the patient, for this will further cloud the issue, escalate the patient's hostility, and add to the materials of his complaints. The willingness to listen and the absence of defensive behavior encourage the patient's adoption of a more accommodating

and constructive style. An empathetic but firm and assured posture should then be taken to focus the patient's attention on the issues of current illnesses and to reduce his fixation on the complaints. Acknowledge his legitimate status of somatic distress, inform the normal results of his physical findings, and avoid rewarding the patient with secondary gains such as medications or disability certificates. Schedule frequent and short visits with time limits (10 to 20 minutes). During the visit, pay full attention to him, listen seriously and empathetically, evaluate his emotional status and life difficulties, and correlate these life stresses with the physical distress when the patient is ready to accept it. Do not promise a cure but promise patience, empathy, and availability. Educate the patient in expressing his emotional difficulties in effective terms without resorting to physical symptoms.

143. **(A)-F, (B)-T, (C)-F, (D)-T, (E)-T.** There is a lag in clinical response of four to six weeks to reach a therapeutic blood level of 150 to 200 mg/mL. Early responses include relief of insomnia and increase of energy; mood depression and sexual dysfunction are often relieved in the later stage.

144. **(A)-T, (B)-T, (C)-T, (D)-T, (E)-T.** Sexual dysfunction is commonly seen in patients with diabetes, hypertension, malnutrition, hypothyroidism, anemia, and depression. Patients recovering from serious illnesses (such as myocardial infarction) often develop sexual dysfunction; this may be due to psychogenic problems, and counseling will help. Recovering cardiac patients on propranolol may develop impotence.

145. **(A)-T, (B)-T, (C)-T, (D)-F, (E)-F.** There is a 5% mortality rate in anorexia nervosa, and hospitalization is advisable. Amitriptyline (Elavil), chlorpromazine (Thorazine), and cyproheptadine (Periactin) have been tried with beneficial results, along with behavior conditioning and family supports.

146. **(A)-F, (B)-T, (C)-T, (D)-T, (E)-F.** In the elderly, long-term use of many drugs may

cause depression. Common drugs used in family practice include antihypertensives (reserpine, methyldopa, clonidine, and hydralazine), estrogens, H2 blockers (cimetidine and ranitidine), steroids, digitalis, propranolol, and benzodiazepines (especially diazepam).

147. **(A)-T, (B)-T, (C)-F, (D)-F, (E)-F.** Reversible causes of dementia account for 10% to 25% of dementia patients, including myxedema, hypercalcemia, pernicious anemia, Wernicke/Korsakoff syndrome, subdural hematoma, normal pressure hydrocephalus, syphilis, chronic meningitis, congestive heart failure, hepatic failure, Cushing syndrome, azotemia, and depression. Sedatives, hypnotics, narcotic pain killers, H2-receptor blockers (cimetidine, ranitidine, and famotidine), cold remedies, and allergy pills can also cause dementia.

148. **(A)-F, (B)-F, (C)-F, (D)-T, (E)-F.** Anorexia nervosa is characterized by weight loss, intense fear of becoming obese, refusal of food intake, extensive exercises, and amenorrhea in the female. Hypokalemic alkalosis and ECG changes (flattened T, ST depression, and QT prolongation) may be noted.

149. **(A)-F, (B)-F, (C)-F, (D)-F, (E)-F.** In 30% of patients with depression, there is hypersecretion of cortisol without suppression (greater than 5 ng/dL) following dexamethasone administration; in 25% of patients with depression, administration of thyrotropin-releasing hormone (TRH) does not increase the TSH by more than 5 ng/mL.

150. **(A)-F, (B)-F, (C)-F, (D)-T, (E)-F.** Sexual behavior has changed rapidly, with many lifestyles being tried which in the past would not have been considered. In studies of couples engaged in switching or those entering group marriages, it has been found that these steps are much more frequently an attempt to cope with and save a marriage that has some problems in it than a first step toward the dissolution of a marriage. A family counseling session is needed to explore the true meaning of "switching" for the husband, and

support should be offered for the couple to work through the problems (including sexual problems) they have had.

151. **(A)-F, (B)-T, (C)-F, (D)-T, (E)-F.** The marriage apparently is in serious trouble and it is likely that without professional help from their family physician they will be unable to modify their malignant interaction. In providing family counseling, the family physician is advised to refrain from siding with either party until the situation is clarified. Even if there is reality in the husband's concern about the finances, it is obvious that this couple is dealing with the stresses confronting them by attacking each other and trying to change each other, rather than by finding some way of working together in a way that would take each one's needs and differences into consideration. The spouses have by now perceived each other as enemies who make life hard to bear. The family physician can point out what each is doing and the consequences of their actions; he can tell them that if they continue this way, the situation will probably continue to deteriorate. The family physician can help them clarify whether the relationship is salvageable and whether a somewhat less destructive way of living together can be found. If the situation gets worse, the couple can be referred to an experienced family counselor for further assistance.

152. **(A)-T, (B)-T, (C)-F, (D)-F, (E)-T.** The common effects of marijuana are reddening of the eyes, euphoria, impaired memory, motor incoordination, depersonalization, time–space distortions, dry mouth and throat, increased hunger, dizziness, increased visual and auditory awareness, sleepiness, spontaneous laughter, increased heart rate, and hallucinations, delusions, and paranoia (high doses).

153. **(A)-T, (B)-T, (C)-T, (D)-T, (E)-T.** Family is the central focus of care in family practice; the family physician needs to be responsive to resolving family problems.

154. **(A)-F, (B)-F, (C)-T, (D)-T, (E)-F.** Most battered women see their family physicians

soon after a battering incident, and the responsive family physician is instrumental in the recovery of the battered woman, who needs immediate protection from the batterer, immediate medical and psychiatric treatment, crisis intervention counseling, and information about available resources for help. Psychotropic drugs should be cautiously used if indicated. They may dull the woman's clear thinking and may be used for suicide attempts. It is important for the family physician to inform these women of available resources for help.

155. **(A)-T, (B)-T, (C)-T, (D)-T, (E)-T.** Family practice encompasses patients of all ages and both sexes. In addition, a family physician may encounter patients within different socioeconomic classes, religious beliefs, and languages. By maintaining an open mind and a proper understanding of different backgrounds, the family physician will be able to improve the communication.

156. **(A)-T, (B)-T, (C)-T, (D)-T, (E)-T.** Effective communications include adequate time for instruction, appropriate written instructions, and supportive and optimistic physician attitudes on compliance. Adequate patient education includes a thorough understanding of the antihypertensive regimen, the desirability of hypertension control, and the need for periodic evaluation of status.

157. **(A)-F, (B)-F, (C)-T, (D)-T, (E)-T.** From 0.5% to 1.0% of patients taking neuroleptic drugs may develop the neuroleptic malignant syndrome, characterized by hyperthermia, muscular rigidity, altered consciousness, and anatomic instability (including tachycardia, labile blood pressure, profuse diaphoresis, cardiac dysrhythmia, and incontinence).

158. **(A)-F, (B)-T, (C)-T, (D)-T, (E)-F.** In neuroleptic malignant syndrome, there is leukocytosis with a shift to the left, marked elevation of serum creatine kinase (may be up to 100,000 U/L), elevated serum aminotransferases, lactase dehydrogenase and alkaline phosphatase, hyponatremia, hyperkalemia, and diffuse slowing on the electroencephalo-

gram. Cerebrospinal fluid (CSF) and computed tomography (CT) scans of the brain are normal.

159. **(A)-T, (B)-T, (C)-F, (D)-F, (E)-T.** The neuroleptic malignant syndrome may also be caused by TCAs and MAOIs; or it may follow withdrawal from hypnotics, levodopa, and amantadine. Complications include aspiration pneumonia, thromboembolism, acute renal failure, disseminated intravascular coagulation, and *Escherichia coli* fascitis. The mortality is 20%. Therapy includes intensive care to maintain cardiopulmonary and renal functions. Dantrodene, bromocriptine, levodopa, amantadine, and electroconvulsive therapy are employed.

160. **(A)-T, (B)-T, (C)-T, (D)-T, (E)-T.** Most problem behaviors of nursing home residents can be avoided if the staff uses approaches that respond to individual needs and moods. Kindness, concern, respect, affection, and lighthearted humor are often effective in quelling troublesome behaviors.

161. **(A)-T, (B)-T, (C)-T, (D)-T, (E)-F.** Obsessive–compulsive behaviors are characterized by obsessive thoughts and by compulsions to touch things or to perform complicated movements. From 50% to 62% of patients also have had ADHD, and 44% of patients are suffering from somnambulism. Their eyes are normal, but their visual–motor coordination and mathematics skills may be poor.

162. **(A)-T, (B)-F, (C)-T, (D)-T, (E)-T.** Characteristic features of Tourette syndrome are coprolalia (involuntary utterance of obscenities), mental coprolalia (thinking about obscenities), copropraxia (involuntary obscene gesturing), echolalia (involuntary repetition of words or sounds heard by the patient), echopraxia or echokinesis (involuntary imitation of the movements of others), and palilalia (involuntary repetition of the patient's own words).

163. **(A)-T, (B)-T, (C)-T, (D)-F, (E)-F.** Haloperidol is useful in 80% of patients. Acute dysto-

nia of haloperidol can be prevented by concomitant use of benztropine (Cogentin) or can be treated by diphenhydramine (Benadryl). Clonidine is useful in 63% of patients. It can be used with haloperidol. Pimozide is as effective as haloperidol, but it may cause cardiotoxicity. Clomipramine and fluoxetine are useful.

164. **(A)-T, (B)-F, (C)-F, (D)-T, (E)-T.** Mescaline may cause extreme nausea, muscle tightness, apprehension, mydriasis, tachycardia, dry mouth, distortion of sensory and time perception, hallucinations, anxiety, mental depression, and exhaustion. The user may commit suicide to escape from terrifying hallucinations or from mental depression and exhaustion.

165. **(A)-F, (B)-T, (C)-F, (D)-T, (E)-T.** Stress causes metabolic changes that increase cardiovascular risk. Concomitants of stress are increased cortisol levels with associated glucose intolerance, increased cholesterol levels, increased platelet adhesion, and impaired lipoprotein ratios. Stress also plays a powerful role in the initiation and continuance of other coronary risk factors, such as cigarette smoking, obesity, and hypertension.

166. **(A)-F, (B)-T, (C)-T, (D)-F, (E)-T.** Akathisia occurs in 20% of psychiatric patients who take neuroleptics, including haloperidol, trifluoperazine (Stelazine), thiothixene (Navene), loxapine (Loxitane), and molindone (Moban). Patients taking prochlorperazine or patients who have been anesthetized with droperidol (Inapsine) can also develop the condition. Treatment is by diphenhydramine, trihexyphenidyl (Artane), or benztropine (Cogentin). Propranolol and diazepam (Valium) may also be helpful.

167. **(A)-F, (B)-F, (C)-F, (D)-F, (E)-F.** During the therapeutic relationship between the physician and the patient, the transference may develop quickly. The physician–patient relationship is basically a fiduciary one, geared entirely to the welfare of the patient. In busi-

ness dealings, bartering goods or services for therapy, transference can leave the patient vulnerable to undue influence, and the physician may easily violate the basic fiduciary obligations. The physician should not abuse the therapeutic relationship to engage in sexual relations with the patient.

168. **(A)-F, (B)-F, (C)-F, (D)-T.**   There is no harm in the physician's (or any other professional helper's) giving advice, making recommendations, educating, etc. However, it is important to know when it will be helpful and when harmful. When the person is in deep conflict and is struggling to find relief by trying to move one way or another, it is most helpful initially to recognize the dilemma the person is confronting. The intention here must be to avoid pushing the patient toward one or another course of action, but to legitimate his right to feel in conflict and to offer help to see if the distress can be relieved in some way. Referral could be the initial action. Somewhat later, as the man makes some progress (perhaps in being more assertive and less tolerant of his wife's behavior), the wife could become involved and the marital problem could become the focus of treatment.

169. **(A)-T, (B)-F, (C)-T, (D)-F.**   The relationship of the physician and patient is usually consensual; the patient knowingly seeks the assistance of the physician, and the physician knowingly undertakes to act in this relation. The relationship may be contractual (oral and written), and the physician may be bound by it. A physician is not bound to render professional service to every person who applies; he may decide whether he will accept a patient. A physician whose custom is to treat only patients who come to his office has the right to refuse to continue treatment away from his office.

170. **(A)-F, (B)-T, (C)-F, (D)-T.**   The general rule of abandonment makes it clear that a physician undertaking to treat a patient generally must give such continued attention as the condition requires unless he is discharged by the patient, or unless he gives the patient rea-

sonable time in which to obtain the services of another physician.

171. **(A)-F, (B)-F, (C)-F, (D)-T.**   The physician is responsible only for the negligent actions of his employee (he has the power to select, discharge, direct, or control his assistants); he is not responsible for the actions of fellow employees.

172. **(A)-T, (B)-T, (C)-T, (D)-F.**   The relationship of physician and patient is consensual. A physician who undertakes to treat someone without his expressed or implied consent is guilty of an unlawful act for which he may be held liable in case of damage. The reason for disclosure of the collateral risks is to give the patient a basis for accepting or rejecting the proposed treatment.

173. **(A)-F, (B)-F, (C)-F, (D)-T.**   Parents' anxiety can be quite great with such "difficult" children, since they do not appear to have the coping ability of the "easier" children. Instead of reaching out to new experiences, they pull back; playing with other children can be a considerable strain for them. Their schedules are much less regular and they react with greater intensity and discomfort to inner and outer stimuli. These children generally need considerable support and cushioning from their environment. Demands should be made only in moderation, and the child should not be pushed to conform to what might otherwise seem to be age-appropriate behavior. Parents can sometimes benefit from assistance in handling these children, since the interaction of the child's difficulties and the parents' anxiety and guilt can more readily lead to problems than with easier children. The family physician is sufficiently familiar with the emotional needs of these children and he can offer such help, although referral is sometimes necessary.

174. **(A)-F, (B)-F, (C)-F, (D)-T.**   The knowledge that they can pass on a disabling and potentially fatal condition to their children throws a family into tremendous conflict. They will tend to cope with that tragedy and the decisions it forces upon them as they do other

difficult life decisions they face. They might tend to act impulsively, use denial, blame each other, or believe that this might not have happened if they were married to someone else. The decision about having other children is bound to be fraught with conflict and requires careful thinking, though in a way that does not minimize the risks and also permits the hopeful aspects to be considered; the family physician should offer to help the family do this. If referral is made, it should not be on the basis that "they need counseling," but rather that they are faced with a difficult decision with which anyone could use help. This approach avoids the pitfall of implying that they need counseling because they cannot handle their own decision, and also avoids the implication that they will be turning the decision over to someone else.

175. **(A)-T, (B)-F, (C)-F, (D)-F.** A suicide attempt is a serious matter. The girl must have been feeling desperate to be pushed to such an extreme. The extent and seriousness of her pathology is at this time not clear, but the fact that she has a set of well-organized complaints is a good sign. It would be much more serious if she complained that she did not want to live because she was hurting the people she loved, or if she appeared disoriented and confused. In any of the latter situations she would need to be referred for psychiatric evaluation immediately, and the possibility of hospitalization would have to be considered. Given the problem as it is presented, psychiatric referral is indicated so that the onus is not put on either side of the conflict. The family physician can briefly explore some of the most pressing complaints, hospitalize the patient, and get the parents to ease off on some of the restrictions.

176. **(A)-F, (B)-F, (C)-T, (D)-F.** Improvement can sometimes be brought about in a situation like this without long-term help. The girl's response indicates that her relationship with the parents is not disrupted. The parents need to be told that their restrictive and punitive measures are serving only to alienate her further and that they should perhaps remove some of the restrictions. Where the girl is getting into

situations that they think might be dangerous, they should discuss with her how to deal with them, since going against the peer group can present considerable difficulty; restrictions should be based on safety rather than on principle of punishment. If at all possible, parents should make less of an issue of chores. The girl can be told that the parents do want to work something out and are willing to meet her halfway. Frequently, parents put much pressure on teenagers because of their anxiety that otherwise teenagers will somehow not develop a sense of responsibility; their way of doing this, however, often undermines the teenager's self-esteem by conveying the message that the youngster is irresponsible and a disappointment.

177. **(A)-F, (B)-F, (C)-T, (D)-T, (E)-T.** Somatizing patients often present with multiple vague complaints involving several organ systems, with stubborn conviction that there are organic causes, and demand tests and drugs for the cure. There are incongruities in the severity of symptoms and the objective findings from numerous work-ups. The patients often are proud of suffering and unwilling to discuss life aside from medical complaints. They often possess multiple drug allergies.

178. **(A)-T, (B)-F, (C)-T, (D)-T, (E)-T.** The patient is often immature, self-centered, emotionally unstable, overreactive, exhibitionistic, seductive, and dramatic. The general mood is characterized by fleetingness and lability.

179. **(A)-T, (B)-F, (C)-F, (D)-T, (E)-T.** Symptoms expressed by malingering patients are contrived, not real; thus, patients are not cooperative to suggested diagnostic or therapeutic procedures, and the claimed disability (this is often the reason for malingering) usually far exceeds objective clinical findings.

180. **(F)**

181. **(F)**

182. **(T)**

183. (T)

184. (T)

185. (T)

186. (T)

ADHD is characterized by inattention, impulsiveness, and hyperactivity. The disorder occurs in around 3% of children, with a male preponderance. The patient's family members are often afflicted with developmental disorders, alcohol abuse, conduct disorders, and antisocial personality. The patient is usually recognized between 4 and 7 years of age and may exhibit low self-esteem, mood lability, low frustration tolerance, and temper outbursts, with school failure. The course may persist throughout childhood. A few may develop antisocial personality and conduct disorder. Those with low IQs have a poor prognosis.

CHAPTER 2

Surgery
Questions

DIRECTIONS (Questions 1 through 45): Each of the numbered items or incomplete statements in this section is followed by answers or by completions of the statement. Select the ONE lettered answer or completion that is BEST in each case.

1. Treatment of frostbite calls for

   (A) topical corticosteroids
   (B) systemic corticosteroids
   (C) oral quinine sulfate
   (D) rewarming with 40°C water
   (E) rewarming with 100°C water   *(Ref. 62)*

2. A 28-year-old male was bitten by a house dog. His left forearm exhibits multiple puncture wounds, and there are several 1- to 2-cm irregular lacerations with ragged edges on his left hand. You will

   (A) suture the puncture wounds
   (B) prescribe oral erythromycin
   (C) irrigate the wounds thoroughly
   (D) inject corticosteroids into the wounds
   (E) administer rabies duck embryo vaccine
   (Ref. 2)

3. To manage a 62-year-old female with a hammertoe on the right foot, you will

   (A) prescribe analgesics
   (B) prescribe nonsteroidal anti-inflammatory drugs (NSAIDs)
   (C) order a custom-made shoe for the right foot
   (D) perform resection of the hammertoe
   (E) inject corticosteroids into the hammertoe
   (Ref. 25)

4. A 7-year-old girl complained that many small brown ants crawled over her right foot and right leg to produce multiple 1- to 2-mm pustules on erythematous bases. You will

   (A) prescribe oral cephalexin (Keflex) for 5 days
   (B) administer ampicillin intramuscularly
   (C) clean the lesions thoroughly with soap and water
   (D) start doxycycline (Vibramycin) orally for 10 days
   (E) inject corticosteroids intradermally at the site of the affected lesions   *(Ref. 2)*

5. A solitary, firm, smooth, discrete, and freely movable breast lesion in a 28-year-old female is probably

   (A) carcinoma
   (B) chronic cystic mastitis
   (C) fibroadenoma
   (D) ductal papilloma
   (E) sclerosing adenosis   *(Ref. 62)*

6. A 25-year-old male suddenly notes chest pain and dyspnea. Vocal and tactile fremitus is reduced, breath sounds are diminished, and the chest film shows absent lung markings on the left side. The most probable diagnosis is

   (A) atelectasis of the left lung
   (B) spontaneous pneumothorax
   (C) pulmonary tuberculosis
   (D) emphysema
   (E) pulmonary embolism   *(Ref. 62)*

7. A 50-year-old heavy smoker is found by routine chest x-ray to have a coin lesion in the right upper lung field. The physical examination is within normal limits, and the purified protein derivative (PPD) is negative. The management of choice is

   (A) antibiotics
   (B) thoracotomy
   (C) observation
   (D) reassurance
   (E) chemotherapy   (Ref. 62)

8. If a patient is allergic to lidocaine (Xylocaine), the choice of local anesthetic is

   (A) bupivacaine (Marcaine)
   (B) procaine (Novocain)
   (C) mepivacaine (Carbocain)
   (D) etidocaine (Duranest)
   (E) hydroquinone (Solaquin)   (Ref. 79)

9. Duodenal obstruction of the newborn can be demonstrated by

   (A) barium enema
   (B) plain film of the abdomen taken in the upright position
   (C) plain film of the abdomen taken in the inverted position
   (D) upper gastrointestinal (GI) series
   (E) intravenous pyelogram (IVP)   (Ref. 62)

10. A 40-year-old female with a history of rheumatic mitral stenosis suddenly complains of pain and numbness over the left leg. The physical examination reveals an absence of pulsation over the pedis dorsalis and an increase of pulsation over the common femoral pulse. The most likely diagnosis is

    (A) thrombophlebitis obliterans
    (B) occlusion of popliteal artery
    (C) embolism of femoral artery
    (D) thrombosis of femoral artery
    (E) thrombosis of aorta   (Ref. 62)

11. A 50-year-old male executive complains of claudication in the left leg with walking, with the pain subsiding at rest. Examination finds a normal pulse in the common femoral artery but absent popliteal and pedal pulses. The surface skin of the left leg is normal. The possible diagnosis is

    (A) phlebothrombosis
    (B) femoral artery occlusion
    (C) Leriche syndrome
    (D) Raynaud's disease
    (E) occlusion of the popliteal artery   (Ref. 62)

12. A 40-year-old teacher suddenly develops abdominal pain. She has been on an ulcer therapy for 5 years. Physical examination reveals a boardlike rigidity of her abdomen. The most likely diagnosis is

    (A) acute pancreatitis
    (B) acute cholecystitis
    (C) ectopic pregnancy
    (D) perforated peptic ulcer
    (E) rupture of appendiceal abscess   (Ref. 62)

13. The most common cause of intestinal obstruction is obstruction secondary to

    (A) neoplasm
    (B) adhesive bands
    (C) hernia
    (D) intussusception
    (E) volvulus   (Ref. 62)

14. A 60-year-old male who has had cholelithiasis without surgery develops progressive jaundice with palpable gallbladder. Occult blood is found in steatorrheic stools. The most likely diagnosis is

    (A) pancreatic head tumor
    (B) stone in the common bile duct
    (C) tumor of the ampulla of Vater
    (D) cancer of the gallbladder
    (E) chronic cholecystitis   (Ref. 62)

15. A 60-year-old diabetic man is found to have dull abdominal pain and progressive jaundice with palpable gallbladder. The most likely diagnosis is

    (A) common bile duct stone
    (B) chronic cholecystitis

(C) hydrops of the gallbladder

(D) carcinoma of the pancreatic head

(E) stone in the gallbladder   *(Ref. 62)*

16. Intussusception can be demonstrated by

(A) barium enema

(B) plain film of the abdomen taken in the upright position

(C) plain film of the abdomen taken in the inverted position

(D) upper GI series

(E) lateral chest film   *(Ref. 62)*

17. A 52-year-old female suffered a human bite laceration on her right hand 1 hour ago. You will

(A) perform primary closure promptly

(B) perform primary closure 5 hours later

(C) request the hand surgeon to perform primary closure immediately

(D) send the patient to the emergency room immediately for primary closure of the laceration wound

(E) thoroughly irrigate the wound without primary closure   *(Ref. 2)*

18. Homicide is the leading cause of death for

(A) white men aged 55 to 74 years

(B) white women aged 55 to 74 years

(C) black men aged 75 years and above

(D) black women aged 15 to 34 years

(E) Hispanic women aged 35 to 54 years

    (Ref. 5)

19. Urban areas generally have higher crime rates than rural areas; the high crime rates in the urban areas are most likely to be associated with

(A) ethnic identity

(B) unemployment

(C) nonstrict judiciary system

(D) liberal public policy

(E) tolerant religious attitudes   *(Ref. 5)*

20. Carcinoid is most frequently found in the

(A) sigmoid colon

(B) ovary

(C) ileum

(D) appendix

(E) jejunum   *(Ref. 62)*

21. An 84-year-old nursing home patient has sustained a stroke with left hemiparesis. To prevent pressure sores, you will order

(A) rotation in 30-degree oblique position every two hours

(B) intravenous cephalosporins

(C) topical full-strength povidone-iodine

(D) use of doughnut cushions at all time

(E) strict vitamin C–restricted diet   *(Ref. 2)*

22. A 35-year-old workaholic executive complains of severe rectal pain awakening him in the middle of the night. The most likely diagnosis is

(A) proctalgia fugax

(B) amaurosis fugax

(C) rectal carcinoma

(D) dysentery

(E) ulcerative colitis   *(Ref. 62)*

23. A 45-year-old farmer has experienced claudication of both lower legs after walking for a few blocks. The patient also complains of coldness of the legs and impotence. On physical examination, the femoral and the pedal pulses are absent. The blood pressure is 140/90 mm Hg. The most likely diagnosis is

(A) Leriche syndrome

(B) Raynaud's disease

(C) Buerger's disease (thromboangiitis obliterans)

(D) sexual dysfunction

(E) diabetes mellitus   *(Ref. 62)*

24. A 12-year-old girl is stung by a wasp on her right forearm. Initially, a small red wheal develops at the site of the sting. Later, there are several hives with swelling and redness at the right forearm. These hives cause intense itching. There are no other systemic symptoms and signs. You will

    (A) refer the patient to a medical entomologist
    (B) send the patient to the emergency room immediately
    (C) hospitalize the patient at the family medicine inpatient service
    (D) prescribe oral antihistamines
    (E) administer wasp antivenin 0.1 cc intramuscularly   (Ref. 2)

25. A 27-year-old ballet dancer has suddenly developed crampy abdominal pain associated with nausea and vomiting. She has had obstipation and has been unable to pass flatus. Three months ago she underwent a prophylactic appendectomy. Physical examination reveals a distended abdomen without definite tenderness. The most likely diagnosis is

    (A) acute cholecystitis
    (B) perforated peptic ulcer
    (C) mechanical small bowel obstruction
    (D) ectopic pregnancy
    (E) paralytic ileus   (Ref. 62)

26. A 15-year-old male sustained a contusion on his right leg 2 hours ago at school. He was treated with ice by the school nurse. On examination, ecchymosis and swelling with pain was found. You would

    (A) start oral antibiotics
    (B) advise elevation of the right leg
    (C) aspirate the swelling area
    (D) incise and drain
    (E) apply topical antibiotics   (Ref. 3)

27. A child suffered an injury to the distal phalanx of his right index finger. Twenty-four hours later, he developed swelling, redness,

pain, and semiflexion of the right finger. The most likely diagnosis is

    (A) acute tenosynovitis
    (B) felon
    (C) acute paronychia
    (D) carbuncle
    (E) flexor tendon injuries   (Ref. 62)

28. The most common cause of accidental deaths is

    (A) motor vehicle accidents
    (B) home accidents
    (C) work accidents
    (D) firearms
    (E) drowning   (Ref. 2)

29. Work accidents occur most commonly among

    (A) physicians
    (B) engineers
    (C) lawyers
    (D) truck drivers
    (E) farmers   (Ref. 2)

30. The most common cause of home accidents is

    (A) burns
    (B) drug poisoning
    (C) electric appliances
    (D) falls
    (E) drowning   (Ref. 2)

31. The most common accidental injury results from

    (A) motor vehicle accidents
    (B) home accidents
    (C) work accidents
    (D) firearms
    (E) drowning   (Ref. 2)

32. Falls among the elderly most commonly occur in

    (A) the home
    (B) the workplace

(C) public institutions

(D) streets

(E) motor vehicles   *(Ref. 2)*

33. The treatment choice of glomus tumor of the finger is

    (A) total excision

    (B) antibiotics

    (C) irradiation

    (D) observation

    (E) NSAIDs   *(Ref. 62)*

34. The treatment choice for hemorrhagic nevus in the back of the foot is

    (A) total excision

    (B) topical antibiotics

    (C) irradiation

    (D) systemic antibiotics

    (E) observation   *(Ref. 62)*

35. The treatment of lymphangitis of the lower extremities is

    (A) total excision

    (B) antibiotics

    (C) irradiation

    (D) laser applications

    (E) cryosurgery   *(Ref. 62)*

36. Imperforate anus can be demonstrated by

    (A) barium enema

    (B) plain film of the abdomen taken in the upright position

    (C) plain film of the abdomen taken in the inverted position

    (D) upper GI series

    (E) splenoportography   *(Ref. 62)*

37. The clinical presentation of third-degree burns is

    (A) painless

    (B) erythema

    (C) lichenification

    (D) blisters

    (E) urticaria   *(Ref. 62)*

38. The suture removal of a laceration on the forehead is scheduled in

    (A) 2 days

    (B) 5 days

    (C) 10 days

    (D) 20 days

    (E) 31 days   *(Ref. 21)*

39. A cutaneous abscess is to be drained when it is

    (A) indurated

    (B) fluctuant

    (C) painful

    (D) itching

    (E) reddened   *(Ref. 81)*

40. Periungual infection is termed

    (A) felon

    (B) paronychia

    (C) ingrown nail

    (D) onychocryptosis

    (E) onychomycosis   *(Ref. 62)*

41. A 45-year-old male executive presents with pain in the sacrococcygeal area after a long drive; palpable tender nodule is most likely due to

    (A) midlife crisis

    (B) hypochondriasis

    (C) pelvic fracture

    (D) pilonidal disease

    (E) hemorrhoid   *(Ref. 62)*

42. A 46-year-old female who had an external hemorrhoid for 4 years, with minimal discomfort and occasional soiling of underclothes, suddenly developed extreme pain during bowel movement. The patient is most likely suffering from

    (A) an internal hemorrhoid

    (B) external skin tags

    (C) a thrombosed hemorrhoid

    (D) an anal fissure

    (E) menopausal syndrome   *(Ref. 62)*

43. A 25-year-old male complains of sudden rectal pain lasting for 40 minutes each day for the past 3 days. The patient is most likely suffering from

    (A) a thrombosed internal hemorrhoid
    (B) a thrombosed external hemorrhoid
    (C) proctalgia fugax
    (D) rectal prolapse
    (E) pilonidal sinus   *(Ref. 62)*

44. A 16-year-old male was stung by several yellow jackets in the park. After a few minutes, he felt a tingling sensation at the site of the stinging on the right leg. In 10 minutes, he felt weak and lightheaded, and a number of itching hives developed on the anterior chest wall. Vital signs are stable and there are no signs of shortness of breath. The patient is very anxious. You will

    (A) perform a tracheotomy
    (B) start propanolol (Inderal) orally
    (C) administer subcutaneous epinephrine
    (D) prescribe oral antihistamines
    (E) begin desensitization shots   *(Ref. 2)*

45. An indirect inguinal hernia is located

    (A) medial to inferior epigastric vessels
    (B) in the linea alba
    (C) lateral to inferior epigastric vessels
    (D) within the umbilicus
    (E) beneath the inguinal ligament   *(Ref. 62)*

DIRECTIONS (Questions 46 through 62): Each question consists of an introduction followed by some statements. Mark T (true) or F (false) after each statement.

46. The following statements are concerned with informed consent:

    (A) A patient refuses your proposed diagnostic procedure; you should not perform the procedure.
    (B) A patient refuses your proposed treatment plan, which is beneficial to the patient; you should proceed with the treatment.

    (C) Parental consent is needed to treat a 6-year-old girl.
    (D) Parental consent is needed to treat a pregnant teenager.
    (E) Telling a patient about all the possible side reactions of the medications prescribed will reduce compliance; thus, it should not be told.   *(Ref. 2)*

47. Heat exhaustion is characterized by

    (A) vertigo
    (B) headache
    (C) nausea
    (D) fainting
    (E) elevated temperature   *(Ref. 2)*

48. Prior to performing a procedure, you need to inform the patient of the

    (A) nature of the procedure
    (B) undesirable results of the procedure
    (C) desirable results of the procedure
    (D) seriousness of the risks associated with the procedure
    (E) available alternatives to the proposed procedure   *(Ref. 2)*

49. Human bites are to be treated by

    (A) observation
    (B) antibiotics
    (C) irrigation
    (D) primary closure
    (E) no treatments are needed   *(Ref. 2)*

50. Anal fissures are often associated with

    (A) gonorrhea
    (B) syphilis
    (C) ulcerative colitis
    (D) Crohn's disease
    (E) rectal carcinoma   *(Ref. 62)*

51. Common clinical presentations of varicose veins include

    (A) leg pain
    (B) swelling

(C) calf cramps

(D) leg ulcers

(E) superficial phlebitis   *(Ref. 62)*

52. Trouble removing a ring may be due to

(A) trauma

(B) arthritis

(C) weight gain

(D) pregnancy

(E) slippery fingers   *(Ref. 82)*

53. Toxic reactions to the local anesthetic lidocaine include

(A) mental confusion

(B) coma

(C) euphoria

(D) numbness

(E) tingling   *(Ref. 67)*

54. Clinical presentations of rupture of the spleen include

(A) left shoulder pain

(B) infectious mononucleosis

(C) blunt trauma

(D) hematemesis

(E) hemoptysis   *(Ref. 62)*

55. Dog bites can be treated with

(A) irrigation

(B) tetanus prophylaxis for susceptibles

(C) oral cephalosporins

(D) rabies surveillance

(E) debridement of devitalized tissues
          (Ref. 62)

56. Common clinical presentations of early-stage cancer of the right colon include

(A) anemia

(B) obstruction

(C) adenocarcinoma

(D) bowel change

(E) weight gain   *(Ref. 62)*

57. The brown recluse spider may cause

(A) hyperreflexia

(B) hemoglobinuria

(C) abdominal cramps

(D) panic disorder

(E) splenomegaly   *(Ref. 75)*

58. The clinical presentations of rupture of the liver include

(A) left shoulder pain

(B) infectious mononucleosis

(C) blunt trauma

(D) hematuria

(E) penetration injury   *(Ref. 62)*

59. Common clinical presentations of acute appendicitis include

(A) decreased serum calcium

(B) rectal tenderness

(C) pneumoperitoneum

(D) leukopenia

(E) cholelithiasis   *(Ref. 62)*

60. Mechanical large bowel obstruction is frequently caused by

(A) volvulus

(B) fecal impaction

(C) adhesions

(D) diverticulitis

(E) carcinoma   *(Ref. 62)*

61. In traumatic arteriovenous fistula, the clinical presentations include a(n)

(A) increase in venous pressure distal to the fistula

(B) increase in diastolic blood pressure

(C) decrease in systolic blood pressure

(D) increase in cardiac output

(E) elevated pulse rate   *(Ref. 62)*

62. Which of the following statements is/are true for familial polyposis of the colon?

    (A) Total colectomy is recommended.
    (B) It is a hereditary disease.
    (C) It will usually develop into colorectal carcinoma.
    (D) A large number of adenomatous polyps will appear in the colon and rectum.
    (E) Cancers of familial polyposis are all polypoid cancers.   *(Ref. 62)*

DIRECTIONS (Questions 63 through 72): The following clinical set problem consists of clinical information presented in the format of questions or incomplete statements followed by a group of numbered options.

**Indicate T if the option is true;
Indicate F if the option is false.**

A 34-year-old female executive complained of abdominal pain of 12-hour duration. The pain started at the epigastrium and shifted to the right lower abdomen. The patient reported that she was anorexic and constipated; she also experienced nausea, but vomiting did not occur. At this time, you would

63. order ECGs

64. refer to a surgeon

65. order a complete blood count

66. order a barium enema

67. order urinalysis

Acute appendicitis was diagnosed, and appendectomy was performed that evening. The next morning, she suddenly developed a fever of 102°F with tachycardia and tachypnea. A few posterior basal rales were heard at the base; other physical examinations were unremarkable. Chest x-rays were essentially normal. The appropriate treatment options include

68. absolute bedrest

69. Tylenol with codeine (35 mg) three tablets every 2 hours

70. gentamycin 1 g IV every 6 hours

71. immediate laparotomy

72. erythromycin 500 mg every 6 hours PO
(Ref. 62)

Answers and Explanations

1. **(D)** Frostbite is treated by rewarming with water 40ºC to 42ºC until thawed. The affected parts are elevated, and trauma should be prevented. Dressings or bandages are avoided; infection is controlled.

2. **(C)** *Pasteurella multocida* is the most common organism causing infection in dog bite wounds. Gram stain reveals many neutrophil leukocytes and small gram-negative pleomorphic coccobacilli with bipolar staining. It is sensitive to penicillins but may be resistant to the first-generation oral cephalosporins (cephalexin [Keflex]) and erythromycin. Doxycycline (Vibramycin) is recommended for patients who are allergic to penicillin. Wounds are prone to infection, and primary closure may not be advised. Rabies prophylaxis is needed when there are recent cases associated with the dog. If a house dog has already received rabies immunization, it can be observed. Tetanus immunization may be needed.

3. **(C)** Hammertoe can be treated by a custom-made shoe to protect the toe. A protective shield with a central aperture of foam rubber can be placed over the hammertoe. Reconstructive surgery is reserved for unresponsive patients.

4. **(C)** The presentations are characteristic for the fire ant bites. Although fire ants are aggressive, the lesions are usually not infected. Antibiotics are not needed in most cases, and corticosteroids are administered only in severe cases.

5. **(C)** Fibroadenomas are most common in persons aged 20 to 35. They present as lobular but not scattered masses with a firm, rubbery consistency and sharply defined edges. Most commonly solitary, they may occasionally be multiple. They are differentiated from cancer by smooth rather than irregular lobulations and by the age group in which they occur. Biopsy is usually required for definite diagnosis.

6. **(B)** Although pneumothorax can be caused by tuberculosis or trauma, the most common type is spontaneous pneumothorax in a healthy young person who suddenly develops chest pain, dyspnea, and decreasing breath sounds. Diagnosis is usually made by chest film showing the collapsed lung. Severe, progressive dyspnea in a patient with a collapsed lung means tension pneumothorax. Treatment consists of inserting a large-bore needle into the pleural space and connecting the open end of the needle with tubing to a water bottle on the floor. This will suffice until a chest tube can be inserted.

7. **(B)** Often, a small mass in the lung is discovered on roentgenographic examination in a person with no pulmonary symptoms. The age of the patient, where he has lived, the history and physical examination, skin tests, and laboratory tests may point toward a statistically likely diagnosis. In the older adult who is a heavy smoker, excision of a coin lesion is usually indicated, because a high percentage are carcinomas proved by biopsy.

8. **(B)** Lidocaine may cause lightheadedness, drowsiness, bradycardia, and hypotension, and these side effects are very similar in the amide group of local anesthetics (such as bupivacaine, mepivacaine, and etidocaine). Patients who are allergic to lidocaine can use ester group anesthetics, which include procaine, tetracaines, and chloroprocaine.

9. **(B)** An upright plain film of the abdomen will show characteristic double bubbles (air in the stomach and duodenum) in duodenal obstruction of the newborn.

10. **(C)** The five Ps of acute occlusion—pain, paralysis, paresthesia, absent pulses, and pallor—are the principal clinical features in arterial embolism. The most common underlying heart diseases are mitral stenosis, atrial fibrillation, and myocardial infarction. The emboli ejected from the heart lodge in the arteries of the bifurcation of the popliteal artery. The pulse proximal to the site of the embolus may be increased. The treatment is immediate embolectomy.

11. **(B)** Occlusion of the femoral artery produces claudication in the leg with moderate exercise but is usually asymptomatic at rest. Occlusion of the popliteal artery develops into severe claudication or rest pain associated with trophic changes in the foot, ultimately resulting in ulceration and gangrene.

12. **(D)** Sudden onset of severe abdominal pain, past history of an ulcer, absolute abdominal rigidity, and the presence of free air under the diaphragm all point to perforated ulcer. A stomach tube should be inserted to avoid further peritoneal soilage, and prompt surgery is in order.

13. **(B)** Probably about 20% of surgical admissions for acute abdomen are for intestinal obstruction. Adhesive bands are the most frequent cause of obstruction for all age groups combined. Strangulated groin hernia is the second most frequent cause, and neoplasm of the bowel is third. These three etiologic agents account for more than 80% of intestinal obstructions. Hernia is the most common

cause of obstruction in childhood. Colorectal carcinoma and diverticulitis coli are prominent etiologic agents in the older age group.

14. **(C)** Tumor of the ampulla of Vater frequently occurs in males in their sixties and seventies. Cholelithiasis has also been implicated as a contributing factor in carcinoma of the gallbladder, but with lower frequency. Rapid onset of jaundice, weight loss, palpable liver, and a gallbladder that is smooth and nontender favor the diagnosis of malignancy in the ampulla of Vater. Anemia with evidence of upper gastrointestinal bleeding (occult blood) and steatorrhea are often seen.

15. **(D)** Carcinoma of the pancreatic head is frequently found in diabetic males over 60 years of age. The patient may be pain free but usually complains of dull aching confined to the midepigastrium; weight loss and progressive jaundice are common, and the liver and gallbladder are usually palpable. Chronic cholecystitis is associated with discrete attacks of epigastric or right upper quadrant pain with jaundice or fever; the gallbladder is rarely palpable. If the cystic duct remains obstructed when the acute cholecystitis subsides, the gallbladder may become distended with clear mucoid fluid to form hydrops of the gallbladder, which will usually cause pain without jaundice. Asymptomatic gallstones are rare, and cholelithiasis is usually manifested by chronic cholecystitis. Choledocholithiasis is usually accompanied by colicky pain and progressive jaundice. In contrast to patients with neoplastic obstruction of the common bile duct or ampulla of Vater, the gallbladder is usually not distended because of associated inflammation (Courvoisier's law).

16. **(A)** Barium enema will demonstrate a filling defect in the ascending colon in intussusception; previously healthy infants 3 to 11 months of age with this defect suddenly develop severe crampy abdominal pain with bloody stool and palpable abdominal mass.

17. **(E)** Human bites are often contaminated with a myriad of microorganisms. The wound

should not be closed primarily; it should be widely opened, excised, and thoroughly irrigated. Broad-spectrum antibiotics should be selected according to culture results and started immediately.

18. **(D)** Homicide is the leading cause of death for both black men and women aged 15 to 34 years. This may be related to poverty, despair, deprivation, and inadequate outlets for stress.

19. **(B)** Unemployment, crowding, and inadequate housing are associated with higher crime rates in urban areas.

20. **(D)** The most common site of carcinoid tumors is the appendix, followed by the small bowel (mostly the ileum). Carcinoid arises from argentaffin cells in the crypts of Lieberkuhn and forms yellowish, firm nodules in the submucosa. The carcinoid syndrome consists of cutaneous flushing, diarrhea, bronchoconstriction, skin rash, and right-sided cardiac valvular disease due to collagen deposition. Urinary 5-hydroxyindoleacetic acid (5-HIAA, a metabolite of serotonin) is usually increased. This is a malignant neoplasm in slow motion.

21. **(A)** Pressure sores can be prevented through family physicians' genuine concerns, careful nursing care, use of air-fluidized beds, adequate nutrition (including adequate provision of vitamin C and zinc), and avoidance of shearing and moisture. A doughnut cushion increases central ischemia and should be avoided. The semi-Fowler position should be avoided to reduce shear over the sacrum. Sheepskin and egg-crate mattresses are popular but not very useful.

22. **(A)** Proctalgia fugax is a severe spasmodic rectal pain lasting a few minutes. The cause is unknown, but it is associated with patients who are overworked and anxious. Sigmoidoscopy is performed and reassurance is offered, with application of analgesic suppositories, heat pads, and warm baths. Diazepam (Valium) may be found to be useful.

23. **(A)** Leriche syndrome (aortoiliac occlusive disease) is an ischemic syndrome resulting from occlusion of the abdominal aorta due to atherosclerosis. It is characterized by claudication and impotence. The physical examination usually discloses absence or diminution of the femoral pulses combined with absence of the popliteal and pedal pulses. Aortography can establish the diagnosis as well as the extent of the occlusive disease. The aortic occlusion may be corrected by directly removing the obstruction by a thromboendarterectomy or by insertion of a prosthetic bypass (Dacron or Teflon) graft.

24. **(D)** Usual management of insect stings includes analgesics for pain and antihistamines for itching. The lesions are seldom infected to become cellulitis, and antibiotics are not usually required. In severe cases, oral corticosteroid may be useful.

25. **(C)** Acute small bowel obstruction is most commonly due to adhesions acquired from an abdominal operation. Simple mechanical obstruction without vascular compromise often presents with nontenderness on palpation. The absence of tenderness does not rule out the diagnosis of acute bowel obstruction. The more proximal the obstruction, the less the distention and the more the vomiting. Paralytic ileus is usually secondary to pancreatitis, peritonitis, renal calculi, or pneumonia. Ectopic pregnancy is a possibility, and further differentiation may be required.

26. **(B)** A contusion (bruise or ecchymosis) is formed by trauma that injures underlying soft-tissue structures while leaving the epidermis intact. Cellular, vascular, and lymphatic damage causes blood and fluids to leak into the tissue, producing swelling and discoloration. The treatment is elevation of the affected part. The lesion is treated with pressure, ice (initially), and warm pack (after 72 hours).

27. **(B)** Felon is infection of the digit pulp at the distal phalangeal level. Erythema, pain, and

tenderness are characteristic findings. The pulp space should be incised for drainage.

28. **(A)** Accidents rank fourth as a cause of death, following heart disease, cancer, and strokes. In 1985, of approximately 91,500 accidental deaths, about half resulted from motor vehicle accidents.

29. **(E)** The largest category of work accidents occurs among agricultural workers.

30. **(D)** Home accidents are commonly sustained by the elderly and children; common causes include falls, fire burns, suffocation of ingested objects, poisoning, and firearms.

31. **(B)** Home accidents rank second among accidental deaths, accounting for 30% of deaths, next only to motor vehicle accidents. Home accidents rank first as a cause of accidental injury; more than 40% of all injuries result from home accidents.

32. **(A)** Falls are a major medical problem in the elderly that lead to fractures, dependency, and often death. The home remains the most common site of fatal accidents in the elderly, followed by highways, hospitals, and nursing homes. Home hazards include floors that are slippery from polish, spills, or urine; rugs that are loose or have holes; chairs with castors; poor lighting; and high steps.

33. **(A)** The glomus tumor is a rare, benign, and extremely painful small tumor of the skin and subcutaneous tissue occurring on the extremities, particularly in the nailbeds of the hands and feet. The tumor is derived from the glomic end-organ apparatus, consisting of arteriovenous anastomoses, which functions normally to regulate the blood flow in the extremity to control the temperature. Total excision is indicated, since the tumor is radioresistant.

34. **(A)** The following characteristics of any pigmented nevus are indications for excision: change in color or pigment distribution, development of erythema, change in size and consistency, change in surface characteristics

(bleeding, erosion, oozing), pain, burning, or lymphadenopathy.

35. **(B)** Lymphangitis, an inflammation of lymphatic pathways manifested by tenderness and streaking erythema of the skin, is frequently caused by hemolytic streptococci and is often associated with swelling of the regional lymph nodes. Treatment is with appropriate antibiotics sensitive to causal organisms.

36. **(C)** A plain film taken in the inverted position for a patient with imperforate anus shows a colonic pouch filled with air. There is the possibility of the existence of fistulas connecting to urinary or reproductive organs.

37. **(A)** First-degree burns cause erythema and pain; second-degree burns cause erythema and blistering; and third-degree burns result in pale or charred skin, thrombosed superficial vessels, and insensitivity to touch or painful stimuli.

38. **(B)** The schedule for suture removal is approximately 2 to 3 days for the eyelid; 3 to 5 days for the face; 5 to 7 days for the scalp; 7 to 10 days for the trunk; 10 to 14 days for the back and hands; and 10 to 21 days for the extremities.

39. **(B)** Abscesses are collections of purulent material within a contained space, walled off by the anatomic barrier and the body's localizing response to infection. An abscess causes tenderness, redness, and swelling. Fluctuance is the principal indicator for drainage. Hot compresses may be helpful in speeding up fluctuation.

40. **(B)** Acute paronychia is the acute onset of painful, bright red swelling of the proximal and lateral nail fold. It may occur spontaneously or may follow trauma or manipulation. Superficial infections present with an accumulation of purulent material behind the cuticle.

41. **(D)** Most patients with pilonidal disease are asymptomatic; many may present with a tender or nontender nodule, and moisture and drainage/bleeding at the sacrococcygeal area, although it can also occur at the umbilicus, the axilla, the clitoris, the interdigital webs of barbers' hands, the interdigital web of the foot of a worker in a hair mattress factory, the sole of the foot, and the anal canal. Abscess, cellulitis, leukocytosis, fever, and malaise can also be produced.

42. **(C)** Manifestations include a painful lump and a tense, tender, bluish mass covering the skin. A radial ellipse of skin is excised to evacuate the clot.

43. **(C)** Proctalgia fugax is more likely to happen in healthy young adults. The pain may awaken the patient at night. It can occur after intercourse as a spasm or a cramp in some women. The patient may obtain relief by a hot sitz bath, pressure application, and sublingual nitrates.

44. **(C)** The anaphylaxis or generalized reactions to the sting of a hymenopteron is injection of 0.3 to 0.5 cc 1:1,000 solution of aqueous epinephrine subcutaneously when the airway is patent. Corticosteroids and antihistamines are not useful for the immediate therapy but are useful for maintenance support. Desensitization therapy may be available for selected patients.

45. **(C)** An indirect inguinal hernia is located lateral to the inferior epigastric vessels. The swelling is oblique and cylindrical, and extends into the scrotum. A direct inguinal hernia is located medial to the inferior epigastric vessels. A femoral hernia is below the inguinal ligament and medial to the femoral vein. The umbilical hernia is in the congenital fascia defect within the umbilicus, while the epigastric hernia is above the umbilicus and is located in the linea alba.

46. **(A)-T, (B)-F, (C)-T, (D)-F, (E)-F.** All procedures and treatments need informed consent except in the following situations: (1) risks generally known, (2) patient asks not to be told, (3) emergency (immediate danger to life or health and no time to obtain consent), (4) not a reasonable need for patient to know, (5) therapeutic privilege (when disclosure will complicate or hinder treatment, cause psychologic harm, or upset the patient to the extent that the patient is unable to make a decision).

47. **(A)-T, (B)-T, (C)-T, (D)-T, (E)-F.** In heat exhaustion, the patient may present with weakness, vertigo, headache, anorexia, nausea, vomiting, fainting, or collapse; skin is cold and clammy, the pupils are dilated, and body temperature is subnormal. Bathe with an alcohol sponge and administer oral saline solution.

48. **(A)-T, (B)-T, (C)-T, (D)-T, (E)-T.** Prior to performing a procedure, sufficient information must be given to the patient for the patient to make a decision (ie, either accept or reject the proposed procedure). Thus, it is imperative to disclose to the patient the benefits and the risks associated with the procedure, the problems of recuperation, the consequence of not performing the procedure, and the available alternatives and their consequences as well as risks.

49. **(A)-F, (B)-T, (C)-T, (D)-F, (E)-F.** Human bites may cause aerobic and anaerobic infections leading to severe necrotizing cellulitis. No primary closures should be done, minor lesions should be cleansed thoroughly, and antibiotics administered. Severe lesions need meticulous debridement. The possibility of spouse or child abuse is to be considered.

50. **(A)-T, (B)-T, (C)-T, (D)-T, (E)-T.** The anal fissure is a crack that occurs in the mucocutaneous lining. It causes pain on defecation and bleeding on the stool surface. Usually, it responds to analgesic ointment. Surgery is needed for chronic patients with severe symptoms.

51. **(A)-T, (B)-T, (C)-T, (D)-T, (E)-T.** Most patients with varicose veins are asymptomatic; varicosities are often exacerbated by childbirth. A few may suffer from burning, pain,

cramping, and swelling following standing for a long period. Recurrent ruptures, phlebitis, and severe symptoms may require surgery.

52. **(A)-T, (B)-T, (C)-T, (D)-T, (E)-F.** To remove the ring, push the ring proximally beyond the proximal interphalangeal joint; apply soap to a piece of ordinary wrapping string. Wrap the string tightly around the finger distal to the ring; pass the proximal end of the string beneath the ring; unwrap the string, drawing the ring distally along the wrapped finger and passing easily over the proximal interphalangeal joint to slip off. If this fails, cut the ring with a circular-blade ring cutter to open it up.

53. **(A)-T, (B)-T, (C)-F, (D)-T, (E)-T.** Lidocaine is the most common local anesthetic agent. The common reasons for allergic reactions are due to intravascular injections and the patient's autonomic responses to the procedure. Systemic toxicity is presented as a feeling of numbness and tingling, mental confusion, and coma.

54. **(A)-T, (B)-T, (C)-T, (D)-F, (E)-F.** The spleen is the organ most commonly injured in blunt trauma. Rupture of the spleen causes generalized abdominal pain with radiation to the left shoulder. Shock may also occur. Often, the patient is asymptomatic at first. Spontaneous splenic rupture may happen in patients with infectious mononucleosis, mostly during the second to fourth weeks of the course. The treatment of splenic rupture is immediate surgery.

55. **(A)-T, (B)-T, (C)-T, (D)-T, (E)-T.** Infections in dog bites are often caused by streptococci, staphylococci, gram-negative bacilli, and anaerobes; thus, oral cephalosporins are a reasonable choice of initial antibiotics until the results of causative microorganisms are available. Health authorities are to be contacted for the risk of rabies to initiate needed rabies vaccine prophylaxis. Healthy domestic dogs with rabies vaccine are to be held for observation for 10 days. A patient bitten by a stray or escaped dog may need human rabies immune globulin and human diploid cell rabies vaccine.

56. **(A)-T, (B)-F, (C)-T, (D)-F, (E)-F.** Colonic cancer is usually adenocarcinoma. Cancer of the right colon is usually characterized by persistent, dull, nagging, right lower quadrant pain, anemia, and a mass in the right abdomen. Colonic cancer will frequently cause weight loss. Late cases of colonic cancer will cause anemia and obstruction.

57. **(A)-F, (B)-T, (C)-F, (D)-F, (E)-F.** The brown recluse spider is indigenous in the Southern United States. It is not aggressive and it bites in self-defense. Bites greater than 2 cm may cause hemolysis, which results in hemoglobinuria. The black widow spider may cause hyperreflexia and abdominal muscle cramps, which may be treated with intravenous calcium gluconate.

58. **(A)-F, (B)-F, (C)-T, (D)-F, (E)-T.** The spleen is the organ most commonly injured in blunt trauma, followed by the intestine and the liver. Traumatic rupture of the liver usually causes shock, abdominal pain, spasm, and rigidity.

59. **(A)-F, (B)-T, (C)-F, (D)-F, (E)-F.** Appendicitis is characterized by acute abdominal pain. Pelvic appendicitis is usually manifested by rectal tenderness. Acute appendicitis will cause moderate leukocytosis (10,000 to 18,000/μL).

60. **(A)-T, (B)-T, (C)-F, (D)-T, (E)-T.** Large bowel obstruction is commonly caused by carcinoma of the bowel, volvulus of the sigmoid colon, and stenosing diverticulitis. However, the most common cause is fecal impaction in the elderly; this may be associated with dietary habits, frequent constipation, and inadequate fluid intake. Although adhesion is the most common cause of small bowel obstruction, it is relatively rare in large bowel obstruction. Abdominal pain and abdominal distention are the prominent picture. Vomiting may not occur until late in the course, with fecal character. Peritonitis may occur following fecal perforation.

61. **(A)-T, (B)-F, (C)-T, (D)-T, (E)-T.** The immediate effects of arteriovenous fistula include a decrease in blood flow to tissues distal to the lesion and an increase in venous pressure. The peripheral vascular resistance is lowered as a result of blood flowing directly through the newly created arteriovenous shunt. This results in a decrease in systolic and diastolic blood pressure, an increase in heart rate, and an increase in cardiac output.

62. **(A)-T, (B)-T, (C)-T, (D)-T, (E)-F.** Familial polyposis is a rare hereditary disease characterized by the appearance, early in life, of large numbers of adenomatous polyps in the colon and rectum. Carcinoma of the colorectum will develop in essentially 100% of patients; thus, total colectomy and cutaneous ileostomy have been advocated. The cancers developed are not all polypoid cancers, however; polypoid, ulcerating, and scirrhous cancers occur in the same proportions as idiopathic colonic cancer.

63. **(F)**

64. **(F)**

65. **(T)**

66. **(F)**

67. **(T)**

68. **(F)**

69. **(F)**

70. **(F)**

71. **(F)**

72. **(F)**

Acute appendicitis is basically a clinical diagnosis; its diagnosis is usually based on detailed history information and physical findings. Localized tenderness at the right lower quadrant (RLQ), particularly at McBurney's point, with rebound tenderness is suggestive of acute appendicitis. Laboratory tests are used for confirming the suspicion; moderate leukocytosis with predominant neutrophils is the most frequent finding and can aid in the diagnosis. Urine is usually normal but may show white or red blood cells. Plain film of the abdomen may show distended loops of small intestine in the RLQ, gas-filled appendix, fecaliths in the RLQ, increased soft-tissue density, and altered right flank stripe. Barium enema may show nonfilling of the appendix. Twenty-five percent of patients undergoing abdominal surgery may develop atelectasis. Treatment consists of clearing the airway by chest percussion, coughing, or nasotracheal suction.

CHAPTER 3

Gynecology
Questions

DIRECTIONS (Questions 1 through 75): Each of the numbered items or incomplete statements in this section is followed by answers or by completions of the statement. Select the ONE lettered answer or completion that is BEST in each case.

1. Which of the following individuals are at higher risk to develop breast cancer?

    (A) women with parity greater than five
    (B) women with late menarche
    (C) women who have surgical menopause at age 30
    (D) women who used estrogen for 15 years
    (E) women whose first parity is in their teens   *(Ref. 11)*

2. A teenage girl comes to you for contraceptive advice. You would

    (A) call her mother immediately
    (B) refuse to see her
    (C) tell her to behave herself and drive her out of the office
    (D) encourage her by prescribing the "pill" without exploring the situation
    (E) explore the situation to determine her need for contraceptives and be ready to support her in solving the problem
    (Ref. 11)

3. A 27-year-old single female requests contraceptive advice. She has had three induced abortions during the past 2 years. You would

    (A) accuse her of manslaughter
    (B) refuse to see her

    (C) discuss the effectiveness and safety of each contraceptive method
    (D) advise her not to use any contraceptives and to resort to induced abortions when she becomes pregnant
    (E) tell her to behave herself and to stop having intercourse   *(Ref. 11)*

4. A 32-year-old female complains of postcoital bleeding. On examination, a small, soft polypoid mass is found protruding from the cervical canal. What is the next step you would take?

    (A) antibiotic treatment
    (B) reassurance only
    (C) irradiation
    (D) acid douches
    (E) excisional biopsy   *(Ref. 11)*

5. Carcinoma in situ of the cervix uteri discovered in pregnancy at the 14th week of gestation should be treated as follows:

    (A) Schiller staining of the cervix and total hysterectomy
    (B) continuation of the pregnancy with biopsies and Pap smears and postpartum reevaluation
    (C) total hysterectomy with bilateral salpingo-oophorectomy
    (D) amputation of the cervix and continuation of the pregnancy
    (E) irradiation   *(Ref. 11)*

6. A 46-year-old female complained of having a frothy and yellowish vaginal discharge for 2 weeks. Examination of the vagina revealed multiple round, red papules and an intensely inflamed cervix. The most likely diagnosis is

   (A) cervical cancer
   (B) myoma uteri
   (C) trichomonal vaginitis
   (D) monilial vaginitis
   (E) normal finding   *(Ref. 11)*

7. Which of the following contraceptive procedures is most likely to increase the risk of pelvic inflammatory disease (PID)?

   (A) oral contraceptives
   (B) condoms
   (C) intrauterine devices (IUDs)
   (D) spermicidal creams
   (E) postcoital contraceptions   *(Ref. 3)*

8. A 25-year-old unmarried college student complains of severe vulvar pruritus and dysuria. Examination reveals a malodorous, frothy, yellow-green discharge. The laboratory study is most likely to show

   (A) multiple flagellate protozoa seen on the wet smear
   (B) multiple brown-black colonies growing on Nickerson's medium
   (C) gram-negative intracellular diplococci on Gram stain
   (D) small gram-negative rods
   (E) positive darkfield examination   *(Ref. 17)*

9. A strawberry-like appearance of the vagina with the presence of small petechial lesions on the cervix strongly suggests the diagnosis of

   (A) streptococcal vaginitis
   (B) pelvic congestion
   (C) trichomonal vaginitis
   (D) monilial vaginitis
   (E) cervical polyp   *(Ref. 17)*

10. A diabetic female patient complains of severe vulvar pruritus with discharge. Examination reveals a fiery red mucosa with a patchy, curdlike, white discharge. The laboratory examination will most likely show

    (A) mobile flagellate protozoa on wet smear
    (B) multiple brown-black colonies growing on Nickerson's medium
    (C) positive Thayer–Martin culture
    (D) gram-negative intracellular diplococci
    (E) positive darkfield examination   *(Ref. 17)*

11. The most appropriate therapy for monilial vaginitis is

    (A) aqueous penicillin, 4.8 million units IM
    (B) oral metronidazole (Flagyl) 250 mg three times daily for the patient and two times daily for her sexual partner, for 10 days
    (C) miconazole vaginal suppository 100 mg for 7 days
    (D) oxytetracycline (Terramycin) vaginal tablets 250 mg inserted at bedtime for ten days
    (E) reassurance that the condition will improve spontaneously in 4 days   *(Ref. 11)*

12. A 35-year-old female complains of dysuria and dribbling after urination. A small suburethral mass is found by digital examination. The compression of the anterior vaginal wall produces purulent discharge at the urethral meatus. The most likely diagnosis is

    (A) venereal urethritis
    (B) abscess of Skene's duct
    (C) carcinoma of the urethra
    (D) urethral diverticulum
    (E) Gartner's duct cyst   *(Ref. 6)*

13. Concerning the diaphragm for contraceptive use, you will instruct the patient that

    (A) the diaphragm should be removed immediately following intercourse
    (B) a new diaphragm should be used for each intercourse
    (C) spermicidal cream is not needed for repeated intercourse

(D) a new diaphragm must be used for repeated intercourse

(E) the use of a diaphragm increases the risk of urinary tract infections   (Ref. 3)

14. Monilial vaginitis is characterized by

(A) vulvar erythema

(B) clear cervical discharge

(C) chronic pelvic pain

(D) vaginal spotting

(E) frothy vaginal discharge   (Ref. 11)

15. Mastitis is commonly due to

(A) breast carcinoma

(B) lactation

(C) traumatic infection

(D) fibroadenoma of the breast

(E) lipoma of the breast   (Ref. 30)

16. Pseudomyxoma peritonei is associated with

(A) cervical carcinoma

(B) myoma uteri

(C) metastatic carcinoma of the uterus

(D) gonococcal tubo-ovarian abscess

(E) ovarian cystadenoma   (Ref. 11)

17. Stein–Leventhal syndrome is characterized by acquired amenorrhea, obesity, and occasional hirsutism. The ovaries show

(A) atrophy

(B) multiple corpora lutea

(C) cortical fibrosis and multiple follicular cysts

(D) germinal-cell hyperplasia and capillary engorgement

(E) cortical stromal hyperplasia   (Ref. 31)

18. Six months ago, a 35-year-old patient was accidentally found to have a small, movable pelvic mass during a routine physical examination without any complaints. Now she suddenly experiences excruciating pain in the right lower abdomen. The most likely diagnosis is

(A) acute pyelonephritis

(B) acute appendicitis

(C) torsion of an ovarian cyst

(D) myoma uteri

(E) diverticulitis   (Ref. 34)

19. Myomas are usually asymptomatic. Which of the following types of uterine myomas frequently cause symptoms?

(A) intramural

(B) submucous

(C) subserous

(D) pedunculated

(E) cervical   (Ref. 31)

20. The treatment of choice for symptomatic adenomyosis in a 40-year-old female with three children is

(A) hormonal therapy

(B) total hysterectomy

(C) total hysterectomy and bilateral oophorectomy

(D) psychotherapy only

(E) repeated curettage   (Ref. 11)

21. The most frequent complications of simple uterine retroversion include

(A) backache

(B) irregular menstruation

(C) leukorrhea

(D) constipation

(E) none of the above   (Ref. 59)

22. A 35-year-old unmarried, nulliparous female complains of lower abdominal pain over both sides just prior to menstruation. She has also noted bleeding from the rectum associated with the menses. On pelvic examination, a small, hard, fibrotic nodule is found. The most likely diagnosis is

(A) rectal carcinoma

(B) myoma uteri

(C) cervical carcinoma

(D) endometriosis

(E) adenomyosis   (Ref. 31)

23. A nulliparous diabetic patient complains of postmenopausal bleeding. The physical examination reveals obesity and hypertension. Pelvic examination shows a normal vulva and cervix, but the uterus is slightly enlarged. The most likely diagnosis is

    (A) cervical polyp
    (B) cervical cancer
    (C) endometrial carcinoma
    (D) myoma uteri
    (E) ovarian tumor   (Ref. 31)

24. For women who are breast feeding, you will recommend which of the following oral contraceptives?

    (A) Ortho-Novum 7/7/7
    (B) Ortho-Novum 10/11
    (C) Micronor
    (D) Ovulen
    (E) Enovid-E   (Ref. 3)

25. The most common reason for removal of the levonorgestrel (Norplant) system is

    (A) foreign-body sensation
    (B) intermenstrual spotting
    (C) mood changes
    (D) weight loss
    (E) cough   (Ref. 3)

26. In a case of chronic PID, the sudden onset of hyperpyrexia, shock, and tachycardia usually indicates

    (A) intestinal obstruction
    (B) torsion of an ovarian cyst
    (C) rupture of a pelvic abscess
    (D) acute appendicitis
    (E) ectopic pregnancy   (Ref. 31)

27. Annual mammogram is recommended for low-risk women

    (A) aged 50 and under
    (B) aged 50 to 70
    (C) aged 70 and above

    (D) of all ages
    (E) aged 18 and under   (Ref. 11)

28. A young woman recently noted lower abdominal pain accompanied by chills and low-grade fever. On examination, the abdomen is spastic and tenderness is elicited by the manipulation of the cervix. Examination of the cervical discharge reveals the causative organism. The most likely diagnosis is

    (A) gonococcal salpingitis
    (B) ectopic pregnancy
    (C) tuberculous salpingitis
    (D) acute appendicitis
    (E) regional ileitis   (Ref. 30)

29. A 25-year-old female is seen for infertility. She has been married for 2 years. Your initial evaluation is within normal limits; you instruct her in the recording of basal body temperature (BBT). She returns in 3 months for further evaluative studies. The BBT chart shows a biphasic curve in the first month and a sustained temperature elevation curve for the second and the third months. The patient possibly has

    (A) hyperestrogenism
    (B) estrogen insufficiency
    (C) PID
    (D) pregnancy
    (E) Stein–Leventhal syndrome   (Ref. 31)

30. A healthy housewife has taken Ortho-Novum 7/7/7 for 2 weeks. She now complains of vaginal spotting. You would now

    (A) discontinue Ortho-Novum 7/7/7
    (B) switch to Ortho-Novum 1/35
    (C) switch to Triphasil
    (D) evaluate the timing of pill taking
    (E) order a work-up for prolactinoma   (Ref. 2)

31. Endometrial biopsy shows secretory phase, indicating

    (A) preovulatory phase
    (B) that menstruation is in progress

(C) that ovulation has occurred

(D) proliferative stage

(E) that no ovulation is possible   *(Ref. 11)*

32. In a normal cycle of 34 days' duration, ovulation occurs

    (A) two weeks before menstrual flow

    (B) two weeks after onset of menstrual flow

    (C) at midcycle

    (D) not at all

    (E) on the first day of menstruation   *(Ref. 11)*

33. The routine Pap smear of an asymptomatic 35-year-old female was abnormal. You would

    (A) offer reassurance

    (B) perform colposcopic biopsy endocervical curettage

    (C) schedule another Pap smear in 3 months

    (D) perform an ultrasound

    (E) schedule a hysterectomy   *(Ref. 11)*

34. A 16-year-old female has a complaint of primary amenorrhea. On assessment of her work-up, you have obtained the following information: height, 5 ft 4 in; weight, 148 lb; normal pelvic examination; normal 17-ketosteroids; normal visual fields; and negative pregnancy test. A normal menstrual period is induced by IM injection of 100 mg progesterone. This supports which of the following interpretations?

    (A) She has adrenal cortical hyperplasia.

    (B) She is producing adequate levels of estrogen.

    (C) She has arrhenoblastoma.

    (D) She has pituitary tumor.

    (E) She has Turner syndrome.   *(Ref. 31)*

35. A 26-year-old housewife has been taking Ortho-Novum 1/35 for 15 months. She has missed two periods, with negative pregnancy tests. You would now

    (A) administer testosterone

    (B) discontinue the pill

    (C) offer reassurance

(D) switch to a progestin-dominant pill

(E) order work-ups for endometrial cancer
    (Ref. 3)

36. The most reliable method of contraception is

    (A) tubal sterilization

    (B) vasectomy

    (C) oral contraceptives

    (D) coitus interruptus

    (E) abstinence   *(Ref. 3)*

37. The vaginal discharge of a normal woman is

    (A) malodorous

    (B) gray colored

    (C) yellowish

    (D) cheese-like

    (E) clear   *(Ref. 11)*

38. An anxious nurse practitioner, who is the mother of a 14-year-old girl, brought her daughter in because of amenorrhea. You found that the patient never started her period; her breasts are well developed, and there are pubic and axillary hair present, with normal configuration of external genitalia. You would now perform

    (A) chromosomal studies

    (B) cervical biopsy

    (C) computerized axial tomography (CAT) of the skull

    (D) urinary gonadotropins

    (E) counseling and support   *(Ref. 31)*

39. A 65-year-old female indicated that she has had a small, pea-sized, whitish ulcer at her left labia minora for a year, with intense itching. She has tried various ointments with little relief, and the ulcer never closed. The most likely diagnosis is

    (A) condyloma lata

    (B) monilial vaginitis

    (C) herpes genitalis

    (D) vulvar cancer

    (E) trichomonal vaginitis   *(Ref. 11)*

40. Bacterial vaginosis, without treatment, may cause

    (A) toxic shock syndrome
    (B) postpartum endometritis
    (C) diabetes mellitus
    (D) mastitis
    (E) fibrocystic breast disease   *(Ref. 11)*

41. A 35-year-old housewife complained of 2 days of painful vaginal bumps. She also experienced burning, tingling, and itching sensations, with dysuria. The examination showed multiple tender, small vesicles and ulcers. The most likely diagnosis is

    (A) bacterial vaginosis
    (B) chancroid
    (C) herpes simplex infection
    (D) chancre
    (E) trichomonal vaginitis   *(Ref. 11)*

42. The contraindications for oral contraceptives include

    (A) age beyond 30 years
    (B) teenage girl
    (C) pregnancy
    (D) smoker
    (E) tuberculosis   *(Ref. 2)*

43. The drug of choice for initial genital herpes is

    (A) oral Zovirax
    (B) oral Herpecin
    (C) topical Zovirax
    (D) topical Herpecin
    (E) IV Adriamycin   *(Ref. 14)*

44. The acute stage of genital herpes is best diagnosed by

    (A) serologic typing of HSV 1
    (B) antibody titer of HSV 3
    (C) culture with Nickerson medium
    (D) Tzanck test
    (E) Schick test   *(Ref. 31)*

45. To perform an annual health screening for an asymptomatic 52-year-old female whose history and physicals are essentially negative, you will order

    (A) an electrocardiogram (ECG)
    (B) chest x-rays, posteroanterior and lateral
    (C) a complete blood count (CBC)
    (D) a mammogram
    (E) a serum estrogen level   *(Ref. 31)*

46. Which of the following is the precursor of vulvar cancer?

    (A) bacterial vaginosis
    (B) leukoplakia
    (C) herpes genitalis
    (D) condyloma acuminata
    (E) Bartholin's cyst degeneration   *(Ref. 59)*

47. A 43-year-old female complains of vaginal spotting for 10 days. She has always experienced abdominal cramping beginning 2 or 3 days before the period and lasting through the entire 6- to 8-day period. The uterus is globular and symmetrically enlarged and tender, with a finely nodular surface. The most likely diagnosis is

    (A) pregnancy
    (B) myoma
    (C) endometrial cancer
    (D) adenomyosis
    (E) endometriosis   *(Ref. 11)*

48. Which of the following tumors may metastasize to the ovary?

    (A) cervical cancer
    (B) endometrial carcinoma
    (C) vulvar cancer
    (D) vaginal cancer
    (E) all of the above   *(Ref. 59)*

49. After menarche, an imperforate hymen may be associated with

    (A) hematometra
    (B) urinary retention
    (C) abdominal pain
    (D) hematocolpos
    (E) all of the above   *(Ref. 59)*

50. Postmenopausal bleeding is most likely caused by

    (A) emotional excitement
    (B) progesterone withdrawal
    (C) depression
    (D) malignancies
    (E) estrogen deficit   *(Ref. 11)*

51. Teenage pregnancies are associated with an increased incidence of

    (A) multiple pregnancies
    (B) low-birth-weight infants
    (C) cesarean sections
    (D) chromosomal trisomies
    (E) postdate pregnancies   *(Ref. 3)*

52. The patency of the fallopian tube is best demonstrated by

    (A) Rubin's test
    (B) hysterography
    (C) hysterosalpingography
    (D) follicle-stimulating hormone (FSH) determination
    (E) endometrial biopsy   *(Ref. 34)*

53. During the secretory phase of a menstrual cycle

    (A) progesterone is secreted by the endometrium
    (B) the surge of the FSH occurs
    (C) the surge of estradiol occurs
    (D) the surge of leuteinizing hormone (LH) occurs
    (E) a low BBT predominates   *(Ref. 11)*

54. During the follicular phase of a menstrual cycle

    (A) the ovary secretes FSH
    (B) the endometrium secretes estradiol
    (C) FSH predominates
    (D) the BBT elevates above 98°F
    (E) progesterone predominates   *(Ref. 11)*

55. Side effects of IUD use include

    (A) leukorrhea
    (B) chronic endometritis
    (C) pelvic pain
    (D) hypermenorrhea
    (E) all of the above   *(Ref. 34)*

56. Which of the following are characteristic of oral contraceptives?

    (A) They increase the total thyroxine concentration in the blood.
    (B) They increase the protein-bound iodine (PBI).
    (C) They increase the risk of thromboembolic disease.
    (D) A high dose of estrogen and progestin alone may inhibit ovulation.
    (E) all of the above   *(Ref. 3)*

57. The diagnosis of trichomonal vaginitis can be established firmly by

    (A) a history of itching
    (B) wet saline smear of the vaginal discharge
    (C) strawberry appearance of the cervix
    (D) yellowish vaginal discharge
    (E) potassium hydroxide (KOH) smear of the vaginal discharge   *(Ref. 11)*

58. Patients complaining of bleeding with intercourse may have

    (A) trichomonas
    (B) cervical polyp
    (C) cervical cancer
    (D) gonorrhea
    (E) all of the above   *(Ref. 14)*

59. A 25-year-old medical transcriptionist is seen because of her inability to conceive in the past year. She is

    (A) fertile
    (B) fecundable
    (C) sterile
    (D) infertile
    (E) unattractive   *(Ref. 34)*

60. Bacterial vaginosis is best diagnosed by

(A) the presence of hyphae

(B) a high concentration of lactobacilli

(C) low pH

(D) the presence of clue cells

(E) a cheese-like discharge   *(Ref. 11)*

61. The drug of choice for endometriosis is

(A) metronidazole

(B) danazol

(C) bromocriptine

(D) ethinyl estradiol

(E) cyclophosphamide   *(Ref. 11)*

62. Oral contraceptives may reduce the incidence of

(A) lung cancer

(B) ectopic pregnancy

(C) breast cancer

(D) cervical cancer

(E) esophageal cancer   *(Ref. 11)*

63. Which of the following is a contraindication for oral contraceptive use?

(A) fibrocystic breast disease

(B) obesity

(C) a history of gestational diabetes

(D) a history of hepatitis B

(E) a history of postpartum thromboembolism   *(Ref. 2)*

64. Hyperprolactinemia is most frequently associated with

(A) diabetes mellitus

(B) hyperthyroidism

(C) long-term use of phenothiazines

(D) peptic ulcer diseases

(E) polycystic ovarian disease   *(Ref. 30)*

65. The most troublesome side reaction for women taking danazol is

(A) hirsutism

(B) weight loss

(C) hypoglycemia

(D) diastolic hypertension

(E) hypercholesterolemia   *(Ref. 11)*

66. A 40-year-old female complains of fishy vaginal discharges for 2 weeks. The most likely diagnosis is

(A) nonspecific vaginitis

(B) *Haemophilus* vaginitis

(C) *Gardnerella vaginalis* vaginitis

(D) anaerobic vaginosis

(E) bacterial vaginosis   *(Ref. 11)*

67. Bromocriptine is most commonly used for

(A) hypertriglyceridemia

(B) hyperprolactinemia

(C) hyperglycemia

(D) hyperuricemia

(E) hypomagnesemia   *(Ref. 59)*

68. In polycystic ovary syndrome

(A) LH is decreased

(B) FSH is decreased

(C) the estrogen level is decreased

(D) the testosterone level is decreased

(E) LH is elevated   *(Ref. 31)*

69. A 67-year-old female comes for a routine check-up without any complaints. You would offer

(A) a pneumococcal vaccine

(B) a vitamin B_{12} shot

(C) a vitamin K injection

(D) chest x-ray surveillance

(E) oral penicillin chemoprophylaxis *(Ref. 2)*

70. In the United States, the prevalence of infertility among couples is

(A) 0%

(B) 2%

(C) 3%

(D) 7%

(E) 14%   *(Ref. 11)*

71. Which of the following microorganisms reaches the fallopian tube through hematogeneous dissemination?

    (A) *Streptococcus*
    (B) *Trichomonas*
    (C) gonococcus
    (D) tubercle bacillus
    (E) *Candida albicans*   *(Ref. 59)*

72. A postmenopausal woman complained of vaginal itching and dyspareunia. The vaginal mucosa appears thin, dry, and pale. The most likely diagnosis is

    (A) monilial vaginitis
    (B) herpes simplex infection
    (C) atrophic vaginitis
    (D) depression
    (E) bacterial vaginosis   *(Ref. 11)*

73. Progesterone may

    (A) increase alveolar P_{CO_2}
    (B) decrease body temperature
    (C) stop lactation
    (D) relax pubic symphysis
    (E) produce natriuresis   *(Ref. 59)*

74. A 35-year-old nulliparous infertile female presents with chronic cyclic pelvic pain, dysmenorrhea, and dyspareunia for 6 months. Pelvic examination reveals tender nodules in the posterior vaginal fornix and pain upon uterine motion. The most likely diagnosis is

    (A) myoma uteri
    (B) endometriosis
    (C) cervical polyp
    (D) acute cervicitis
    (E) ectopic pregnancy   *(Ref. 11)*

75. Hydrothorax is often associated with

    (A) serous cystadenoma of the ovary
    (B) bilateral polycystic ovaries
    (C) pseudomucinous cystadenoma of the ovary
    (D) ovarian fibroma
    (E) myoma uteri   *(Ref. 16)*

DIRECTIONS (Questions 76 through 109): Each question consists of an introduction followed by some statements. Mark T (true) or F (false) after each statement.

76. Estrogen produces

    (A) breast development
    (B) secretory endometrium
    (C) proliferative endometrium
    (D) pubic hair growth
    (E) elevation of cholesterol   *(Ref. 59)*

77. Endometrial polyps are characterized by

    (A) metrorrhagia
    (B) dysfunctional bleeding
    (C) menorrhagia
    (D) dyspareunia
    (E) postmenopausal bleeding   *(Ref. 11)*

78. Climacterium is characterized by

    (A) hot flashes
    (B) dysfunctional bleeding
    (C) dyspareunia
    (D) low FSH
    (E) low LH   *(Ref. 1)*

79. IUDs

    (A) are used in mass programs in developing societies
    (B) cause irreversible fertility
    (C) are 70% effective
    (D) may inhibit libido
    (E) may cause pelvic pain   *(Ref. 11)*

80. Important risk factors for endometrial cancer include which of the following?

    (A) obesity
    (B) hypertension
    (C) first-birth order
    (D) diabetes mellitus
    (E) use of estrogen   *(Ref. 11)*

81. The choice of contraception for a woman with a history of ectopic pregnancy includes

    (A) oral contraceptives
    (B) intrauterine device
    (C) diaphragm
    (D) condom
    (E) foam and jelly   (Ref. 3)

82. Menarche is characterized by

    (A) anovulatory cycle
    (B) dysfunctional bleeding
    (C) hot flashes
    (D) monophasic BBT
    (E) puberty   (Ref. 31)

83. A female patient who appears for her routine annual examination at a family physician's office should receive which of the following procedures?

    (A) rectovaginal examination
    (B) breast examination
    (C) measurement of height and weight
    (D) percussion of the lung fields
    (E) electroencephalogram (EEG)   (Ref. 3)

84. The ovarian granulosa cell tumor may produce

    (A) menorrhagia
    (B) clitoris enlargement
    (C) atrophic vaginitis
    (D) breast pain
    (E) pseudoprecocious puberty   (Ref. 11)

85. A 47-year-old housewife complains of profuse, prolonged vaginal spotting at varied intervals during the last 6 months. The patient may have

    (A) ectopic pregnancy
    (B) abortion
    (C) uterine myoma
    (D) dysfunctional uterine bleeding
    (E) endometrial carcinoma   (Ref. 11)

86. Toxic shock syndrome is frequently associated with

    (A) contraceptive pills
    (B) tampon use
    (C) delivery
    (D) diaphragm
    (E) soft-tissue abscesses   (Ref. 30)

87. The benefits of estrogen replacement therapy include

    (A) prevention of endometrial cancers
    (B) relief of hot flashes
    (C) alleviation of vaginal atrophy
    (D) prevention of osteoporosis
    (E) increased high-density lipoprotein
                                          (Ref. 11)

88. The prolonged use of oral contraceptives may increase the risk of

    (A) myocardial infarction
    (B) thromboembolism
    (C) stroke
    (D) subarachnoid hemorrhage
    (E) hypertension   (Ref. 2)

89. Rectovaginal fistulas may result from

    (A) cervical cancer invasion
    (B) radiotherapy for cervical cancer
    (C) hemorrhoidectomy
    (D) lymphogranuloma inguinale
    (E) birth injury   (Ref. 32)

90. Vesicovaginal fistulas are often caused by

    (A) repair of the cystocele
    (B) radiotherapy of cervical cancer
    (C) invasion of cervical cancer
    (D) radical hysterectomy
    (E) hemorrhoid   (Ref. 11)

91. Monilial vaginitis is frequently seen in women with

    (A) pregnancy
    (B) long-term systemic antibiotic therapy

(C) diabetes

(D) oral contraceptive use

(E) pruritus vulvae   *(Ref. 11)*

92. Methotrexate has which of the following side effects?

(A) bone marrow suppression

(B) gastrointestinal (GI) disturbances

(C) hepatitis

(D) oral ulcers

(E) polycythemia   *(Ref. 32)*

93. Urethrovaginal fistulas are often caused by

(A) irradiation

(B) repair of urethrocele

(C) repair of cystocele

(D) lymphogranuloma venereum

(E) lymphogranuloma inguinale   *(Ref. 11)*

94. Prolonged use of oral contraceptives is associated with an increased incidence of

(A) breast cancer

(B) cervical dysplasia

(C) hepatocellular adenoma

(D) cervical cancer

(E) ovarian cancer   *(Ref. 3)*

95. *Chlamydia trachomatis* is implicated to cause

(A) cervicitis

(B) urethritis

(C) conjunctivitis

(D) bartholinitis

(E) mastitis   *(Ref. 2)*

96. Recurrent abortions may be associated with

(A) cervical incompetence

(B) cytomegalovirus infection

(C) hyperthyroidism

(D) diabetes mellitus

(E) leiomyoma   *(Ref. 11)*

97. Next to age, the strongest risk factor in breast cancer is

(A) abundant fat intake

(B) positive family history

(C) nulliparity

(D) early menarche

(E) late menopause   *(Ref. 11)*

98. Infertility may be caused by

(A) psychogenic conflict

(B) tubal obstruction

(C) submucous myomas

(D) hyperthyroidism

(E) ovarian tumor   *(Ref. 11)*

99. Concerning infertility

(A) 90% of causes are due to the male partner

(B) 90% of causes are due to the female partner

(C) infertility evaluation should be family-oriented

(D) pregnancy may occur in 15 to 20% of couples just by infertility work-ups

(E) causes of infertility may be found in 85 to 90% of patients   *(Ref. 32)*

100. Hysterectomy is indicated for

(A) chronic trichomonal vaginitis

(B) symptomatic leiomyomas

(C) cervical polyp

(D) symptomatic adenomyosis

(E) endometrial polyp   *(Ref. 11)*

101. Clinical presentations of the PID include

(A) normal sedimentation rate

(B) leukopenia

(C) Gram stain of endocervix shows gram positive cocci

(D) temperature of 102°F

(E) anorexia   *(Ref. 11)*

102. Complications of PID include

    (A) tubo-ovarian abscess
    (B) increased fecundity
    (C) ectopic pregnancy
    (D) chronic pelvic pain
    (E) Fitz-Hugh–Curtis syndrome   (Ref. 30)

103. Initial managements of nonspecific vulvo-vaginitis in children involve

    (A) 1% clotrimazole vaginal cream, 6 g per application at bedtime for 7 days
    (B) metronidazole PO, 2 g stat dose
    (C) metronidazole PO, 250 mg tid for 7 days
    (D) avoidance of bubble baths
    (E) sitz baths   (Ref. 59)

104. Managements of monilial vaginitis include

    (A) change to a different brand of oral contraceptives if the patient is on oral contraceptives for more than six cycles
    (B) oral doxycycline 100 mg bid for 10 days
    (C) oral metronidazole 2 g stat for the sexual partner
    (D) nystatin 100-mg vaginal suppository at bedtime for 1 week
    (E) clotrimazole 100-mg vaginal suppository at bedtime for 1 week   (Ref. 11)

105. Which of the following regimens are used for the empiric ambulatory management of pelvic inflammatory diseases?

    (A) cefoxitin PO stat + probenecid PO stat + doxycycline PO stat
    (B) cefoxitin PO stat + probenecid IM stat + doxycycline IM stat
    (C) cefoxitin IM stat + probenecid IM stat + doxycycline PO for 10 days
    (D) cefoxitin IM stat + probenecid PO stat + doxycycline PO for 10 days
    (E) cefoxitin IM stat + probenecid PO stat + doxycycline IM stat   (Ref. 11)

106. Which of the following statements are true/false for vaginitis?

    (A) Trichomonal vaginitis is a sexually transmitted disease, and the sexual partner must be treated as well.
    (B) Microscopic examination of the vaginal discharge with KOH preparation will identify the causal organism of trichomonal vaginitis.
    (C) A white, cheese-like discharge is characteristic of *Gardnerella* vaginitis.
    (D) Vaginitis caused by *Chlamydia trachomatis* is best treated by oral metronidazole combined with nystatin vaginal suppositories.
    (E) Clue cells are diagnostic for atrophic vaginitis.   (Ref. 11)

107. Supernumerary nipples and accessory breasts may develop following which disease processes?

    (A) cystic lesions
    (B) mastitis
    (C) lactation
    (D) carcinomas
    (E) abscesses   (Ref. 59)

108. The side effects of metronidazole (Flagyl) include

    (A) diarrhea
    (B) fruit taste
    (C) nausea
    (D) headache
    (E) anorexia   (Ref. 30)

109. Risk factors for osteoporosis include

    (A) menopause
    (B) cigarette smoking
    (C) sedentary life style
    (D) white race
    (E) estrogen replacement therapy   (Ref. 7)

DIRECTIONS (Questions 110 through 121): The following clinical set problem consists of clinical information presented in the format of questions or incomplete statements followed by a group of numbered options.

    Indicate T if the option is true;
    Indicate F if the option is false.

A 24-year-old female computer programmer complained of lower abdominal pain of 10 days' duration. The pain was crampy, intermittent, and aggravated by intercourse. She has never been pregnant and has used an IUD for 2 years. She missed her menstrual period for 6 days, and she was also annoyed by a malodorous, yellowish, mucous vaginal discharge. You should now

110. prescribe triple-sulfa vaginal cream

111. prescribe oral nystatin for 10 days

112. instruct the use of alkaline douches twice a day for 2 weeks

113. perform culdocentesis

114. order laparoscopy

A clinical diagnosis of PID has been established. If untreated, the likely complications include

115. infertility

116. ectopic pregnancies

117. breast cancers

118. endometrial carcinomas

Appropriate managements include

119. removal of IUD

120. total hysterectomy

121. counseling of the protective sexual activities

(Ref. 3)

Answers and Explanations

1. **(D)** Women who have a positive family history and contralateral breast cancer are at higher risk. Women who are also at risk include the following: nulliparous, older primigravida, early menarche, late menopause, and chronic use of high-dose estrogen (more than 10 years).

2. **(E)** There is no ready answer to teenage contraception. The solution is determined by the individual problem, which should be clarified by exploration. Simply complying with the request or denying it usually is of little help to the girl who is really seeking help for the total problem. Contraceptive counseling is provided to determine the need and appropriateness of contraception.

3. **(C)** It is unlikely that a woman who has been having intercourse regularly (three pregnancies in the past 2 years) will stop simply because she is told it is wrong. Her problem is that she has already made the decision to have coitus and is in desperate need of contraception (her motivation is high if she has resorted to induced abortions three times). This patient is highly fertile, and she possibly needs contraceptives with low pregnancy risk (ie, oral contraceptives). Any patient undergoing induced abortion who does not want pregnancies in the near future should be on pills. However, the decision has to be made by the patient.

4. **(E)** This is most probably a case of cervical polyp. Excision is in order, and the tissue should be submitted for histologic examination to be certain of its benign nature and to rule out cervical cancer in particular.

5. **(B)** The pregnancy may be allowed to continue and to terminate vaginally at term with subsequent postpartum reevaluation.

6. **(C)** Trichomonal vaginitis is often asymptomatic. It is characterized by a profuse, purulent, malodorus vaginal discharge accompanied by vulvar pruritus. An appearance of "strawberry" cervix may be noted.

7. **(C)** The most commonly used contraceptive worldwide is the IUD, which is recommended for monogamous, parous females in the United States. It increases the risk of PID.

8. **(A)** Trichomoniasis is characterized by pruritus and frothy, yellow-green or clear discharge. Diagnosis is made by the presence of the flagellate in the wet smear.

9. **(C)** This appearance of the vagina is quite characteristic of *trichomonal vaginitis*. The mucous membrane is reddened, and the posterior fornix often presents a granular or strawberry-like appearance, which is almost pathognomonic. Small petechial erosions may be seen on the cervix.

10. **(B)** Monilial vaginitis is characterized by the typical cheesy or curd-like, adherent discharge. Multiple brown-black colonies of 1 to 2 mm will grow on Nickerson's medium in 48 hours without incubation.

11. **(C)** Monilial vaginitis is treated with an oral agent (fluconazole 150 mg single dose) or topical drugs (butoconazole 2% cream 5 mg

for 3 days; miconazole, ticonazole 6.5% ointment 5 mg single dose; terconazole 0.8% cream 5 mg for 3 days; and clotrimazole 500 mg single vaginal tablet).

12. **(D)** The characteristic findings of a suburethral mass, which on compression produces purulent exudate from the urethral meatus, is diagnostic of a urethral diverticulum. Carcinoma of the female urethra may develop in urethral diverticulum but is not as localized and mostly occurs in older age groups. Gartner's duct cysts do not communicate with the urethra. Venereal urethritis is a diffuse process. Abscess of Skene's duct is extremely rare and generally occupies a position much closer to the external urinary meatus.

13. **(E)** The diaphragm must be used with spermicidal cream. The diaphragm is to be inserted 2 hours before intercourse and left for 6 hours after intercourse. The same diaphragm can be used for the repeated intercourse with new application of the spermicidal cream. The diaphragm can be used repeatedly.

14. **(A)** Monilial vaginitis is characterized by vulvar pruritus associated with vaginal discharges that resemble cottage cheese. A presumptive diagnosis is often made if the pH of the discharge is normal (less than 4.5) and the saline preparation is normal. A fungal culture is recommended for diagnosis.

15. **(B)** Mastitis is fairly common in the puerperium on the lactating breast. Mastitis seldom occurs prior to the end of the first week after delivery and often is seen for the first time 3 or 4 weeks postpartum. The usual symptoms are mild chills, fever, and breast soreness. Soon, erythema and local heat develop over the infected and indurated segment of the breast. Tender, ipsilateral, axillary adenopathy is common. The infection is usually staphylococcal in origin and can be treated with antibiotics. If breast abscess develops, incision and drainage are frequently performed.

16. **(E)** Pseudomyxoma peritonei is an unusual condition characterized by the transformation of peritoneal mesothelium to mucus-secreting epithelium. Pseudomyxoma peritonei occurs in association with ovarian mucinous cystadenomas, carcinoma, colon cancer, and appendiceal mucoceles. Huge amounts of mucinous material are secreted, and bowel obstruction and death can occur.

17. **(C)** Stein–Leventhal (polycystic ovary) syndrome is characterized by bilaterally enlarged polycystic ovaries, amenorrhea (or oligomenorrhea), infertility, obesity, and hirsutism. Grossly, the ovary is described as bilaterally enlarged and gray in color, with a firm, smooth cortex and a thickened, fibrosed tunica. Beneath the surface are multiple cystic follicles and no evidence of corpora lutea.

18. **(C)** The most frequent complication of ovarian cyst is torsion or twisting of the pedicle, and the acute symptoms (pain and rigidity) thus precipitated are frequently the first indication of the presence of an ovarian tumor. This complication is more common in small or moderate-sized tumors than in large ones. When the cyst is on the right side, it often mimics acute appendicitis and often the diagnosis is made upon operation. The complication of torsion of an ovarian cyst is frequently peritonitis; treatment is immediate surgery.

19. **(B)** Submucous myomas comprise only 5% of all myomas, but are much more likely than other types of myomas to cause profuse bleeding and thus require hysterectomy, although their size is usually small.

20. **(B)** In the patient in her early forties who has completed her childbearing function, total hysterectomy is not looked on with disfavor. Preservation of the ovaries is desirable in premenopausal patients.

21. **(E)** Uncomplicated uterine retroversion is usually symptomless. Backache is one of the most common complaints in female patients and is usually an orthopedic backache. Back-

ache may be associated with retroversion of the uterus only in a severe case.

22. **(D)** Although patients with endometriosis may be asymptomatic, the classic symptomatology includes acquired dysmenorrhea, hypermenorrhea, polymenorrhea, cyclic bowel disturbances with painful defecation and rectal bleeding, and bladder irritability with hematuria. The physical finding is usually a hard, fixed, fibrotic nodule, usually noted as a beaded or "shotty" thickening in the uterosacral ligament, cul-de-sac, or posterior surface of the lower uterine wall or cervix. These patients are often unmarried or infertile.

23. **(C)** Two thirds of endometrial carcinoma occurs in women beyond menopause. Obesity, hypertension, diabetes, and sterility or poor fertility are associated with endometrial carcinoma. Any patients with postmenopausal bleeding should first be tested for cancer of the uterus, either of the cervix or of the body. Cervical cancer can usually be detected by careful inspection and office smears and biopsy. Once the vagina and cervix have been eliminated as sources of the bleeding, an intrauterine source may be safely assumed, and fractional dilatation and curettage should be in order.

24. **(C)** For lactating women, the progesterone-only pills (minipills such as Ovrette and Micronor) are recommended. Depo-Provera injections are also commonly used.

25. **(B)** Many adolescent patients are enthusiastic about the Norplant system for its 5 years of contraceptive protection. However, following the implantation, many soon request removal due to common side reactions, including menstrual irregularities (intermenstrual spotting and amenorrhea), headache, weight gain, and depression.

26. **(C)** Perforation of adnexal abscess causes pelvic or generalized peritonitis with severe abdominal pain (usually referred to the side of rupture), tachycardia, shock, and subnormal temperature that rises rapidly to 107°F to 108°F. Pelvic examination may fail to demonstrate the previously palpable adnexal mass. Surgical exploration is immediately in order.

27. **(B)** For women under 50, biennial screening is advocated by the American Cancer Society. For women older than 50, annual physical examination with mammography is recommended.

28. **(A)** Gonococcus is responsible for many PIDs. Confirmation of the diagnosis is usually obtained by identifying the gram-negative intracellular diplococci on a stained smear of the urethral, vaginal, or cervical discharge, of secretions milked from Skene's glands in the paraurethral area, or of material from rectal crypts obtained via anoscopy. A definite diagnosis is made by culture on Thayer–Martin medium.

29. **(D)** The irregular monophasic curve of BBT is characteristic of anovulatory cycle; biphasic temperature curve is indicative of ovulation and normal progesterone effect; and the sustained temperature elevation following ovulatory curve (biphasic) is the indication for pregnancy. Conception while the patient is maintaining a record of her BBT curve occurs fairly frequently during the course of an infertility investigation.

30. **(D)** Spotting is common during the initial three cycles, and this breakthrough bleeding should subside within 3 months. However, when spotting occurs in the first cycle, it most likely is due to inconsistency in taking pills each day. Advise the patient to take the pill at the same time daily. If bleeding continues and is heavy, switch to pills with more progestin (Nordette, Triphasil). If spotting continues for two to three cycles, supplement with estrogen (Premarin 0.625 mg).

31. **(C)** Endometrial biopsy is the most accurate diagnostic technique of ovulation.

Phase	Day of Menstrual Cycle	Hormone
Proliferative (preovulation) Follicular	6–14	FSH, estrogen
Secretory (ovulation) Luteal	15–28	FSH, estrogen, progesterone, and LH
Menstrual	1–5	FSH, estrogen, and progesterone (low titer)

32. **(A)** Ovulation usually occurs 14 days before the menstrual flow. However, in younger women, ovulation will possibly occur 10 days before the menstrual flow.

33. **(E)** An abnormal Pap smear calls for repeated Pap smear in 3 to 6 months. If the repeated two consecutive tests are negative, a low-risk patient may return to yearly Pap smears. If the repeated test is again abnormal, a colposcopically directed biopsy and a human papilloma virus (HPV) test are to be performed. However, an individualized approach is needed (many family physicians may perform colposcopic biopsy and endocervical curettage if the patient is at high risk for HPV).

34. **(B)** With an initial evaluation of normal pelvic findings, including normal vaginal estrogenic smear and normal arborization of cervical mucus, normal gonadotropins (and 17-ketosteroids), and normal skull x-rays (normal visual field), a clinical test with IM injection of 100 mg progesterone (or 10 mg of medroxyprogesterone acetate daily for 10 days) can be employed after a negative pregnancy test. The withdrawal response to progestin administration indicates that the patient has a functional end organ (uterine endometrium) and normal production of estrogen. A heavy dose of "tincture of time" will solve the problem.

35. **(D)** Decreased menstrual flow and even amenorrhea are common problems after 1 to 2 years of use. Pregnancy is to be ruled out and progestin-dominant pills (Nordette, Lo/Ovral) administered. If this does not help, increase the estrogen content to 50 μg or supplement with Premarin.

36. **(E)** The average pregnancy rate for vasectomy, tubal ligation, oral contraceptives, and IUDs are around 0.2% to 2%; condom is 12%; diaphragm, sponge, foams, and jellies are 18% to 21%; coitus interruptus and fertility awareness are 10%; abstinence is 0%.

37. **(E)** The vaginal discharge of a normal woman is clear, flocculent, odorless, and has a pH of 3.8 to 4.2. The predominant organisms are lactobacilli (95%).

38. **(E)** Since the secondary sexual characteristics are well developed and there is no evidence of other constitutional problems, further diagnostic studies do not seem warranted at this time. Moreover, ordering laboratory studies may increase the girl's anxiety and emotional stress and may further delay menarche, contrary to the therapeutic objective you have tried to accomplish. The diagnosis in this adolescent girl is normal variation of sexual development. This should be explained in detail to both the girl and her mother to alleviate their anxiety and to correct their fantasies (such as the possibility of pregnancy without menarche). They should be informed that if the patient at age 17 is still without menarche, a further diagnostic work-up will be necessary then. Also, it will be more appropriate for the clinician to prepare the girl for the upcoming menarche to alleviate possible fears and surprise.

39. **(D)** About 4% of female genital tract malignancies are vulvar malignancies. It is one of the most easily diagnosed malignancies because of its visibility on the external body surface. It has a high cure rate if detected early. However, it is the most poorly managed female malignancy due to patient's delay (embarrassment).

40. **(B)** Common complications of bacterial vaginosis are postpartum endoenteritis and posthysterectomy septicemia. Other complications include preterm labor, preterm birth, premature rupture of membranes (PROM), amniotic fluid infection, chorioamnionitis, and PIDs.

41. **(C)** Grouped vesicles with small ulcers are most likely due to genital herpes. Culture is almost 100% positive during the vesicle stage (89% during the pustular stage and 33% in patients with ulcers).

42. **(C)** The contraindications for oral contraceptives include thromboembolic disease, strokes, pregnancy, hyperlipidemia, coronary artery diseases, hepatic adenoma, impaired hepatic function, history of obstructive jaundice, and breast cancers.

43. **(A)** Initial genital herpes is treated with 400 mg of oral Zovirax (acyclovir) three times a day for 7 to 10 days. The recurrent infections of genital herpes may heal speedily by administration of oral acyclovir.

44. **(D)** Genital herpes is diagnosed by detailed history and characteristic physical findings. Confirmation is done by Tzanck test (multinucleate giant cells by Giemsa stain), viral culture, modified viral culture, Pap smear, and direct immunofluorescence test. Serologic tests are not very useful.

45. **(D)** For women over 50 years, annual mammography, annual occult blood, and annual sigmoidoscopy are indicated. Serum cholesterol and serologic tests for syphilis are recommended. ECG, chest x-rays, urinalysis, and CBC are ordered for high-risk groups or for symptomatic patients. Pap smears are performed every 3 years if previous three consecutive annual smears were negative.

46. **(B)** Elderly patients with the following conditions are at high risk of developing vulvar cancer: diabetes mellitus, glucose intolerance, adenocarcinoma of the breast, adenocarcinoma of the endometrium, intraepithelial car-

cinoma of the vagina or the cervix, obesity, arteriosclerosis, hypertension, early menopause, nulliparity, leukoplakia, syphilis (condyloma lata), lymphogranuloma inguinale, lymphogranuloma venereum, and hyperplastic, hyperkeratotic vulvitis. Leukoplakia is considered to be the precursor of epidermoid carcinoma of the vulva.

47. **(D)** Dysmenorrhea, menorrhagia, and an enlarged, firm, tender uterus in a 43-year-old woman is very likely due to adenomyosis, and hysterography and magnetic resonance imaging (MRI) are ordered to aid in the diagnosis of this condition. However, the differential diagnosis includes submucous myoma, endometrial cancer, endometriosis, myoma uteri, pelvic congestion syndrome (Taylor syndrome, continuous pelvic pain and menometrorrhagia in the emotional patient), and salpingitis. These entities often can be differentiated from adenomyosis by laparoscopy, dilatation and curettage (D&C), and ultrasonography.

48. **(E)** The ovary is one of the frequent sites of metastasis from almost any site. Cancers of all pelvic organs metastasize to the ovary, and the spread is usually bilateral. Five percent of endometrial carcinomas and 1% of cervical carcinomas metastasize to the ovary. The metastasis of vulvar and vaginal cancers to the ovary is usually in the late stage.

49. **(E)** The imperforate hymen is rarely discovered before puberty. The frequent symptoms after menarche are cyclic abdominal pain, urinary retention with flank pain, and the accumulation of the blood in the vagina, uterus, and tubes (hematosalpinx).

50. **(D)** Postmenopausal bleeding is commonly caused by malignancies, endometrial dysplasia, estrogen administration, atrophic vaginitis, and cervical polyps.

51. **(B)** Teenage pregnancies are associated with an increased incidence of low-birth-weight infants, maternal complications (gonorrhea and syphilis), toxemia, anemia, malnutrition, and perinatal mortality.

52. **(C)** Tubal patency is demonstrated by hysterosalpingography and laparoscopy. Hysterosalpingography is preferable to Rubin's test for infertility evaluation because it provides information on the structure and function of the uterus and tube.

53. **(D)** The secretory phase is characterized by the LH surge, ovulation, and progesterone production by the ovary. Progesterone produces gland secretion, stromal edema, and a decidual reaction. The BBT is elevated above 98°F during this phase. The duration of this phase is fairly constant (12 to 16 days, usually 14 days).

54. **(C)** The follicular phase is characterized by the development of the ovarian follicles, which produce estrogen (estradiol). The FSH predominates during this phase.

55. **(E)** Side effects of IUD use include breakthrough bleeding, leukorrhea, pelvic pain (dysmenorrhea), hypermenorrhea, psychiatric disturbances, PID, and chronic endometritis. Uterine perforation, ectopic IUD, peritonitis, and intestinal obstruction have been experienced.

56. **(E)** Both an estrogen alone and progestin alone will prevent ovulation if large enough doses are given; the effect is apparently at the level of the hypothalamus or higher nerve centers. Small doses of progestins change endometrial metabolism and the type and amount of cervical mucus to prevent pregnancy. The oral pills seem certainly to increase the risk of thromboembolic disease. Oral pill users will have an increase in PBI and total thyroxine concentration in the blood due to the effect of estrogen on the binding capacity of globulin.

57. **(B)** A saline smear of vaginal secretions may reveal clue cells due to common association with bacterial vaginosis. The number of leukocytes is increased, and motile, pear-shaped trichomonads are present.

58. **(E)** Abnormal uterine bleeding is deviation from the woman's normal menstrual pattern, an increase of two pads or more per day, or menses that last three or more days longer than usual. Although cervical polyp characteristically causes postcoital bleeding, other conditions may also occur.

59. **(D)** Fifty percent of normal couples may conceive within three months; after one year of unprotected intercourse 80% of women in the reproductive age may achieve pregnancy; 90% of women may conceive in two years. When the patient did not conceive during the past year, detailed menstrual, contraceptive, and sexual (frequency of coitus) histories should be taken to determine the possible causes and take appropriate action. Common causes include coitus during the safe period, use of contraceptives, emotional stress, tubal obstructions (such as tuberculous or gonococcal salpingitis), endometrial or ovarian defects (such as endometriosis and polycystic ovaries), and the male partner's inadequate sperm.

60. **(D)** Bacterial vaginosis can be established by finding three of the four following signs: thin, homogeneous discharge that adheres to the vaginal walls; an elevated pH >4.5; a positive KOH "whiff" test; and the presence of clue cells on microscopic examination.

61. **(B)** Danazol (Danocrine) is a synthetic androgen that suppresses the pituitary–ovarian axis by inhibiting the output of gonadotropins from the pituitary gland. Daily dosage of 400 mg may be responsive for painful symptoms, and the patient may achieve pregnancy by a continuing therapy every 9 to 12 months.

62. **(B)** Noncontraceptive benefits of oral contraceptives include reduction of benign breast disease, reduction in functional ovarian cysts, reduced incidence of PID, reduced incidence of ectopic pregnancy, reduced ovarian and endometrial cancer, reduced incidence of rheumatoid arthritis, and reduction of iron deficiency anemia.

63. **(E)** The contraindications for oral contraceptives include thromboembolism, cerebrovascular disease, coronary artery disease, abnormal genital bleeding, pregnancy, breast cancers, endometrial cancers, malignant melanoma, and hepatocellular adenoma. Oral contraceptives may be protective for patients with fibrocystic disease.

64. **(C)** Hyperprolactinemia is characterized by amenorrhea and galactorrhea with an increased serum prolactin level beyond 400 ng/mL. It is commonly caused by side reactions of the drugs (such as phenothiazines, reserpine, methyldopa, and oral contraceptives), primary hypothyroidism, and pituitary adenomas.

65. **(A)** Danazol (Danocrine) is used for endometriosis; its troublesome side reactions are due to androgenic effects, including acne, amenorrhea, hirsutism, weight gain, decrease in breast size, deepening of voice, and oily skin. Its hypoestrogenic activity includes hot flashes, vaginal dryness, and emotional lability. It may also cause muscle cramps and impair glucose tolerance.

66. **(E)** Bacterial vaginosis is the currently accepted name for the disease. In the past it has been labeled as nonspecific vaginitis, *Haemophilus* vaginitis, corynebacterium vaginitis, *Gardnerella vaginalis* vaginitis, and anaerobic vaginosis.

67. **(B)** Bromocriptine (Parlodel) is an ergot alkaloid that stimulates the prolactin inhibition factor of the hypothalamus in reducing prolactin secretion to abolish amenorrhea. It may be able to control the growth of a pituitary prolactinoma. Its side reactions include giddiness and nausea.

68. **(E)** In polycystic ovary syndrome, LH is constantly elevated over FSH (FSH is usually in a low-normal range).

69. **(A)** A pneumococcal vaccine is protective against 80 to 90% of *Streptococcus pneumoniae*, which causes bacteremic pneumococcal dis-

ease. Side reactions include myalgias, low-grade fever, arrhythmia, and pain for 1 to 2 days.

70. **(E)** Voluntary childlessness is increasing, and one in seven couples is infertile.

71. **(D)** The fallopian tubes constitute the initial seat of genital tuberculosis, which is usually secondary to extragenital tuberculosis (mostly pulmonary tuberculosis, although usually inactive) by hematogenous dissemination. Pyogenic acute salpingitis usually follows childbirth, abortion (septic or puerperal), or pelvic surgery (vaginal hysterectomy) when streptococci or staphylococci travel from a cervical or corporeal focus to the tube via veins and lymphatics of the broad ligament. Gonococci reach the tube via cervical focus by the mucous membrane, frequently with occlusion of the tubal lumen and subsequent sterility. Trichomonads are usually confined to vaginal mucosa to cause trichomonal vaginitis and are rare causes of salpingitis. *Candida albicans* causes monilial vaginitis in susceptible patients, including diabetics, pregnant women, and patients on oral contraceptives or broad-spectrum antibiotics.

72. **(C)** Due to estrogen deficiency, the patient may develop atrophic vaginitis, which is characterized by atrophy of external genitalia with loss of vaginal rugae. The vaginal mucosa is friable. The vaginal secretions contain parabasal epithelial cells and many leukocytes. Topical estrogen is effective. Hormone replacement therapy is needed to prevent recurrence.

73. **(E)** Progesterone stimulates the development of lobules and alveoli in the breast. It supports the secretory function of the breast during lactation. Progesterone increases BBT at the time of ovulation, lowers alveolar P_{CO_2} during the luteal phase, and induces natriuresis. Relaxin may relax the pubic symphysis and pelvic joints.

74. **(B)** Endometriosis is prevalent in around 7% of women of reproductive years. Diagno-

sis often requires laparoscopic visualization. Endometriosis may implant at the bowel or uterus. It can also cause ovarian torsion or even chemical peritonitis. Treatment modalities include amenorrhea induction, oral contraceptives, gonadotropin-releasing hormone agonists, danazol, and surgery.

75. **(D)** Meigs' syndrome is characterized by ovarian fibroma, hydrothorax, and ascites.

76. **(A)-T, (B)-T, (C)-T, (D)-F, (E)-F.** The growth of the duct system of the breast is stimulated by estrogen. Nipple erectility and pigmentation of the areola are also estrogen dependent. The development of acinar buds from the breast milk ducts and the formation of lobules and alveoli are stimulated by progesterone. Under the influence of estrogen, the endometrium proliferates, and under the effects of progesterone and estrogen, the secretory phase develops. Estrogen lowers cholesterol and increases libido. The androgen stimulates pubic and axillary hair growth.

77. **(A)-T, (B)-T, (C)-T, (D)-F, (E)-T.** Endometrial polyps are frequently associated with bleeding (metrorrhagia) and offensive discharge. In postmenopausal women, endometrial polyps are often associated with malignancy, and excision is recommended.

78. **(A)-T, (B)-T, (C)-T, (D)-F, (E)-F.** Climacterium is characterized by vasomotor disturbances (hot flashes), irritability, and musculoskeletal symptoms (osteoporosis). It is diagnosed by the elevated FSH and LH, denoting ovarian failure. Menopause usually occurs at a median age of 51 years.

79. **(A)-T, (B)-F, (C)-F, (D)-F, (E)-T.** IUDs are used in mass programs in developing societies for their long-term protection and low pregnancy rate (0.4 to 2.8 per 100 women in 12 months of use). The fertility is restored immediately after IUD removal. IUDs may cause expulsion, pain, bleeding, and PIDs, and are suitable for monogamous women.

80. **(A)-T, (B)-T, (C)-F, (D)-T, (E)-T.** Obesity, hypertension, and diabetes mellitus are known risk factors in the development of endometrial cancer. Prolonged unopposed estrogen administration also increases the risk.

81. **(A)-T, (B)-F, (C)-T, (D)-T, (E)-T.** The absolute contraindications to using an IUD include pregnancy and active pelvic infections; the relative contraindications include recurrent pelvic infections, acute cervicitis, a history of ectopic pregnancy, valvular heart diseases (may lead to subacute bacterial endocarditis), and uterine abnormalities (cervical stenosis, a uterus smaller than 6 cm, endometriosis, endometrial polyps, bicornuate uterus, uterine myomata, endometrial hyperplasia, and severe dysmenorrhea and hypermenorrhea).

82. **(A)-T, (B)-T, (C)-F, (D)-T, (E)-T.** Menarche is the initial period, usually from age 8 to 16 years. Anovulatory cycle is seen in the first 1 to 2 years after menarche. The bleeding is irregular in amount and duration in accordance with the prior stimulation and the withdrawal of estrogen. During the anovulatory cycle, the BBT will show a monophasic curve, which indicates the failure of ovulation.

83. **(A)-T, (B)-T, (C)-T, (D)-T, (E)-F.** Although routine physicals of female patients are frequently directed toward the performance of Pap smears and sometimes are limited to only pelvic and abdominal organs, examination of the breasts and general survey of the entire physical make-up are essential as the basis of continuity of care quality practice. Three consecutive yearly negative Paps may be followed by repeated Paps every 3 years.

84. **(A)-T, (B)-F, (C)-F, (D)-T, (E)-T.** The granulosa cell tumor produces estrogen to cause pseudoprecocious puberty in children (early breast development, appearance of pubic and axillary hair, and vaginal bleeding); menorrhagia, amenorrhea, breast pain, and fluid retention in patients during menstrual years;

and postmenopausal dysfunctional bleeding. It is associated with endometrial hyperplasia and cancer.

85. **(A)-T, (B)-T, (C)-T, (D)-T, (E)-T.** Dysfunctional bleeding occurs frequently in the premenopausal age group. However, uterine neoplasms, both benign and malignant, also occur commonly in women of this age and must be ruled out. Rarely, complications of pregnancy, pelvic infections, adenomyosis, myomas, and endometrial polyps may also occur. If dysfunctional bleeding is ascertained, Provera administration may be useful.

86. **(A)-F, (B)-T, (C)-T, (D)-T, (E)-T.** Toxic shock syndrome is characterized by high fever of 102°F, diffuse macular rashes, vomiting, lethargy, and orthostatic syncope. It is associated with the use of tampons, diaphragms, and possibly contraceptive sponges. It is also associated with soft-tissue abscesses, osteomyelitis, and postdelivery. It is caused by an exotoxin produced by *Staphylococcus aureus*.

87. **(A)-F, (B)-T, (C)-T, (D)-T, (E)-T.** The benefits of estrogen replacement therapy include alleviation of menopausal symptoms (hot flashes, vaginal dryness, dyspareunia, urethral atrophy, irritability, and depression), prevention of osteoporosis, and decreased risk of coronary artery disease (decreased low-density lipoproteins, decreased cholesterol, decreased very-low-density lipoproteins, and increased high-density lipoproteins). However, estrogen may increase triglyceride and increase the risk of endometrial cancers, and there is possibly a low risk of development of breast cancers.

88. **(A)-T, (B)-T, (C)-T, (D)-T, (E)-T.** The prolonged use of oral contraceptives is associated with general cardiovascular diseases, including myocardial infarction, thromboembolism, stroke, subarachnoid hemorrhage, and hypertension. However, the evidence of association is not universally accepted.

89. **(A)-T, (B)-T, (C)-T, (D)-T, (E)-T.** Rectovaginal fistula is the most common form of vaginal fecal fistula. The possible causes include birth injury, irradiation, vaginal surgery (vaginal puncture for pelvic abscess), hemorrhoidectomy, cancer, and lymphogranuloma inguinale. The treatment is observation and surgery.

90. **(A)-T, (B)-T, (C)-T, (D)-T, (E)-F.** Vesicovaginal fistulas are the most common type of urinary fistulas and usually result from surgical procedures. Vesicovaginal fistulas from radical hysterectomy are relatively rare.

91. **(A)-T, (B)-T, (C)-T, (D)-T, (E)-T.** Women with the complaint of pruritus vulvae are most likely to be patients who have monilial vaginitis. Others are during pregnancy, diabetics, or those who have received broad-spectrum antibiotics (tetracyclines) or are on oral contraceptives.

92. **(A)-T, (B)-T, (C)-T, (D)-T, (E)-F.** Methotrexate is a toxic drug that is used for choriocarcinoma. Minor problems such as dermatitis, alopecia, and simple nausea and vomiting are common. Severe possibilities include bone marrow suppression, renal or hepatic complications, stomatitis, and GI ulcerations.

93. **(A)-T, (B)-T, (C)-T, (D)-T, (E)-T.** Urethrovaginal fistulas are less likely from obstetric injury than postoperation or postirradiation. Lymphogranuloma venereum or inguinale may cause urethrovaginal fistulas. It is also seen in the excision of a suburethral diverticulum.

94. **(A)-T, (B)-T, (C)-T, (D)-T, (E)-F.** Prolonged use of oral contraceptives is associated with an increased risk of breast cancer, cervical dysplasia and cancer, and hepatocellular adenoma. The risk of developing endometrial and ovarian cancers is reduced.

95. **(A)-T, (B)-T, (C)-T, (D)-T, (E)-F.** *Chlamydia trachomatis* is implicated for mucopurulent cervicitis, salpingitis, urethritis, bartholinitis, endocervicitis, perihepatitis, conjunctivitis, epididymitis, proctitis, and PIDs. Erythromycin and tetracyclines are recommended for treatment.

96. **(A)-T, (B)-T, (C)-T, (D)-T, (E)-T.** Spontaneus abortion occurs in 15% of all pregnancies. The most common cause of spontaneous abortion is a chromosomal abnormality of the fetus. However, genetic, anatomic, infectious, autoimmune, and endocrine factors may be associated.

97. **(A)-F, (B)-T, (C)-F, (D)-F, (E)-F.** Any positive family history increases the risk of breast cancer. If the postmenopausal mother or sisters had breast cancer, the risk is not increased significantly; if the premenopausal mother or sisters had bilateral breast cancers there is a 40 to 50% increase of breast cancer risk.

98. **(A)-T, (B)-T, (C)-T, (D)-T, (E)-T.** Infertility may be caused by abnormalities of the cervix (15% of infertile women, including polyps and endocervicitis), tubal occlusions (30% of infertile women, including gonorrheal salpingitis, PID, and adenomyosis), endocrine dysfunction (anovulatory cycle, hypothyroidism, hyperthyroidism, adrenogenital syndrome), submucous myomas of the uterus, and emotional conflicts. Before psychogenic characteristics can be diagnosed, the possibility of organic causes first should be ruled out and the specific emotional or psychogenic characteristics identified for therapeutic purposes. The psychogenically infertile woman consciously verbalizes a wish for a child but unconsciously rejects pregnancy because of her deep conflict in femininity. She may be "tired" or "ill" whenever intercourse is to be conducted during the fertile period.

99. **(A)-F, (B)-F, (C)-T, (D)-T, (E)-T.** A family-oriented (couple-oriented) approach is important in the management of infertility. Both male and female partners should be involved in the infertility study. Many times, infertility is solely due to male factors; in 50 to 60% of the infertile couples, the male factor is the important causal factor. When only the woman (instead of the couple) visits your office complaining of infertility, you should always insist on the evaluation of the male partner, unless he refuses. Conception frequently occurs during the infertility work-ups and many "infertile" women may even become pregnant just after the initial consultation visit. The primary-care practitioner is often the most useful therapeutic agent to facilitate conception through the process of a positive transference reaction from the patient and the family. The patient should be educated that your diagnostic and therapeutic approaches are scientifically and logically based and are empathetically and humanely delivered. The success is due to your devoted effort and the cooperative effort of the patient and family.

100. **(A)-F, (B)-T, (C)-F, (D)-T, (E)-F.** The uterus may be viewed by many women as the badge of femininity, and hysterectomy may be viewed as associated with loss of femininity; loss of reproductive function (even though the woman may have already completed her reproductive cycle) may be viewed by many women as inadequacy and may generate a sense of uselessness. Women near menopause may experience insecurities (empty-nest syndrome), and hysterectomy may add to the psychologic stress. Hysterectomy for adenomyosis is usually an elective procedure. The patient should be counseled in detail about the hysterectomy (indications, benefits, and consequences), and she should be allowed to take time in working through her anxiety and concern before reaching the decision for hysterectomy to minimize emotional stresses postoperatively.

101. **(A)-F, (B)-F, (C)-F, (D)-T, (E)-T.** Clinical presentations of PIDs include lower abdominal pain, leukorrhea, vaginal spotting, fever, anorexia, dysuria, tender cervix, leukocytosis, and elevated sedimentation rate. Gonococcus and chlamydia are the most common microorganisms.

102. **(A)-T, (B)-F, (C)-T, (D)-T, (E)-T.** The major complication of PID is infertility. Chronic salpingitis may develop with chronic lower abdominal pain, fever, and irregular uterine bleeding. Fitz-Hugh–Curtis syndrome is a perihepatitis resulting from gonococcal septicemia.

103. **(A)-F, (B)-F, (C)-F, (D)-T, (E)-T.** Vulvovaginitis in children is managed by sitz baths, loose-fitting clothes, and avoidance of bubble baths and harsh soaps to improve perineal hygiene. Pinworms, moniliasis, foreign bodies, and gonorrhea need to be ruled out. Topical estrogen creams can be used for refractory cases.

104. **(A)-F, (B)-F, (C)-F, (D)-T, (E)-T.** Monilial vaginitis is commonly treated with topical nystatin or clotrimazole. Diabetic patients need tight glucose control; oral antibiotics, steroids, and oral contraceptives are to be avoided.

105. **(A)-F, (B)-F, (C)-F, (D)-T, (E)-F.** Most cases of PID are caused by *Chlamydia trachomatis* and *Neisseria gonorrhoeae*. The remaining ones are often caused by *Escherichia coli*, group B streptococci, and anaerobes. Empirical ambulatory treatments include cefoxitin (Mefoxin) IM and oral probenecid, followed by doxycycline (Vibramycin) PO for 10 to 14 days. However, culture of the causative organisms is often needed to select the best antibiotics.

106. **(A)-T, (B)-F, (C)-F, (D)-F, (E)-F.** KOH preparation is used to detect monilial vaginitis, which is characteristically cheese-like in appearance. *C. trachomatis* vaginitis is treated by erythromycin or tetracyclines. Clue cells are seen in bacterial vaginosis, which is treated by oral or topical metronidazole.

107. **(A)-T, (B)-T, (C)-T, (D)-T, (E)-T.** Supernumerary nipples and accessory breasts are reported to occur in 1 to 2% of the population. The condition occurs equally in males and females. It may cause cosmetic discomforts and diseases, which may need attention. Its association with urogenital anomalies is not entirely clear.

108. **(A)-T, (B)-F, (C)-T, (D)-T, (E)-T.** Metronidazole is effective against *Trichomonas vaginalis*, histolytica, and *Bacteroides fragilis*. It is also used for *Giardia lamblia* infections abroad. The most common side reaction is GI upset, including nausea, headache, anorexia, vomiting, abdominal cramps, diarrhea, epigastralgia, constipation, and metallic taste. Leukopenia, cystitis, urticaria, dizziness, peripheral neuropathy, and convulsions may also develop.

109. **(A)-T, (B)-T, (C)-T, (D)-T, (E)-F.** Risk factors for osteoporosis are (1) sex: F/M; (2) race: white/black; (3) age: bone mass decreases with increasing age; (4) menopause: rapid loss of bone following menopause; (5) body weight: bone mass is positively correlated with body weight; (6) activity (work or exercise): increased bone mass with lifelong physical activity; (7) diet: high sodium, protein, and phosphate diets implicated in osteoporosis; (8) cigarette smoking; and (9) alcohol. Estrogen replacement therapy is useful for preventing osteoporosis.

110. **(F)**

111. **(F)**

112. **(F)**

113. **(F)**

114. **(F)**

115. **(T)**

116. **(T)**

117. **(F)**

118. **(F)**

119. **(T)**

120. **(F)**

121. **(T)**

There are about a half-million cases of PIDs a year in the United States. Diagnosis is primarily on the clinical findings, which include: abdominal tenderness, adnexal tenderness, and cervical motion tenderness; fever (greater than 38°C); pelvic mass; positive gonococcal culture; leukocytosis and pus on culdocentesis. Laparoscopic diagnosis is performed for differential diagnosis of ectopic pregnancy, appendicitis or ruptured abscess. The most common etiologic agents are gonococci (treated initially by penicillin G or ampicillin) and *C. trachomatis* (treated initially by tetracyclines). Rarely, it may be caused by tuberculosis (mostly in postmenopausal women). Appropriate measures include the identification and treatment of sexual contacts, antibiotic therapy, continuity of care, and emotional supports. Health education of the sexually active woman is urgently needed for preventive efforts.

CHAPTER 4

Obstetrics
Questions

DIRECTIONS (Questions 1 through 61): Each of the numbered items or incomplete statements in this section is followed by answers or by completions of the statement. Select the ONE lettered answer or completion that is BEST in each case.

1. A 35-year-old primigravida presents at term with a history of regular uterine contractions of increasing frequency for the past 5 hours. The interval between contractions is now 5 minutes. The abdominal examination reveals the following: The first maneuver reveals a hard, round, readily ballottable object occupying the fundus. The second maneuver identifies the back on the left side of the abdomen and the small parts on the right. The third maneuver identifies an irregular, freely movable structure above the superior strait; the fourth maneuver confirms absence of engagement of the presenting part. The fetal presentation is likely to be

   (A) left occipitotransverse
   (B) breech
   (C) twin
   (D) occipitoposterior
   (E) right occipitotransverse   *(Ref. 19)*

2. Lower leg edema during the last trimester of pregnancy is largely due to

   (A) complete venous obstruction
   (B) lymphatic stenosis
   (C) intra-abdominal tumor
   (D) increased venous pressure due to partial obstruction
   (E) arterial obstruction in the pelvis   *(Ref. 14)*

3. The most common cause of postpartum hemorrhage is

   (A) multiple gestation
   (B) uterine atony
   (C) macrosomia
   (D) multiparity
   (E) hemophilia   *(Ref. 19)*

4. At the end of 28 weeks of gestation (seven lunar months), the fetus weighs (in grams)

   (A) 15
   (B) 600
   (C) 1000
   (D) 1800
   (E) 2500   *(Ref. 19)*

5. The approximate frequency of occurrence of twins is

   (A) 1:10
   (B) 1:20
   (C) 1:40
   (D) 1:80
   (E) 1:160   *(Ref. 19)*

6. Initial prenatal care during the first trimester for a new patient includes

   (A) chest x-rays
   (B) abdominal x-rays
   (C) intravenous pyelogram (IVP)
   (D) Rh-factor determination
   (E) all of the above   *(Ref. 3)*

7. Implantation of the fertilized ovum usually occurs

   (A) within 24 hours after ovulation
   (B) 2 to 3 days following ovulation
   (C) 6 to 7 days following ovulation
   (D) 10 to 12 days following ovulation
   (E) exactly 14 days following ovulation

   (Ref. 19)

8. Alpha-fetoprotein (AFP) screening is best to be conducted at the gestational age of

   (A) prior to 10th week
   (B) 16th to 18th week
   (C) 21st to 25th week
   (D) 26th to 28th week
   (E) after 30th week   *(Ref. 3)*

9. Missed abortion means

   (A) the fetus was delivered prematurely
   (B) a dead fetus remained in the uterus for a period of time
   (C) inevitable abortion
   (D) the patient has recovered from the abortion
   (E) habitual abortion   *(Ref. 19)*

10. The best evidence of progress in labor is gained by assessing

    (A) descent
    (B) dilatation
    (C) descent and dilatation
    (D) the degree of pain
    (E) the rapidity of the fetal heartbeat

    (Ref. 19)

11. The most common fetal presentation and position at term is

    (A) right occipitotransverse (ROT)
    (B) left occipitotransverse (LOT)
    (C) right occipitoanterior (ROA)
    (D) left occipitoanterior (LOA)
    (E) left occipitoposterior (LOP)   *(Ref. 19)*

12. Identical twins are usually

    (A) of the same sex
    (B) of the same body weight
    (C) of the same height
    (D) the result of several intercourses just before conception
    (E) of two chorions and two amnions

    (Ref. 19)

13. One minute after birth, a pink infant is found to have a pulse of 98 with slow, irregular respirations; he sneezes when a catheter is placed in his nostril and demonstrates weak flexion of the extremities, which are blue in color. His 1-minute Apgar score is

    (A) 2
    (B) 3
    (C) 4
    (D) 6
    (E) 10   *(Ref. 19)*

14. The umbilical cord in the neonate normally contains

    (A) two veins and one artery
    (B) two arteries and one vein
    (C) one vein and one artery
    (D) two arteries and two veins
    (E) none of the above   *(Ref. 19)*

15. The largest diameter of the fetal head is the

    (A) occipitomental (OM)
    (B) occipitofrontal (OF)
    (C) biparietal (BP)
    (D) bitemporal (BT)
    (E) suboccipitobregmatic (SOB)   *(Ref. 19)*

16. All patients who develop acute infection of the kidneys during pregnancy should

    (A) have postpartum urinalysis
    (B) be treated with antibiotics for 6 months without urinalysis
    (C) not become pregnant again for a year

(D) have surgery done in 6 months

(E) have pyelograms done the day following delivery   (*Ref. 19*)

17. A pregnant woman at term with a 4-cm dilated cervix is found to have marginal placenta previa with mild bleeding. The appropriate management is

(A) cesarean section

(B) rupture of the membrane

(C) internal podalic version

(D) use of an inflatable intrauterine rubber bag

(E) use of Willett's scalp traction forceps
(*Ref. 19*)

18. Anticipatory measures should be instituted for which of the following pregnant women who are at increased risk for postpartum hemorrhage?

(A) pregnant women who are on non-steroidal anti-inflammatory drugs

(B) pregnant women with von Willebrand's disease

(C) pregnant women who developed pregnancy-induced hypertension

(D) pregnant women with previous cesarean section who plan to deliver vaginally

(E) all of the above   (*Ref. 19*)

19. A 43-year-old female (G6 P5) in her 32nd week of gestation experienced the sudden onset of severe pelvic pains and dark, partly clotted blood (about half a bowl) discharging from her vagina. In the emergency room, a tube of blood without anticoagulant failed to clot, the abdomen was boardlike, and the fetal heart tones were absent. The most likely diagnosis is

(A) placenta previa

(B) choriocarcinoma destruens

(C) normal pregnancy

(D) abruptio placentae

(E) rupture of placental vessels   (*Ref. 19*)

20. A 32-year-old female, gravida 3, para 2, presents in the emergency room with gushing, bright red vaginal bleeding without abdominal pain in her ninth month of gestation. The blood clots well, and her blood pressure is 120/80 mm Hg. The most probable diagnosis is

(A) hydatidiform mole

(B) abruptio placentae

(C) marginal sinus bleeding

(D) placenta previa

(E) induced abortion   (*Ref. 19*)

21. A multiparous pregnant woman is expected to deliver a full-term baby vaginally. At the 36th week of gestation during a normal prenatal vaginal examination, you find a complete placenta previa. You will deliver the baby by

(A) rupture of the membrane

(B) induction of labor

(C) forceps delivery

(D) the normal vaginal route

(E) cesarean section   (*Ref. 19*)

22. The most common cardiovascular change in a normal pregnancy is

(A) a 30-mm increase in the systolic blood pressure

(B) a fall in the diastolic blood pressure of 10 mm Hg

(C) a decrease of 20 beats per minute in the heart rate

(D) a decrease of 1.5 L/min of the cardiac output

(E) development of a diastolic rumbling murmur at the apex   (*Ref. 19*)

23. A 24-year-old healthy female is 12 weeks pregnant. You would order

(A) electroencephalogram (EEG)

(B) ultrasound of uterus

(C) hematocrit

(D) computed tomography (CT) scan of head

(E) hysterography   (*Ref. 19*)

24. Hydatidiform mole is most common in

    (A) the United States
    (B) the United Kingdom
    (C) Scandinavia
    (D) Eastern Europe
    (E) the Orient   (Ref. 19)

25. Average duration of labor in primigravidas is

    (A) 30 minutes
    (B) 50 minutes
    (C) 5 hours
    (D) 10 hours
    (E) 15 hours   (Ref. 19)

26. The expected amount of amniotic fluid at term (in mL) is between

    (A) 1500 and 1800
    (B) 2000 and 2500
    (C) 200 and 500
    (D) 20 and 50
    (E) 800 and 1100   (Ref. 19)

27. In Down syndrome, the maternal

    (A) AFP is increased
    (B) human chorionic gonadotropin (hCG) is increased
    (C) hCG is decreased
    (D) unconjugated estriol is increased
    (E) aminocaproic acid is decreased   (Ref. 2)

28. Thyroid changes in pregnancy include

    (A) a decrease of thyroxine-binding globulin (TBG)
    (B) a decrease in protein-bound iodine (PBI)
    (C) palpable thyroid gland
    (D) a fall in basal metabolic rate (BMR)
    (E) lowered iodine uptake   (Ref. 19)

29. A 23-year-old unmarried, pregnant college girl (G1 P0) in her 18th week of gestation presents with a 3-day history of right calf aches. The physical examination reveals right calf swelling and tenderness. The use of Doppler has confirmed the diagnosis of a deep-vein thrombophlebitis. The treatment of choice is

    (A) dextran
    (B) heparin
    (C) coumadin
    (D) indocin
    (E) high-dose salicylates   (Ref. 19)

30. A 20-year-old known diabetic is found to be pregnant. This is her first pregnancy, and she is currently at her eighth week of gestation. She is greatly overweight and on one dose of 35 units neutral protamine Hagedorn (NPH) and a weight-reduction, 1000-calorie diet. Records of the urine testings reveal persistent negative glucose, but off and on positive readings for ketones, especially during the early morning. The best course of action is to

    (A) split the NPH dose
    (B) increase the NPH dose to 54 units
    (C) start a 600-calorie diet
    (D) start an 1800-calorie diet
    (E) administer oral hypoglycemics   (Ref. 19)

31. A 24-year-old pregnant woman with Graves' disease is best treated with

    (A) radioactive iodine
    (B) subtotal thyroidectomy
    (C) low-dose propylthiouracil (PTU)
    (D) high-dose PTU
    (E) Inderal (propranolol)   (Ref. 19)

32. A 25-year-old woman who delivered a normal full-term infant 5 days ago has fever, pleuritic pain, pelvic tenderness, and arterial hypoxemia. Management of this patient should consist of

    (A) immediate ligation of the inferior vena cava
    (B) administration of aspirin
    (C) administration of heparin
    (D) intermittent positive pressure breathing (IPPB)
    (E) antibiotics   (Ref. 19)

33. During her fourth month of pregnancy, a patient comes for follow-up prenatal care. You find that the uterus is enlarged to the level of the umbilicus. You may suspect that the patient has

    (A) twins
    (B) myoma uteri
    (C) ectopic pregnancy
    (D) hydramnios
    (E) hydatidiform mole   (Ref. 19)

34. The most frequent cause of amenorrhea in young female adults is

    (A) primary ovarian failure
    (B) hypothyroidism
    (C) pituitary failure
    (D) psychoneurosis
    (E) pregnancy   (Ref. 19)

35. The period during pregnancy when large dosages of abdominal irradiation are most likely to cause serious abnormality in the newborn is

    (A) the first 3 months
    (B) months 3 through 6
    (C) months 6 through 9
    (D) before conception
    (E) no hazardous effect during pregnancy   (Ref. 14)

36. During "flu" season, a 25-year-old pregnant woman develops fever and sore throat and then suddenly develops acute dyspnea and nonproductive cough. She is found to be extremely hypoxic. She most likely has

    (A) pneumococcal pneumonia
    (B) staphylococcal pneumonia
    (C) influenza viral pneumonia
    (D) *Pseudomonas* pneumonia
    (E) streptococcal pharyngitis   (Ref. 14)

37. Which of the following conditions enters into the differential diagnosis of pregnancy?

    (A) hematometra
    (B) myoma
    (C) ovarian cysts
    (D) pseudocyesis
    (E) all of the above   (Ref. 14)

38. The average duration of labor in multigravidas is

    (A) 13 hours
    (B) 50 minutes
    (C) 20 minutes
    (D) 8 hours
    (E) 2 hours   (Ref. 14)

39. During a routine prenatal care visit of a 6-month pregnant woman, asymptomatic bacteriuria is found. The best approach is

    (A) reassurance
    (B) IVP
    (C) antibiotics
    (D) low-sodium diet
    (E) exercise   (Ref. 15)

40. The leading cause of maternal mortality is

    (A) puerperal complications
    (B) toxemia
    (C) ectopic pregnancy
    (D) hemorrhage
    (E) abortion   (Ref. 14)

41. You are the urgent-care doctor at the family health center. An adolescent female walks in at 4:59 P.M., requesting a pregnancy test. You would

    (A) order a urine pregnancy test
    (B) order a serum beta hCG
    (C) perform a pelvic exam
    (D) perform a complete history and physical
    (E) request a parental consent   (Ref. 3)

42. Which of the following educational approaches is most likely to reduce teenagers' pregnancy behaviors?

    (A) magazine articles
    (B) television stories
    (C) newspaper advertisements
    (D) church lectures
    (E) peer counseling   (Ref. 3)

43. Pregnant women with chemical diabetes are best treated by

    (A) cesarean section at 32nd week
    (B) induction of labor at 33rd week
    (C) strict glucose control of plasma glucose below 105 mg/dL
    (D) short-acting oral hypoglycemics
    (E) increased insulin dosage according to glycosuria   (Ref. 19)

44. Giant babies are most likely to be delivered by a

    (A) diabetic mother
    (B) hypertensive mother
    (C) mother with twin pregnancy
    (D) mother with breech pregnancy
    (E) cigarette-smoking mother   (Ref. 19)

45. Hydramnios is most likely to be associated with

    (A) essential hypertension
    (B) gestational hypertension
    (C) diabetes mellitus
    (D) urinary tract infection
    (E) diabetes insipidus   (Ref. 19)

46. The treatment choice of an ectopic pregnancy is

    (A) IV oxytocin
    (B) observation only
    (C) immediate laparotomy
    (D) systemic corticosteroids
    (E) IV cephalosporins   (Ref. 11)

47. Which of the following laboratory tests is most useful in the work-up of an ectopic pregnancy?

    (A) white blood count (WBC) and differentials
    (B) hemoglobin and hematocrit
    (C) urine hCG determination
    (D) hCG serum beta-subunit determination
    (E) serum prolactin level   (Ref. 11)

48. Which of the following conditions is associated with an ectopic pregnancy?

    (A) cervical polyps
    (B) endosalpingitis
    (C) polycystic ovaries
    (D) previous premature labor
    (E) vasectomy in the male partner   (Ref. 11)

49. Sheehan syndrome may produce

    (A) amenorrhea with hypertension
    (B) amenorrhea and acromegaly
    (C) amenorrhea with visual disturbance
    (D) amenorrhea with hypometabolism
    (E) amenorrhea and galactorrhea   (Ref. 19)

50. Factors that may play a role in breech presentations are

    (A) prematurity
    (B) placenta previa
    (C) fetal malformation
    (D) abnormalities of the uterus
    (E) all of the above   (Ref. 19)

51. Acceptable indications for cesarean section in breech presentation include

    (A) cephalopelvic disproportion
    (B) fetal distress
    (C) elderly primigravidas
    (D) early delivery of a mother with diabetes
    (E) all of the above   (Ref. 19)

52. Which of the following individuals are most likely to develop an ectopic pregnancy?

    (A) users of an intrauterine device (IUD)
    (B) users of oral contraceptives
    (C) users of condoms
    (D) homosexuals
    (E) users of contraceptive diaphragms   (Ref. 19)

53. Among the following, the most useful procedure for the management of the postdates pregnancy is

    (A) nonstress test
    (B) pelvic ultrasonography

(C) amniocentesis

(D) cervical mucus test

(E) ABO and Rh typing   *(Ref. 19)*

54. Which of the following is recommended for the pregnant woman?

    (A) chlordiazepoxide (Librium)

    (B) alcohol

    (C) cigarettes

    (D) folic acid

    (E) marijuana   *(Ref. 85)*

55. The recommended daily caloric allowance added to pregnancy is

    (A) 100 calories

    (B) 300 calories

    (C) 500 calories

    (D) 700 calories

    (E) 1000 calories   *(Ref. 19)*

56. Pregnancy-induced hypertension is most likely to develop in patients with

    (A) hyperuricemia

    (B) primigravida

    (C) diabetes insipidus

    (D) depression

    (E) common cold   *(Ref. 19)*

57. Urban teenage pregnancy is most likely to be associated with

    (A) Down syndrome in the baby

    (B) diabetes mellitus in the baby

    (C) low birth weight in the baby

    (D) postdated baby

    (E) giant baby   *(Ref. 5)*

58. Urban teenage childbearers are more likely to

    (A) enroll in professional education

    (B) interrupt education

    (C) pursue graduate education

    (D) engage in a high-income profession

    (E) have fewer children   *(Ref. 5)*

59. When you suspect a postdates pregnancy, you will

    (A) schedule a cesarean section

    (B) induce labor

    (C) take a detailed menstrual history

    (D) order a contraction stress test

    (E) institute continuous fetal monitoring at an obstetric ward   *(Ref. 19)*

60. At the 40th week of gestation, you will

    (A) offer counseling and support

    (B) order a contraction stress test

    (C) order a nonstress test

    (D) induce labor

    (E) order a pelvic ultrasonography   *(Ref. 19)*

61. Postterm pregnancy is frequently associated with

    (A) low-birth-weight infants

    (B) polyhydramnios

    (C) infants with high intelligence

    (D) rapid growth during the first year of life

    (E) meconium aspiration syndrome   *(Ref. 19)*

DIRECTIONS (Questions 62 through 83): Each question consists of an introduction followed by some statements. Mark T (true) or F (false) after each statement.

62. Predisposing causes for puerperal infection include

    (A) prolonged labor

    (B) excessive blood loss

    (C) excessive number of vaginal examinations during labor

    (D) premature rupture of membrane

    (E) retained placenta   *(Ref. 19)*

63. Urinary estriols are often low in

    (A) diabetic pregnancies

    (B) placental insufficiency

    (C) anencephaly

    (D) early fetal death

    (E) hydatidiform mole   *(Ref. 19)*

64. Complications of twinning include

    (A) maternal anemia
    (B) placenta previa
    (C) shortness of breath
    (D) low fetal birth weight
    (E) twin-to-twin transfusion syndrome

    (Ref. 19)

65. Patients at high risk of developing gestational diabetes mellitus include

    (A) previous macrosomia (greater than 9 lb)
    (B) obesity
    (C) previous unexplained miscarriage
    (D) polyhydramnios
    (E) Asians   *(Ref. 19)*

66. Presumptive signs of pregnancy include

    (A) breast tingling
    (B) lassitude and somnolence
    (C) amenorrhea
    (D) nausea and vomiting
    (E) vaginal discharges   *(Ref. 19)*

67. Methotrexate is used for

    (A) termination of pregnancy
    (B) ectopic pregnancy
    (C) pregnancy-induced hypertension
    (D) diabetes in pregnancy
    (E) gestational trophoblastic disease *(Ref. 11)*

68. In regard to macrocytic anemia of pregnancy, which of the following is accurate?

    (A) It occurs most commonly in the third trimester of pregnancy.
    (B) It responds to folic acid.
    (C) The anemia disappears spontaneously on interruption or termination of the pregnancy.
    (D) Splenomegaly presents in about one third of cases.
    (E) It is always due to iron deficiency.

    (Ref. 19)

69. Which of the following changes occurs in the urinary system during normal pregnancy?

    (A) decrease in renal blood flow
    (B) decrease in glomerular filtration
    (C) glycosuria
    (D) dilatation of the urethra
    (E) urinary frequency   *(Ref. 19)*

70. Common causes of shoulder presentations include

    (A) placenta previa
    (B) twins
    (C) hydramnios
    (D) contracted pelvis
    (E) abnormal shape of uterus   *(Ref. 19)*

71. Which of the following clinical presentations are characteristic in the inevitable abortion?

    (A) vaginal bleeding
    (B) passage of conception products
    (C) closed cervix
    (D) hematemesis
    (E) leaking amniotic fluids   *(Ref. 19)*

72. The clinical characteristics of hyperemesis gravidarum include

    (A) weight gain
    (B) dry mouth
    (C) vomiting
    (D) tachycardia
    (E) hypotension   *(Ref. 19)*

73. Complications of induced abortions include

    (A) vaginal bleeding
    (B) uterine perforation
    (C) retained conception products
    (D) infection
    (E) retained blood clots   *(Ref. 19)*

74. Elevated AFP may be associated with

    (A) colon cancers
    (B) neural tube defects

(C) ovarian cancers

(D) cervical cancers

(E) pleurisy   *(Ref. 19)*

75. A 24-year-old female patient with stable asthma becomes pregnant. You would

    (A) advise the patient to engage in vigorous exercises

    (B) allow her to continue cigarette smoking

    (C) prescribe dextromethorphan cough preparation when she has cold symptoms

    (D) continue methylxanthine therapy

    (E) reassure the patient that her asthma will improve by pregnancy   *(Ref. 19)*

76. A 27-year-old hypertensive patient becomes pregnant. You would start with

    (A) nifedipine

    (B) captopril

    (C) guanethidine

    (D) methyldopa

    (E) hydralazine   *(Ref. 19)*

77. The PUPPP syndrome

    (A) produces fetal anomaly

    (B) elevates hCG level

    (C) usually occurs during the third trimester

    (D) produces all violet-colored eruptions

    (E) produces eruptions that appear mostly on the face   *(Ref. 19)*

78. The method of therapeutic abortion at 25 weeks of gestation is

    (A) menstrual extraction

    (B) dilatation and curettage (D&C) of the endometrial cavity

    (C) suction curettage of the endometrial cavity

    (D) injection of a 50% hypertonic glucose solution into the amniotic cavity

    (E) 20% sodium chloride intravaginally every 4 hours   *(Ref. 19)*

79. Older pregnant women are at higher risk to develop

    (A) genital herpes

    (B) twin pregnancy

    (C) breech presentation

    (D) placenta previa

    (E) abruptio placentae   *(Ref. 19)*

80. The fetal death syndrome is frequently associated with

    (A) syphilis

    (B) gonorrhea

    (C) chromosome abnormalities

    (D) cervical cancer in situ

    (E) myoma uteri   *(Ref. 19)*

81. Clinical manifestations of the fetal death syndrome include

    (A) excessive uterine growth compared to gestational age

    (B) regression of the pregnancy signs and symptoms

    (C) quickening

    (D) fetal heart tone cannot be auscultated by the stethoscope

    (E) maternal weight gain ceases   *(Ref. 19)*

82. RhoGAM is indicated for

    (A) a baby whose Rh type is negative

    (B) a mother whose antibody screen for anti-Rho(D) is positive

    (C) an Rh-negative mother with first-born Rh-negative son

    (D) a mother whose Rh type is positive

    (E) an Rh-negative mother with immunization to Rh-C   *(Ref. 19)*

83. Leiomyomas in pregnancy

    (A) occur in 50% of pregnancies

    (B) decrease in size during pregnancy

    (C) may cause pain by degeneration

    (D) always require cesarean sections

    (E) may cause postpartum hemorrhage

                                   (Ref. 19)

DIRECTIONS (Questions 84 through 92): The following clinical set problem consists of clinical information presented in the format of questions or incomplete statements followed by a group of numbered options.

Indicate T if the option is true;
Indicate F if the option is false.

A 23-year-old unmarried hypertensive patient (G1 P0) with 12-week gestation visited your office for the first time, requesting prenatal care. She has had essential hypertension for 2 years, controlled by thiazide diuretics and methyldopa (Aldomet). Physical examinations were essentially unremarkable. She indicates that she is interested in natural childbirth in the birthing room. You would now

84. arrange for a therapeutic abortion to reduce the risk of carrying through a pregnancy with hypertension

85. tell her that you object strongly to natural childbirth and ask her to seek care elsewhere

86. explain to her that there may be a time when natural childbirth is not in her best interest

87. discontinue thiazide diuretics and methyldopa during her pregnancy

88. refuse to see her because you do not like unmarried pregnant women

The possible complications of essential hypertension during pregnancy include

89. preeclampsia

90. cerebral hemorrhage

91. macrosomia

92. erythroblastosis fetalis   (Ref. 19)

Answers and Explanations

1. **(B)** Leopold's maneuvers will usually show the following in breech presentation: longitudinal lie, firm lower pole, limbs to one side, and hard head at fundus. Fetal heart is best heard above the umbilicus. Breech presentation is usually confirmed by pelvic examination.

2. **(D)** Venous pressure in the upper extremities remains fairly constant throughout pregnancy; in the lower extremities it rises progressively, beginning about the 12th week, and at term the pressure may reach a level as high as 10 to 20 cm of water above normal. The rise is due primarily to pressure of the gravid uterus on the adjacent pelvic veins, a factor that contributes to the development of ankle edema, varicose veins, and hemorrhoids.

3. **(B)** Postpartum hemorrhage is still a leading cause of maternal death. Approximately 8% of pregnancies are complicated by postpartum hemorrhage, with an estimated blood loss of more than 500 mL in the first 24 hours after delivery. All the options listed may cause postpartum hemorrhage, but the most common cause is uterine atony.

4. **(C)**

At End of Lunar Month	Fetal Weight (g)
3	14
6	600
7	1000
8	1800
9	2500
10	3400

5. **(D)** The frequency of the birth of twins is 1 of 100 white births, 1 of 80 black births, and 1 of 155 births in Japan. It varies widely in race.

6. **(D)** During the first visit for prenatal care, the laboratory tests include hematocrit, syphilis serology, rubella immunity, hepatitis B surface antigen, analysis, Pap smears, and blood typing and Rh-factor determination.

7. **(C)** Fertilization occurs probably within 24 hours after ovulation, and implantation occurs at the blastocyst stage 6 or 7 days after ovulation.

8. **(B)** The measurement of AFP is for the screening of neural tube defects. The maternal serum AFP is measured at the gestational age of 10 to 18 weeks.

9. **(B)** Missed abortion is the failure of the uterus to expel its contents within 8 weeks after the death of the embryo or fetus. The dead fetus may be retained for months or years. Disseminated intravascular coagulation, with resultant incoagulability of the blood, may occur after lengthy retention of a dead fetus in the uterus, particularly after the fourth month of gestation. Therapeutic abortion is often needed.

10. **(C)** The progress of labor is the result of the tendency for each uterine contraction to push the fetus downward through the pelvis and of the resistance of the soft tissue and the bony pelvis to its descent. This progress is best appreciated by assessing cervical dilata-

tion, descent, and position and recording on a labor graph to detect obvious deviations from the normal course. The degree of descent is gauged by the station of the presenting part, which is its relationship to the plane of the ischial spines. If the presenting part is at the level of the spines, it is at station 0; if it is 1 cm above the spines, it is at station −1. If the lowest level of the presenting part is above station −3, it is said to be floating. If the presenting part is 1 cm below the plane of the spines, it is at station +1. When the presenting part reaches station +3, it usually is resting on the pelvic floor. A sigmoid curve can be plotted for the relationship of passage of time of labor to the cervical dilatation. The curve shows latent and active phase (starting from 2 and 4 cm dilatation); deceleration sets in toward the end of the first stage (full dilatation of the cervix—10 cm).

11. **(B)** The most common presentation and position is LOT; 95% of presentations are by head, and 40% of these are LOT. Therefore, 38% of all births are LOT to start. The presenting part is the vertex, the area bounded by the bregma, the parietal eminences, and the posterior fontanelle. The denominator is the occiput.

12. **(A)** Twinning may result from the simultaneous fertilization of two ova (fraternal or dizygotic twins) or from the abnormal development of a single ovum (identical or monozygotic twins). Identical twins are always of the same sex; fraternal twins may be of the same or of different sexes. Identical twins usually have two amnions, one chorion, and one placenta. Fraternal twins have two amnions, two chorions, and two placentas. A twin infant is about 700 g lighter than a singleton infant at birth. Congenital malformations, prematurity, and stillbirths are more common in twins. Twinning is associated with toxemia, hydramnios, abnormal presentation, maternal anemia, and maternal circulatory and respiratory disturbances.

13. **(D)**

Sign	Apgar Score		
	0	1	2
Heart rate	Absent	Below 100	Over 100
Respiratory effort	Absent	Slow, irregular	Good crying
Response to catheter in nostril	None	Grimace	Cough or sneeze
Muscle tone	Limp	Some flexion of extremities	Active motion
Color	Blue, pale	Body pink, extremities blue	Completely pink

The highest possible score, 10, indicates an optimal condition; most normal infants are scored between 7 and 10. Those who are moderately depressed will usually have scores between 4 and 7 (as with the above infant); they will usually respond to stimuli and can be resuscitated without difficulty. Those with scores below 4 are severely depressed and require immediate treatment.

14. **(B)** The umbilical cord (funis) extends from the navel of the fetus to the placenta. It transmits fetal venous blood from the fetus through two arteries to the placenta, returning arterial blood by one vein from the placenta. Its diameter ranges from 1 to 2.5 cm and its length from 30 to 100 cm. The right umbilical vein usually disappears early, leaving only the original left vein. A common vascular anomaly is the absence of one umbilical artery, a condition often associated with other severe fetal anomalies, such as esophageal atresia and imperforate anus. The absence of one umbilical artery has been noted in 1% of the cords of singletons and in 5% of the cords of at least one twin.

15. **(A)** The OM is the largest diameter (13.5 cm), extending from the most prominent portion of the occiput to the chin. This is the anteroposterior diameter presented to the maternal pelvis with brow presentations. The diameter of the BT (8 cm), the smallest diameter of the fetal head, is the greatest distance between the two temporal sutures. The BP (9.25 cm) is the greatest transverse diameter

of the head from one parietal bone to the other. This is customarily the greatest transverse diameter that must traverse the maternal pelvis. The SOB (9.5 cm) extends from the middle of the large fontanel to the undersurface of the occipital bone, just where it joins the neck. This is the anteroposterior diameter presented to the maternal pelvis with occipital presentations and is the one most commonly seen. With the biparietal diameter, it forms a nearly circular plane and presents the smallest possible circumference, 29 cm. The OF (11.5 cm) extends from the most prominent portion of the occipital bone to the root of the nose, seen in sinciput presentations.

16. **(A)** The urine should be examined for the presence of infection during the early puerperium and again after involution in all women who have had acute pyelonephritis during pregnancy. If the infection has been recurrent or if bacteriuria persists, pyelograms should be made 2 or 3 months after delivery in an attempt to demonstrate a lesion that could have caused the attacks or any damage that may have been produced by the infection.

17. **(B)** When the placenta is lateral or only slightly over the os (marginal placenta previa) and the cervix has dilated enough to admit one or two fingers, rupture of the membrane may permit the head to press the placenta against the uterine wall and stop the bleeding. When the child is not viable, the Braxton Hicks version (internal podalic version), the inflatable intrauterine rubber bag, and Willett's scalp traction forceps may be used.

18. **(E)** Antepartum risk factors include previous postpartum hemorrhage, previous uterine rupture, previous uterine surgery, cesarean section, D&C, past placenta previa, placenta increta or placenta percreta, known uterine malformations, leiomyomata or adenomyosis, coagulation disorders, and multiparity. Peripartum risk factors include use of oxytocin (Pitocin, Syntocinon) for augmentation or induction of labor; overdistention by multiple fetuses or hydramnios; use of forceps or other intravaginal manipulations, such as internal podalic version; placenta previa; abruptio placentae; preeclampsia; thromboembolic disease; sepsis; fetal demise; and ruptured or inverted uterus.

19. **(D)** Abruptio placentae is the early separation of the placenta from its normal implantation site in the upper segment of the uterus before the birth of the baby. It frequently occurs in women of high parity (more than five children) and it recurs in about 10% of patients who had abruptio placentae in previous pregnancies. A clotting defect (fibrinogenopenia, intravascular coagulation) frequently develops, with complete placental separation. Some patients may develop acute tubular necrosis or bilateral renal cortical necrosis to cause anuria. The principle of treatment is to control bleeding, to replace the blood loss, and to empty the uterus.

20. **(D)** The cause of placenta previa is unknown and it occurs more frequently in multiparas, increasing with the degree of parity. The differential diagnosis of abruptio placentae and placenta previa is summarized as follows.

Placenta Previa	Abruptio Placentae
Bleeding is painless	Bleeding accompanied by pain
Bright red blood	Blood is usually dark
Shock comparable with bleeding	Profound shock
Slight bleeding at onset, usually recurs	Profuse initial bleeding
Soft, nontender, contracting uterus	Firm, tender, tetanically contracted uterus
Easily felt fetus; fetal heartbeat present	Difficult to feel fetus; fetal heartbeat irregular or absent
Placenta may be felt	Placenta cannot be felt
No evidence of toxemia	May be associated with toxemia; blood pressure low due to bleeding
Normal urine	Proteinuria or anuria
Blood clots normally	Clotting defect present

21. **(E)** In almost every instance, even though the baby is dead, the patient with complete placenta previa should be delivered by cesarean section. It is seldom necessary to delay termination if the pregnancy is of at least 36 weeks' duration. Cesarean section is the best method for terminating pregnancy with incomplete placenta previa. If the fetus is dead, the cervix is soft and patulous, and only the edge of the placenta can be felt; if bleeding is minimal, vaginal delivery is possible. Vaginal delivery usually increases the hazard for the infant because compression of the placenta by the presenting part obstructs fetal vessels, leading to severe anoxia. If a large enough area of fetal circulation is eliminated, the infant will die of anoxia.

22. **(B)** During a normal pregnancy, cardiac output increases 1.5 L/min, which, in turn, increases stroke volume and heart rate. The heart rate is raised by 10 to 15 beats per minute. There is no change in systolic blood pressure with a fall of diastolic pressure of 10 mm Hg. In 10% of women in late pregnancy, there is a profound fall in blood pressure in the supine position (supine hypotension syndrome). There is a rise of venous pressure in the lower extremity. Electrocardiogram (ECG) may show left axis deviation with systolic ejection murmurs at the left sternal border.

23. **(C)** Essential laboratory studies in the normal pregnant woman include determination of the hemoglobin or hematocrit, blood type, Rh factor, serological test for syphilis, urine tests for protein and sugar, and a screening cytologic examination of cervical secretions, gonorrhea, chlamydia, antibody screenings, rubella titer, and hepatitis B surface antibody.

24. **(E)** Hydatidiform mole is a neoplastic proliferation of the trophoblast in which the terminal villi are transformed into vesicles filled with clear, viscid material. Although it is usually benign, it has malignant potentialities and precedes the development of choriocarcinoma. It is uncommon in the United States, occurring once in 2500 pregnancies. In the Orient, it was estimated to occur once in 200 pregnancies in the Philippines and once in 100 (82 to 120) pregnancies in Taiwan.

25. **(D)** The median duration of labor in primigravidas is 11 hours, and the mode 6 to 7 hours.

26. **(E)** The amniotic fluid increases rapidly to an average volume of 50 mL at 12 weeks' gestation and 400 mL at midpregnancy; it reaches a maximum of about a liter at 36 to 38 weeks of gestation. The volume decreases to 600 mL by 43 weeks.

27. **(B)** In Down syndrome, the hCG is increased, the unconjugated estriol level is decreased, and the AFP level is decreased.

28. **(C)** During pregnancy, TBG doubles and PBI increases. The pregnant woman shows hyperplasia of the thyroid gland, increased iodine uptake, and a 20% rise in BMR.

29. **(B)** Untreated patients with deep-vein thrombophlebitis in pregnancy may be at increased risk of developing pulmonary embolism. Heparin does not cross the placenta and is the drug of choice, whether used in a continuous intravenous infusion or in every-four-hour bolus doses. Coumadin agents cross the placenta and have been associated with teratogenic effects (similar to chondrodysplasia punctata with nasal bone hypoplasia and bone stippling). Low-dose subcutaneous heparin is used primarily for prophylaxis with prior phlebitis. Dextran has little beneficial effect. Indocin has been shown to be associated with premature closure of the ductus arteriosus. Salicylate may cause fetal hemorrhage, and prolonged use of high-dose salicylate (as in patients with rheumatoid arthritis) may cause a postmaturity state.

30. **(D)** A well-balanced diet of at least 1800 calories (with needed folic acid and iron supplementation) is needed during pregnancy to achieve an acceptable weight gain of 25 to 27 lb in meeting nutritional requirements of the pregnant woman and her baby. Strict weight reduction is to be avoided during pregnancy, as it will lead to starvation ketosis, which

may be harmful to the fetus. Following the administration of an 1800-calorie diet, blood testing is indicated to assess the adequacy of the insulin dose.

31. (C) Surgical procedure may cause recurrent laryngeal nerve paralysis, parathyroid removal, and anesthetic effects on the fetus. Radioactive iodine is contraindicated during pregnancy due to the fetal radiation exposure. PTU crosses the placenta, and high-dose (or regular-dose) PTU may cause a hypothyroid infant (goitrous cretin). The patient should be controlled with low-dose PTU and the mother maintained in mild hyperthyroidism to minimize the effects of PTU on the fetus. Inderal may induce labor and may cause fetal bradycardia.

32. (C) The treatment of pulmonary embolism is anticoagulation, using heparin or coumadin. Urokinase and streptokinase may be used.

33. (E) Patients with hydatidiform mole usually complain of vaginal bleeding without significant pelvic discomfort in the fourth or fifth month of pregnancy. The uterus is usually soft and of doughy consistency. The enlargement of the uterus is often out of proportion to the calculated duration of pregnancy.

34. (E) Any patient presenting with amenorrhea is presumed to be pregnant until proved otherwise.

35. (A) Irradiation before 2 to 3 weeks of gestation or after 30 weeks of gestation is not likely to produce gross abnormalities. Irradiation between 4 and 11 weeks of gestation would lead to severe abnormalities of many organs in most or all fetuses. Thus, during the first trimester, radiographic diagnostic procedures for pregnant women should be reserved only for cases of absolute necessity.

36. (C) The incubation period is from 24 to 72 hours, and 1% of patients with influenza will develop pneumonia. Bacterial pneumonia is frequently a complication for pregnant patients. However, the definite diagnosis of influenza viral pneumonia is frequently made

by serial determination of complement-fixing and hemagglutination-inhibiting antibody titers.

37. (E) In myoma, menses are not absent, the uterine size usually does not increase steadily, and a pregnancy test is usually negative. In ovarian cysts, no presumptive or positive signs of pregnancy can be determined, and a pregnancy test is usually negative. In pseudocyesis (spurious pregnancy), subjective signs of pregnancy may develop, with abdominal size increased by fat, tympanites, or ascites, but a pregnancy test is usually negative.

38. (D) The median duration in a multipara is 6 hours, and the mode is 4 hours; the average duration is 6 to 8 hours.

39. (C) If untreated, it may increase the risk of developing pyelonephritis in later stage of pregnancy, mostly during the third trimester.

40. (A) The maternal mortality in 1987 was around 7:100,000; the five leading causes, in descending order, were puerperal complications, toxemia, ectopic pregnancy, hemorrhage, and abortion.

41. (E) To provide general health care to a minor requires parental consent. A pregnancy test is considered to be a component of general health care. However, if the pregnancy test is positive, the minor no longer needs parental consent.

42. (E) Many teenage pregnancies are unintended, and most of them are preventable through contraceptive use. Adolescents are heavily influenced by peer pressure for their social behaviors including unprotected intercourse. Thus, peer counseling is the most powerful method to reduce pregnancy behaviors.

43. (C) Most chemical diabetes can be treated by diet alone, and pregnancies can be delivered at term. In insulin-dependent diabetes, the patient needs strict fetal monitoring at 34 to 36 weeks of gestation to decide on labor induction or cesarean section. During the postpartum period, insulin requirements are reduced.

44. **(A)** The diabetic pregnancy is associated with macrosomia, respiratory distress syndrome, hypoglycemia, hyperbilirubinemia, hypocalcemia, hyaline membrane disease, and neural tube defects in infants.

45. **(C)** Diabetes mellitus in pregnancy is often associated with hydramnios, hypertension, and preeclampsia (if vascular sclerosis or renal damage exists).

46. **(C)** Laparotomy is indicated when the patient is hemodynamically unstable. Laparoscopy is used for hemodynamically stable patients. Methotrexate is used as medical therapy.

47. **(D)** Quantitative beta-hCG measurements are the diagnostic cornerstone for ectopic pregnancy. The hCG enzyme immunoassay is an accurate screening test for detection of ectopic pregnancy.

48. **(B)** The following conditions increase the likelihood of an ectopic pregnancy: endosalpingitis, tubal atresia, endometriosis, appendicitis, salpingoplasty, and tumors that press and distort the tube.

49. **(D)** Pituitary necrosis (Sheehan syndrome) consists of postpartum hemorrhage or puerperal infection, no lactation, atrophic genital organs, amenorrhea, loss of pubic and axillary hair, and hypometabolism.

50. **(E)** The breech is the presenting part in 25% of cases before 30 weeks; therefore, prematurity is an important factor. Multiple pregnancies, fetal malformation, hydrocephalus, hydramnios, lax uterus and pendulous abdomen, abnormal shape of pelvic brim or uterus (partial uterine septa), and placenta previa are all associated with breech presentations.

51. **(E)** Outcome for infants will be improved by performing cesarean section for any breech presentation in which easy, uncomplicated delivery cannot be anticipated. Frequent indications for cesarean section include pelvic contraction, a large fetus, a primigravida over 35 years of age, fetal distress (abnormal fetal heart rate), and dysfunctional labor. Cesarean section may also be used for women with medical problems (eg, diabetes).

52. **(A)** The use of contraceptives prevents pregnancy and will also prevent ectopic pregnancy; however, individuals with IUDs have an increased risk of ectopic pregnancy; and individuals receiving tubal ligations who get pregnant are at a higher risk of developing ectopic pregnancy.

53. **(A)** In the management of the postdates pregnancy, the nonstress test and/or the contraction stress test are performed to assess fetal well-being. When there is no fetal distress without obstetric complications, spontaneous labor can be expected, or labor can be induced when the cervix ripens. When the matured fetus is in distress or when the pregnancy reaches the 44th week, consider cesarean section.

54. **(D)** Although there is little evidence that marijuana is a teratogen, there is no long-term study on marijuana use during pregnancy and the child's behavioral development. It is prudent not to recommend marijuana use during pregnancy. Benzodiazepines are possibly associated with the increased risk of oral clefts, fetal dysmorphism and growth, and central nervous system aberrations. Although the association is not strong and the study results are contradictory, it is best not to recommend the use of benzodiazepines during pregnancy. Smoking may increase the risk of abortion, and alcohol use is associated with fetal alcohol syndrome. It is best not to use alcohol or cigarettes during pregnancy.

55. **(B)** Pregnant women require an additional 300 calories a day, a total of 2400 calories, to maintain fetal growth.

56. **(B)** Pregnancy-induced hypertension is associated with teenage and elderly primigravidas and multiparas who have multiple gestations, fetal hydrops, diabetes, chronic hypertension, and renal disease.

57. **(C)** Characteristics of urban teenage pregnancies include: (1) 14% of infants born to mothers below the age of 15 years are low-birth-weight infants; 11% are low-birth-weight infants if the mother's age is 16 to 18 years; low-birth-weight infants increase infant mortality 20-fold and are associated with deafness, blindness, and neurologic defects; (2) increased rate of toxemia; and (3) children of teenage pregnancies may encounter more difficulties in their lives.

58. **(B)** Teenage childbearers are more likely to have lower educational attainment, lower income, larger family size (more unplanned children), increased divorce rate, and government assistance.

59. **(C)** The most common cause of postdates pregnancy is delayed ovulation; a careful history of prior menstrual cycles will aid in determining whether or not a pregnancy is truly postdated.

60. **(A)** Although the estimated date of delivery is 40 weeks from the beginning of the last menstrual period, normal term lasts 40 ± 2 weeks (38 through 42 weeks).

61. **(E)** Postterm pregnancy is often associated with macrosomia, oligohydramnios, meconium aspiration syndrome, dysmaturity (increased mortality and behavioral disturbances during infancy), congenital anomalies (anencephaly, hydrocephalus), adrenal hypofunction, hypoglycemia, and polycythemia.

62. **(A)-T, (B)-T, (C)-T, (D)-T, (E)-T.** Puerperal infection is more common in women who are exhausted and dehydrated from prolonged labor, bleed excessively without replacement and are already anemic, have experienced traumatic deliveries, whose placental fragments are retained, who received excessive vaginal examinations and unsterile intrauterine manipulation during labor and are nulliparous, are under 20 years of age, and whose membranes ruptured prematurely.

63. **(A)-T, (B)-T, (C)-T, (D)-T, (E)-T.** The estriol level fails to rise in molar pregnancy, anencephaly, placental sulfatase deficiency, placental insufficiency, toxemia, diabetes, and prematurity. In late pregnancy, the level falls slowly or abruptly with fetal death.

64. **(A)-T, (B)-T, (C)-T, (D)-T, (E)-T.** The twin-to-twin transfusion syndrome is the most serious problem of local shunting of blood. The recipient twin is plethoric, edematous, and hypertensive, causing glomerulotubal hypertrophy and ascites. The donor twin is small, pallid, and dehydrated, causing growth retardation, malnutrition, and hypoxemia.

65. **(A)-T, (B)-T, (C)-T, (D)-T, (E)-F.** Pregnant women who have a positive family history for diabetes mellitus or who have had previous gestational diabetes mellitus and previous pregnancies that resulted in unexplained stillbirths are at high risk to develop gestational diabetes. Those pregnant women with persistent glycosuria are also at a higher risk. Pima Indians and Micronesians are at a higher risk, but not Asians.

66. **(A)-T, (B)-T, (C)-T, (D)-T, (E)-T.** Presumptive signs of pregnancy include cessation of menstruation, fatigue, nausea and vomiting, breast changes (tingling, enlargement, increased pigmentation, secondary areolae, veins, more prominent follicles of Montgomery, and striae), leukorrhea, abdominal striae, linea nigra (a line of pigmentation in the lower midline of the abdomen, ascending as pregnancy progresses), urinary frequency, and discoloration of the vagina and cervix (Chadwick's sign—color changes in the vagina and cervix from pink to bluish, increasing to a deep purplish hue). Although these presumptive signs are not conclusive, they do offer presumptive evidence of pregnancy. They are valuable evidence, but never proof.

67. **(A)-T, (B)-T, (C)-F, (D)-F, (E)-T.** Methotrexate is a folic acid analogue that inhibits dehydrofolate reductase to reduce deoxyribonucleic acid (DNA) synthesis. It is used for gestational trophoblastic disease (gestational choriocarcinoma, chorioadenoma destruens, and hydatidiform mole) and ectopic pregnancy (although linear salpingostomy remains to be the most common therapy). It is also used for the treatment of breast cancer, epidermoid cancers of the head and neck, mycosis fungoides, lung cancers, non-Hodgkin's lymphoma, psoriasis, and rheumatoid arthritis. It has also been used to terminate pregnancy in other countries. Its side reactions include alopecia, dermatitis, elevated liver enzymes, and pneumonitis.

68. **(A)-T, (B)-T, (C)-T, (D)-T, (E)-F.** The macrocytic anemia of pregnancy is due to deficiency of folic acid. The iron-deficiency state is manifested with microcytic hypochromic anemia.

69. **(A)-F, (B)-F, (C)-T, (D)-T, (E)-T.** During normal pregnancy, renal blood flow increases 25% during the first and second trimesters, and glomerular filtration increases 50% until the last 2 or 3 weeks of gestation. Ureteral dilatation is common, especially on the right side. Dilatation of the kidney pelvis favors a diagnosis of pyelonephritis. Urinary frequency is common early in pregnancy because of bladder compression by the enlarging uterus and again in late pregnancy if the fetal head enters the pelvic cavity. Urinary frequency is also due to hyperemia of the bladder mucosa associated with pelvic venous congestion. Glycosuria is common because of increased glomerular filtration.

70. **(A)-T, (B)-T, (C)-T, (D)-T, (E)-T.** Shoulder presentation is more common in multiparas than in primiparas and in premature than in mature labors. Twins, hydramnios, placenta previa, contracted pelvis, undue mobility or unusual shape of the fetus, or abnormal shape of the uterus (eg, subseptate uterus) will frequently cause shoulder presentation.

71. **(A)-T, (B)-F, (C)-F, (D)-F, (E)-T.** Inevitable abortion occurs during the first 20 weeks of pregnancy. It is characterized by vaginal bleeding and lower abdominal cramping pain. The cervix is dilated and there is leakage of amniotic fluids, but the conception products are not passed. Suction curettage is required. Rh immune globulin is administered if patient is Rh negative.

72. **(A)-F, (B)-T, (C)-T, (D)-T, (E)-T.** Hyperemesis gravidarum occurs at 2 to 4 months of pregnancy. It produces severe nausea and vomiting, and weight loss and dehydration may develop.

73. **(A)-T, (B)-T, (C)-T, (D)-T, (E)-T.** Induced abortions may cause fever, pelvic pain, vaginal discharges, vaginal bleeding, and shock. Upright abdominal x-ray may reveal free air or intraperitoneal fluid. In addition, cervical laceration may also develop.

74. **(A)-F, (B)-T, (C)-T, (D)-F, (E)-F.** Elevated AFP at 16 to 18 weeks of pregnancy may denote neural tube defects. Amniocentesis with elevated AFP and acetylcholinesterase will increase the specificity. Elevated AFP is also associated with defects of abdominal wall, fetal death, threatened abortion, twin gestation, ovarian cancers, hepatoma, teratocarcinoma and embryonal carcinoma (testicular tumor).

75. **(A)-F, (B)-F, (C)-F, (D)-T, (E)-F.** Asthma is present in 0.4% to 1.3% of pregnant patients. Fifty percent of pregnant patients show no change in asthma, 25% improve, and 25% get worse. It is difficult to predict, so reassurance is premature. Prevent allergen exposure, avoid strenuous exercise and asperity, and treat viral upper respiratory infection vigorously without antihistamines and dextromethorphan and iodide cough preparations. Theophylline is the first-line medication; beta-adrenergic agonists, glucocorticoids, and cromolyn can also be used when necessary.

76. **(A)-F, (B)-F, (C)-F, (D)-T, (E)-T.** During pregnancy, nifedipine (calcium-channel

blocker), captopril (angiotensin-converting enzyme inhibitor), guanethidine (ganglionic blocker), guanabenz (centrally acting alpha-2-adrenergic receptor agonist) are not recommended. Hydralazine 25 mg daily or methyldopa 250 mg tid daily is the conventional treatment. Propranolol is not recommended, and metoprolol (Tenormin) should be used with caution. Diuretics must be closely monitored for plasma volume contractions.

77. **(A)-F, (B)-F, (C)-T, (D)-F, (E)-F.** The pruritic urticarial papules and plaques of pregnancy (PUPPP syndrome) are the most common skin conditions occurring during the third trimester. The pruritic papules are red, unexcoriated, and mostly in the abdomen and thighs, not in the face or extremities. The hCG is normal, and immunofluorescence reveals no immunoglobulin or complement. The syndrome is self-limited, and it disappears within 2 weeks after delivery.

78. **(A)-F, (B)-F, (C)-F, (D)-F, (E)-F.** Therapeutic abortions should be done as early as possible. Menstrual extraction is done before a period is missed; D&C and suction curettage are recommended before 20 weeks. Second trimester induced abortions are done by amnioinfusion with 20% saline solution or by intravaginal prostaglandin E2.

79. **(A)-F, (B)-F, (C)-F, (D)-T, (E)-F.** Advanced maternal age is associated with increased maternal mortality, increased perinatal mortality, placenta previa, Klinefelter syndrome, Down syndrome, and eclampsia. The advanced maternal age does not increase the incidence of abruptio placentae. Gestational diabetes is more likely to occur in pregnant women over the age of 25 years. Breech presentation is correlated with small fetal size.

80. **(A)-T, (B)-F, (C)-T, (D)-F, (E)-F.** Fetal death syndrome is frequently associated with chromosome abnormalities, syphilis, herpes gestations, methadone withdrawal, preeclampsia, recurrent pyelonephritis, sickle cell anemia, and malpresentation.

81. **(A)-F, (B)-T, (C)-F, (D)-F, (E)-T.** Fetal death is detected by a failure of uterine growth with regression of pregnancy signs and by the stopping of fetal movement. Fetal heartbeats are inaudible by a Doppler device. The diagnosis is established by real-time ultrasonography.

82. **(A)-F, (B)-F, (C)-F, (D)-F, (E)-F.** RhoGAM is the Rh-D immunoglobulin and is indicated for the Rh-negative non-Rh–sensitized mother with Rh-positive or Rh-unknown baby.

83. **(A)-F, (B)-F, (C)-T, (D)-F, (E)-T.** Leiomyomas occur in about 3% of pregnancies due to difficulty in detecting small fibroids in the pregnant uterus. Leiomyomas grow in response to estrogen stimulation due to a greater number of estrogen receptors in leiomyomas, but growth during pregnancy is infrequent. Complications include pain secondary to degeneration or torsion, difficulty in estimating gestational age, and postpartum hemorrhage. Leiomyomas are associated with fetal abnormalities (eg, congenital torticollis), ectopic pregnancy, premature rupture of membrane, abortions, and uterine inversion. Serial ultrasound follow-ups are needed to determine location of myomas and to assess fetal growth. Cesarean sections are employed for obstetric indications.

84. **(F)**

85. **(F)**

86. **(T)**

87. **(F)**

88. **(F)**

89. **(T)**

90. **(T)**

91. **(F)**

92. (F)

Traditional family structure is changing. A family physician may see more unmarried females determined to start a single-parent family. These females are badly in need of comprehensive and continuous total health care from their family physicians. Patients with essential hypertension during pregnancy are at a higher risk to develop preeclampsia and eclampsia, left ventricular failure, cerebral hemorrhage, malignant encephalopathy, abruptio placentae, and a baby of low birth weight. These patients require frequent prenatal care, and the patients should be informed of occasional needs of surgical intervention rather than natural childbirth. During pregnancy, antihypertensive medical regimens are continued, and outcomes are usually excellent. Most patients are treated with central adrenergic blockers (eg, methyldopa). Some clinicians may withdraw diuretics to avoid hypokalemia, which may cause fetal arrhythmia. Diuretics may rarely cause jaundice or thrombocytopenia in the fetus. Arteriolar dilators such as hydralazine are used when preeclampsia supervenes.

DIRECTIONS (Questions 1 through 98): Each of the numbered items or incomplete statements in this section is followed by answers or by completions of the statement. Select the ONE lettered answer or completion that is BEST in each case.

1. A 25-year-old female comes to your office because of malaise for 4 weeks, fever for 2 weeks, generalized pain in her joints, and swelling of her vulva. Physical examination reveals a mass in the right inguinal region discharging pus and associated with very marked engorgement of the vulva. Laboratory data showed hemoglobin 12 g/100 mL, white blood count (WBC) 12,000 with 55% segmented neutrophils, 45% lymphocytes; and total protein 7.4 g/100 mL, with albumin 3.4 g/100 mL and globulin 4.0 g/100 mL. The most likely diagnosis is

    (A) chancroid
    (B) syphilis
    (C) lymphogranuloma venereum
    (D) tuberculous lymphadenitis
    (E) granuloma inguinale   (Ref. 55)

2. Acute labyrinthitis is characterized by

    (A) resting nystagmus
    (B) diplopia
    (C) neck stiffness
    (D) decreased ankle jerks
    (E) dropped mouth angles   (Ref. 3)

3. Hearing loss in presbycusis is

    (A) unilateral
    (B) conductive type
    (C) commonly seen in young adults
    (D) low-frequency loss
    (E) gradual in onset   (Ref. 2)

4. An 8-year-old girl has had a scaly, itching rash on the dorsal aspect of her toes each winter for the past 3 years. Her father has athlete's foot, her mother has hay fever, and one maiden aunt has psoriasis. The most likely diagnosis is

    (A) dermatophytosis
    (B) atopic dermatitis
    (C) psoriasis
    (D) candidiasis
    (E) contact dermatitis from shoes   (Ref. 55)

5. A middle-aged female patient has had dry skin on the soles of her feet for many years and her toenails are undermined with crumbly material. During the past few summers, she has had circumscribed, itchy, and scaly patches of dermatitis about her ankles. Steroid creams aggravate rather than help, but the rash disappears in the winter. What is your diagnosis?

    (A) psoriasis
    (B) atopic dermatitis
    (C) *Trichophyton rubrum* infection
    (D) lichen planus
    (E) pityriasis rosea   (Ref. 55)

6. Prostatic cancer is to be screened routinely by

   (A) digital rectal examination
   (B) serum prostate-specific antigen (PSA)
   (C) transrectal ultrasound
   (D) urinalysis
   (E) none of the above   *(Ref. 15)*

7. Acanthosis nigricans may be associated with

   (A) hypertension
   (B) microcytic anemia
   (C) cancer of the stomach
   (D) pneumonia
   (E) pericarditis   *(Ref. 55)*

8. A 23-year-old female complains of nasal discharge, nasal obstruction, and pain in the face. The pain is throbbing in nature and is referred to the supraorbital area. The pain is worsened by head movements, walking, or stooping. On examination, tenderness is elicited over the antrum, which fails to transilluminate clearly. The most likely diagnosis is

   (A) frontal sinusitis
   (B) dental infection
   (C) chronic tonsillitis
   (D) maxillary sinusitis
   (E) chronic hypertrophic rhinitis   *(Ref. 10)*

9. An insidious, indolent, inflammatory disease of a salivary gland with sinus tract formation would suggest

   (A) Mikulicz's disease
   (B) syphilis
   (C) tuberculosis
   (D) actinomycosis
   (E) sarcoidosis   *(Ref. 13)*

10. Unilateral nasal discharge in children suggests

   (A) papilloma
   (B) vasomotor rhinitis
   (C) foreign bodies
   (D) juvenile angiofibroma
   (E) nasal polyps   *(Ref. 28)*

11. Squamous cell carcinoma is most frequently associated with

   (A) keratoacanthoma
   (B) actinic keratosis
   (C) solar keratosis
   (D) keloids
   (E) neurofibromatosis   *(Ref. 27)*

12. A 42-year-old man is found to have a new 1.0-cm mole on the anterior surface of his right thigh. A wide surgical resection is performed, and the diagnosis of melanoma is made. The tumor's depth of penetration was 0.75 mm. There is no clinical evidence of lymph node or distant metastases. The most appropriate management would be

   (A) prophylactic right inguinal lymph node dissection
   (B) prophylactic dissection of the right inguinal and pelvic lymph nodes
   (C) bacillus Calmette–Guérin (BCG) immunotherapy
   (D) adjunctive chemotherapy
   (E) continuity of care   *(Ref. 55)*

13. A 30-year-old housewife complains of long-standing nasal obstruction; profuse, clear, watery nasal discharge; conjunctival infection; and annoying sneezing. Physical findings of the lungs and heart are essentially negative. The nasal mucosa appears to be thickened and edematous, with bluish-tinged inferior turbinates. The microscopic examination of the nasal secretion may reveal

   (A) neutrophilia
   (B) numerous staphylococci
   (C) numerous *Escherichia coli*
   (D) eosinophilia
   (E) numerous spirochetes   *(Ref. 28)*

14. A 20-year-old male has had tonsillitis for 10 days with some improvement. Two days ago, he noted that the right side of the throat was becoming increasingly painful, and he was having trouble swallowing; he also noted that his voice was becoming muffled and he had an earache. His temperature is now

102°F. On examination, trismus is present and the buccal mucosa is dirty. The right tonsil is pushed downward and medially. The uvula resembles a white grape. This clinical picture is most commonly caused by

(A) *Staphylococcus*

(B) Vincent's organism

(C) *Streptococcus*

(D) herpes simplex

(E) actinomycosis   *(Ref. 28)*

15. In the traumatic rupture of the tympanic membrane, you would

(A) encourage the patient to swim every day

(B) prescribe antibiotic eardrops for three weeks

(C) instruct the patient to use earplugs during showering

(D) instruct the patient to clean the ear canal four times a day with cotton-tipped swabs

(E) instruct the patient to irrigate the ear canal twice a day

                 (Ref. 2)

16. A patient suddenly feels the need to tilt his head toward his left shoulder in order to see "comfortably." He possibly has a lesion involving which of the following cranial nerves?

(A) II

(B) III

(C) IV

(D) V

(E) VI   *(Ref. 56)*

17. A patient with a sudden ptosis notes that his eye is turned outwards. You examine the eye and find that the pupil reacts normally. The most likely diagnosis is

(A) carotid aneurysm

(B) diabetic neuropathy

(C) hypertension

(D) trauma

(E) strabismus   *(Ref. 56)*

18. In spontaneous, extensive subconjunctival hemorrhage, the treatment should consist of

(A) internal corticosteroids

(B) topical corticosteroids

(C) internal antibiotics

(D) topical antibiotics

(E) reassurance   *(Ref. 1)*

19. A 72-year-old female complains that her "traveling rheumatism" has now affected her head. She has had pain on chewing and anorexia for 2 months. She has a tender area on her right temple. The most probable diagnosis is

(A) temporal arteritis

(B) tension headache

(C) migraine headache

(D) acute rheumatic fever

(E) climacteric syndrome   *(Ref. 56)*

20. A patient with bilateral cataracts appearing at age 30 who has signs of premature aging and diabetes most likely has

(A) Thomson syndrome

(B) Werner syndrome

(C) Waardenburg syndrome

(D) Cogan syndrome

(E) naphthalene poisoning   *(Ref. 56)*

21. Diabetes mellitus is associated with

(A) lichen planus

(B) pemphigus

(C) granuloma annulare

(D) scleroderma

(E) lupus erythematosus   *(Ref. 55)*

22. Which of the following is most likely to lead to secondary (hemorrhagic, thrombotic) glaucoma?

(A) central retinal artery occlusion

(B) branch artery occlusion

(C) branch retinal vein occlusion

(D) internal carotid artery occlusion

(E) central retinal vein occlusion   *(Ref. 56)*

23. A 49-year-old man calls you to say that he has just had three episodes of blindness in his right eye. These episodes all occurred within 2 days of one another, lasted 6 to 7 minutes, and then cleared—first in the inferior field of vision and then in the superior field of vision. Retinal findings in the involved eye show yellow flecks at two bifurcations of the inferior temporal arteriole. The most likely pathology is

(A) atheromatous occlusion of the right internal carotid artery
(B) sclerosis of the retinal vessels
(C) embolization of the retinal vessels of calcific particles from a diseased aortic valve
(D) cholesterol emboli that probably originated from the right carotid siphon
(E) an ulcerating atheroma in the wall of the right carotid bifurcation   (Ref. 56)

24. One of your strabismus patients with accommodative esotropia is being treated with echothiophate iodide drops. You discover an incarcerated inguinal hernia, which requires immediate care. What is your advice to the surgeon and anesthesiologist?

(A) increase the preoperative dose of atropine over the usual amount
(B) use Fluothane (halothane) as a general anesthetic and not ether
(C) avoid succinylcholine for abdominal wall relaxation
(D) monitor the temperature closely for suspected malignant hyperpyrexia
(E) use an intravenous fluid such as Ringer's lactate because of increased acidosis   (Ref. 29)

25. A patient with a perforating wound involving the uveal tract in one eye developed uveitis in the other eye 2 weeks later. The most likely diagnosis is

(A) secondary glaucoma
(B) acute bacterial uveitis
(C) acute viral uveitis

(D) sympathetic uveitis
(E) arteriosclerosis   (Ref. 56)

26. A 10-year-old boy with itching eruptions over the nasolabial angles on the face was found to have progressive protrusion of the right eye and headache. The most likely diagnosis is

(A) orbital cellulitis
(B) cavernous sinus thrombosis
(C) acute conjunctivitis
(D) hordeolum
(E) Horner syndrome   (Ref. 13)

27. A 45-year-old male suddenly develops headache, blurred vision, and excruciating eye pain; he vomits frequently. The most likely diagnosis is

(A) acute conjunctivitis
(B) acute glaucoma
(C) corneal ulcer
(D) acute iritis
(E) episcleritis   (Ref. 56)

28. Pellagra may cause

(A) vaginitis and cervicitis
(B) psychosis and photosensitivity
(C) hypertension and angina
(D) dry cough
(E) night sweats   (Ref. 9)

29. Paranasal sinusitis is caused primarily by

(A) a deviated nasal septum
(B) frequent otitis media
(C) obstruction of the sinus ostia
(D) tonsillar hypertrophy
(E) obstruction of the eustachian tube   (Ref. 10)

30. A 2-month-old Chinese-American boy was brought to your office for a well-baby visit. The mother was very anxious about a dusky blue spot at the boy's buttock. You would

(A) perform a biopsy
(B) reassure the mother

(C) prescribe nystatin cream

(D) initiate griseofulvin therapy

(E) institute laser therapy   *(Ref. 24)*

31. A 52-year-old female has sustained a right knee sprain. You will

(A) perform total right knee replacement surgery

(B) prescribe a cane held on the right side of the body

(C) prescribe a cane held on the left side of the body

(D) apply burned herbs on the right knee area

(E) inject Rocephin (ceftriaxone) 250 mg IM   *(Ref. 2)*

32. Hyperlateralization of the knee joint most likely will cause rupture of the

(A) anterior cruciate ligaments

(B) medial meniscus

(C) lateral meniscus

(D) posterior cruciate ligament

(E) lateral collateral ligament   *(Ref. 4)*

33. A 48-year-old woman has suffered from rheumatoid arthritis for 20 years. Recently, she developed mild hypertension, general edema, proteinuria, and splenomegaly. Hyaline casts and a few red blood cells (RBCs) were found in the urine. The most likely diagnosis is

(A) gout

(B) secondary amyloidosis

(C) nephrotic syndrome

(D) liver cirrhosis

(E) acute glomerulonephritis   *(Ref. 2)*

34. An 18-year-old athlete complained of swelling and pain in his left thigh for three weeks. The pain prevented him from participating in athletic activities. An x-ray showed faint calcification. The most likely diagnosis is

(A) myositis ossificans

(B) osteoarthritis

(C) rheumatoid arthritis

(D) sprain

(E) normal physical   *(Ref. 63)*

35. Thickening of frontal and temporal bones is seen in a skull x-ray. The patient is probably suffering from

(A) gargoylism

(B) hydrocephalus

(C) pituitary tumor

(D) no disorder

(E) hyperthyroidism   *(Ref. 22)*

36. A 60-year-old man falls down with his hand outstretched. His injury is possibly

(A) fracture of the clavicle

(B) supracondylar fracture of the humerus

(C) fracture of the shoulder

(D) Colles' fracture

(E) fracture of the shaft of the humerus   *(Ref. 39)*

37. A 20-year-old male has been suffering from chronic backache with stiffness. On examination, the lumbar curve is flattened, with limited back motion. X-ray of the spine shows erosion and sclerosis of the sacroiliac joints. The most likely diagnosis is

(A) ankylosing spondylitis

(B) rheumatoid arthritis

(C) osteoporosis

(D) acute lumbosacral sprain

(E) psoriatic arthritis   *(Ref. 2)*

38. The most common complaint of patients with Sjögren syndrome is dry eyes manifested by symptoms of chronic conjunctival irritation. The diagnosis is established most definitely by

(A) the finding of salivary gland enlargement

(B) the finding of a dry tongue and a dry mouth with much dental decay

(C) the demonstration of hypergammaglobulinemia and a reactive latex fixation test for rheumatoid factor

(D) a biopsy of the inner surface of the lip

(E) sialography   *(Ref. 56)*

39. A 7-year-old boy stopped riding his bicycle because of pain in his left knee. During the next 4 weeks, he was observed to limp with any activity and continued to complain of pain in his left knee. There was no history of trauma to the knee and no obvious lesion on inspection. The most likely diagnosis is

    (A) a dislocated internal meniscus of the left knee
    (B) osteoid osteoma of the femur
    (C) early osteomyelitis
    (D) leukemia
    (E) osteochondrosis of the femoral head
    (Ref. 2)

40. An elderly patient develops within 6 weeks a bulky tumor on his face the size of the end of your thumb. It has rounded, bulging sides and a central core filled with keratin. The most likely diagnosis is

    (A) squamous cell carcinoma
    (B) basal cell carcinoma
    (C) keratoacanthoma
    (D) common wart
    (E) seborrheic keratosis
    (Ref. 55)

41. Vitiligo is often associated with

    (A) hypothyroidism
    (B) hypertension
    (C) bacterial vaginosis
    (D) tinea pedis
    (E) acute pancreatitis
    (Ref. 55)

42. A 40-year-old male has developed flank pain, albuminuria, and hematuria. On physical examination, there are smooth masses palpable in both flanks, with tenderness. Blood pressure is 160/100 mm Hg. The most likely diagnosis is

    (A) nephrosclerosis
    (B) hydronephrosis
    (C) glomerulonephritis
    (D) essential hypertension
    (E) polycystic kidneys
    (Ref. 15)

43. A 30-year-old male patient has vomited out everything he has ingested for 4 days. The urine specific gravity is 1.014. He possibly has

    (A) poor renal function
    (B) good renal function
    (C) diabetes insipidus
    (D) normal renal function
    (E) diabetes mellitus
    (Ref. 15)

44. A patient received a severe blow over the left flank region. Two hours later, he developed gross hematuria. The first procedure you would order is

    (A) surgical exploration
    (B) cystogram
    (C) infusion urography
    (D) renal angiogram
    (E) electrocardiogram (ECG)
    (Ref. 15)

45. Erythrasma is best diagnosed by

    (A) urinalysis
    (B) hemoglobin determination
    (C) serum potassium level
    (D) viral culture of the lesion
    (E) Wood's lamp
    (Ref. 55)

46. A young man complains of fever, chills, burning, and micturition urgency. There is no hematuria. Rectal examination reveals an exquisitely tender, enlarged mass. The most likely diagnosis is

    (A) acute urethritis
    (B) acute prostatitis
    (C) internal hemorrhoids
    (D) acute pyelonephritis
    (E) acute glomerulonephritis
    (Ref. 15)

47. A 35-year-old male complains of headache, pressure sensation, and facial pain under his right eye for 1 week. The pain increases when he bends over. There is tenderness at the right cheek. The most likely diagnosis is

    (A) ethmoid sinusitis
    (B) maxillary sinusitis

(C) sphenoid sinusitis

(D) orbital cellulitis

(E) frontal sinusitis   *(Ref. 2)*

48. Tinea versicolor is caused by

(A) pityrosporum orbiculare

(B) *Streptococcus pneumoniae*

(C) *Staphylococcus aureus*

(D) *Candida albicans*

(E) cytomegalovirus   *(Ref. 55)*

49. A 25-year-old male presents with erythematous, ovoid, itching lesions on the trunk for 10 days. The patient noted that the largest patch first developed at the abdominal wall, then spread all over the trunk. The long axes of the eruption follow the lines of the cleavage. The most likely diagnosis is

(A) tinea versicolor

(B) secondary syphilis

(C) atopic dermatitis

(D) pityriasis rosea

(E) lichen planus   *(Ref. 55)*

50. A merchant marine sailor whose route was mainly the Pacific and Indian Oceans came to the office complaining of progressive weakness of his left hand accompanied by wasting and anesthesia. On examination, his left ulnar nerve was grossly thickened. There was a red-brown, indolent, pigmented swelling of his right ear. Other parts of the physical examinations are essentially normal. Complete blood count (CBC), urinalysis, and tuberculin test results are all negative. The most likely diagnosis is

(A) syphilis

(B) leprosy

(C) tuberculosis

(D) rheumatoid arthritis

(E) multiple sclerosis   *(Ref. 24)*

51. A 23-year-old male has had 2 years of nasal discharges and sneezing attacks. The symptoms can occur any time of day, but it is worse on arising in the morning. There is no

seasonal variation of the symptoms. Cytology of nasal mucosal smears show eosinophilia. The most likely diagnosis is

(A) allergic rhinitis

(B) atrophic rhinitis

(C) common cold

(D) nonallergic rhinitis with eosinophilia syndrome

(E) acute bacterial rhinitis   *(Ref. 13)*

52. In a 1-day-old infant, mucoid ocular discharge, conjunctival hyperemia, and swollen eyelids are most frequently due to

(A) gonococcal infection

(B) infection due to *Haemophilus influenzae*

(C) inclusion conjunctivitis

(D) congenital toxoplasmosis

(E) instillation of silver nitrate   *(Ref. 56)*

53. A 45-year-old man has developed chronic, pruritic, red-brown and red-blue, well-defined plaques in the chest wall. You would now

(A) order chest x-rays

(B) perform skin biopsy

(C) perform bone marrow aspiration

(D) order serum electrophoresis

(E) perform wood light examination

(Ref. 55)

54. Your 48-year-old male patient was found to have mild hypertension. You prescribed hydrochlorothiazide 25 mg OD. Following 3 months of good control of blood pressure, he presents to your office with pruritic, flat-topped, polygonal, shiny to scaly, violaceous papules on his right forearm. The most likely diagnosis is

(A) lupus erythematosus

(B) acquired immune deficiency syndrome (AIDS)

(C) urticaria vulgaris

(D) lichen planus

(E) impetigo   *(Ref. 55)*

55. A 50-year-old female complains of a sharp pain and swelling of the right submandibular region for 5 days. An x-ray of the right submandibular region reveals several calcified areas. The most likely diagnosis is

(A) mixed tumor

(B) infectious mononucleosis

(C) salivary calculi

(D) cancers of submandibular glands

(E) acute parotitis   *(Ref. 77)*

56. A 19-year-old sexually active female presents with hemorrhagic crusting of her lips with oral erosions, fever, malaise, and a generalized skin eruption consisting of round, raised plaques with tense blisters. The most likely diagnosis is

(A) secondary syphilis

(B) gonococcemia

(C) herpes simplex

(D) lymphogranuloma venereum

(E) venereal warts   *(Ref. 55)*

57. A 10-year-old girl complains of oliguria. Her blood pressure is 80/40 mm Hg, urinalysis is normal, blood urea nitrogen (BUN) is 60, and creatinine is 1.0. The most likely diagnosis is

(A) acute poststreptococcal glomerulonephritis

(B) volume depletion

(C) urolithiasis

(D) chronic glomerulonephritis

(E) hemolytic uremic syndrome   *(Ref. 2)*

58. A 60-year-old female has had a hearing impairment in her left ear for almost 15 years. Intermittently, there was severe pain on the left side of her face. During the office visit for her upper respiratory infection, you noticed a swelling coming out from the external ear. Following manipulation, profuse bleeding developed. The most likely diagnosis is

(A) acoustic neuroma

(B) pyogenic abscess

(C) glomus jugulare tumor

(D) cholesteatoma

(E) foreign body in the left ear canal   *(Ref. 13)*

59. A 21-year-old female with acne was taking isotretinoin (Accutane) 10 mg bid for the past 2 weeks with little improvement. Now she plans to get pregnant. You would

(A) continue isotretinoin for another 2 months with the same dosage

(B) stop isotretinoin

(C) increase isotretinoin dosage to 20 mg bid

(D) add oral tetracyclines

(E) extend the isotretinoin treatment for a year   *(Ref. 55)*

60. A 6-year-old boy complains of right earache following swimming in a pool. You would

(A) prescribe oral decongestants

(B) prescribe oral polymyxin B

(C) prescribe oral corticosteroids

(D) prescribe polymyxin B eardrops

(E) examine both ear canals   *(Ref. 28)*

61. A 55-year-old patient was well on retiring after heavy alcohol intake but was unable to walk on arising. His right great toe was red and swollen, with exquisite tenderness. Among the following, the most specific test for the diagnosis is

(A) polarizing light microscopy of the synovial fluid

(B) erythrocyte sedimentation rate

(C) WBC

(D) serum uric acid level

(E) serum urea level   *(Ref. 2)*

62. A 27-year-old female bank teller complains of an irritated, red left eye. On physical examination, there is a moderate injection of the larger conjunctival vessels, watery discharge, and a palpable preauricular lymph node. The most likely diagnosis is

(A) retinal detachment

(B) subconjunctival hemorrhage

(C) chronic simple glaucoma

(D) acute viral conjunctivitis

(E) acute iritis   *(Ref. 56)*

63. A young patient suddenly develops weakness of the left side of his face accompanied by severe pain inside the left external ear. The otoscopic examination reveals vesicular eruption on the left eardrum. The most likely diagnosis is

(A) herpes simplex

(B) otomycosis

(C) pemphigus vulgaris

(D) pemphigoid

(E) Ramsay–Hunt syndrome   *(Ref. 55)*

64. Pain and swelling of the submandibular region due to eating are most likely caused by

(A) mixed tumor

(B) thyroid nodule

(C) trigeminal neuralgia

(D) salivary calculi

(E) paranasal sinusitis   *(Ref. 13)*

65. Many males have concern over penis size. The size of the penis is important for which *one* of the following reasons?

(A) A small penis provides insufficient stimulation to the female during intercourse.

(B) A large penis cannot be easily accommodated by female genitalia in the aroused state.

(C) Penis size is directly related to body size.

(D) Penis size has important psychological implications.

(E) Penis size in the nonerect state is directly related to penis size in the erect state.
                                          (Ref. 35)

66. Impotence in males is most commonly due to

(A) phimosis

(B) psychological factors

(C) vitamin A deficiency

(D) vasectomy

(E) contraceptive use by the female partner
                                          (Ref. 2)

67. Lice infestations are best treated by

(A) 1% hydrocortisone cream

(B) 0.025% triamcinolone lotion

(C) nystatin ointment

(D) oral griseofulvin

(E) pyrethrin lotion   *(Ref. 55)*

68. A 25-year-old male complains of trismus for 3 days. Physical examination reveals the deviation of the uvula to the right. There are swelling, redness, and exudates around the left tonsil. The most likely diagnosis is

(A) acute tonsillitis

(B) exudative tonsillitis

(C) infectious mononucleosis

(D) upper respiratory infection

(E) peritonsillar abscess   *(Ref. 2)*

69. Stevens–Johnson syndrome is commonly caused by

(A) penicillin

(B) phenytoin

(C) methyldopa

(D) ibuprofen

(E) theophylline   *(Ref. 55)*

70. A 42-year-old female presents with a painful, reddened 1.0-cm swelling at her left axillar area for 3 months. One month ago, the patient noted a purulent discharge burst in the overlying skin. The most likely diagnosis is

(A) hidradenitis suppurativa

(B) sebaceous cyst

(C) lymphadenitis

(D) breast cancer

(E) cat-scratch disease   *(Ref. 55)*

71. A 46-year-old Oriental female presents with a brownish, hyperpigmented, scaling plaque at the medial aspect of her right ankle for 2 years. The itching sensation was somewhat relieved by over-the-counter medications but the symptom recurs. The lesion was thick and lichenified. The most likely diagnosis is

    (A) psoriasis
    (B) contact dermatitis
    (C) lichen simplex chronicus
    (D) mycosis fungoides
    (E) tinea circinata   (Ref. 55)

72. Sarcoidosis is associated with

    (A) tinea versicolor
    (B) pemphigus
    (C) erythema nodosum
    (D) acne vulgaris
    (E) rosacea   (Ref. 63)

73. Presbycusis is characterized by

    (A) low-pitched tinnitus
    (B) air-conduction loss
    (C) sudden paroxysmal onset
    (D) unilateral hearing loss
    (E) high-frequency hearing loss   (Ref. 28)

74. Seborrheic keratoses are associated with

    (A) malignant melanoma
    (B) AIDS
    (C) psoriasis
    (D) autosomal dominance
    (E) acne vulgaris   (Ref. 55)

75. Otitis media with effusion is best treated by

    (A) oral corticosteroids
    (B) nasal corticosteroids
    (C) otic corticosteroids
    (D) nonsedating antihistamines
    (E) observation   (Ref. 66)

76. Tinea capitis is best treated by

    (A) topical 1% gentian violet
    (B) oral griseofulvin

    (C) oral nystatin
    (D) topical nystatin
    (E) topical clotrimazole   (Ref. 55)

77. A 25-year-old female has had multiple linear, itching vesicles on her right index finger for 6 weeks. Her palms are sweaty, temperature is normal, and thyroid is not enlarged. The most likely diagnosis is

    (A) dyshidrotic eczematous dermatitis
    (B) herpes zoster
    (C) pemphigus vulgaris
    (D) contact dermatitis
    (E) tinea manus   (Ref. 27)

78. A 42-year-old female has taken good control of her hypertension by taking captopril 25 mg tid. During the past 2 weeks, she has found multiple painful bullae inside her mouth, and in the past few days, new bullae have spread at the back. A few of them have ruptured and erosion has developed. The most likely diagnosis is

    (A) contact dermatitis
    (B) porphyria
    (C) herpes zoster
    (D) pemphigus foliaceus
    (E) dermatitis herpetiformis   (Ref. 55)

79. Erysipelas is caused by

    (A) diabetes mellitus
    (B) *S. aureus*
    (C) group A streptococci
    (D) hyperlipidemia
    (E) syphilis   (Ref. 55)

80. A 46-year-old female diabetic presents with a sharply marginated, brownish-red rash on the groin. The most likely diagnosis is

    (A) erythrasma
    (B) erysipelas
    (C) tinea versicolor
    (D) tinea cruris
    (E) seborrheic dermatitis   (Ref. 55)

81. A 50-year-old female with a history of dental abscess complains of fever, chills, severe jaw pain, and swelling of the left neck. Opening the mouth is painful, the floor of the mouth is indurated, and the tongue is difficult to move as directed. The patient is most likely suffering from

    (A) quinsy
    (B) tongue cancer
    (C) herpangina
    (D) thrush
    (E) Ludwig's angina   *(Ref. 77)*

82. A 65-year-old male developed severe chest pain in the left side of the chest for 4 days. Two days ago, a group of vesicles developed in the same area. The most likely diagnosis is

    (A) angina pectoris
    (B) myocardial infarction
    (C) pleurisy
    (D) herpes zoster
    (E) pneumonia   *(Ref. 55)*

83. A 27-year-old homosexual male presents with multiple oval, violaceous nodules on the left leg for 3 weeks. You would

    (A) prescribe steroid cream
    (B) perform biopsy
    (C) prescribe antibiotic ointment
    (D) schedule for excision
    (E) initiate sulfa drugs   *(Ref. 55)*

84. A 6-year-old boy is noticed to have a right retractile testicle. You will

    (A) order ultrasound of the right testicle
    (B) perform biopsy of the right testicle
    (C) start chorionic gonadotropin injections
    (D) schedule for orchiopexy of the right testicle
    (E) provide continuous total health care for regular follow-ups   *(Ref. 15)*

85. A 4-month-old boy is found to have a scrotal mass that increases in size with crying. The amount of the fluid varies the size with position changes. The most likely diagnosis is

    (A) varicocele
    (B) epididymitis
    (C) communicating hydrocele
    (D) testicular teratoma
    (E) sarcoma of the scrotum   *(Ref. 15)*

86. A 42-year-old obese female has had multiple tiny, pedunculated, nonitching, nonpainful, papillomatous, brown-colored lesions on the side of the neck for 8 months. The most likely diagnosis is

    (A) lichen planus
    (B) impetigo
    (C) acrochordon
    (D) neurofibromatosis
    (E) molluscum contagiosum   *(Ref. 55)*

87. A 35-year-old female presents with erythematous, sharply outlined, nonitching macular eruptions on the face in a butterfly pattern. The most likely diagnosis is

    (A) scleroderma
    (B) contact dermatitis
    (C) eczema
    (D) systemic lupus erythematosus
    (E) erythema multiforme   *(Ref. 55)*

88. A 5-month-old girl was brought by her mother for an irregularly shaped, violaceous plaque at her left cheek since birth. The most likely diagnosis is

    (A) rosacea
    (B) Sturge–Weber syndrome
    (C) acne vulgaris
    (D) solar keratosis
    (E) verruca vulgaris   *(Ref. 27)*

89. A 43-year-old female alcoholic presents with erythematous papulopustules on the nose and cheeks for 3 weeks. The most likely diagnosis is

    (A) systemic lupus erythematosus
    (B) carcinoid syndrome
    (C) rosacea
    (D) Sturge–Weber syndrome
    (E) acne vulgaris   (Ref. 55)

90. A 17-year-old female presents with distal oncolysis in her left index finger. The most likely diagnosis is

    (A) nutritional anemia
    (B) tinea unguium
    (C) *Candida* infection
    (D) paronychia
    (E) psoriasis vulgaris   (Ref. 55)

91. A 17-year-old male was accompanied by his mother to your office. He was found to be mentally retarded, and there were tiny, freckle-like macules in the left axillar area since childhood; there were many pedunculated, brownish nodules appearing on the trunk for 5 years. The most likely diagnosis is

    (A) neurofibromatosis
    (B) familial hypercholesterolemia
    (C) xanthoma tendineum
    (D) tuberous sclerosis
    (E) cytomegalovirus infection   (Ref. 55)

92. Gluten-sensitive enteropathy is associated with

    (A) alopecia areata
    (B) ichthyosis vulgaris
    (C) dermatitis herpetiformis
    (D) contact dermatitis
    (E) eczematous dermatitis   (Ref. 55)

93. Solar lentigo can best be treated by

    (A) oral erythromycin
    (B) topical erythromycin
    (C) cryotherapy

    (D) oral acyclovir
    (E) IV acyclovir   (Ref. 55)

94. Solar keratosis is most likely to occur in

    (A) physicians
    (B) lawyers
    (C) teachers
    (D) farmers
    (E) office managers   (Ref. 27)

95. A 30-year-old male presents with multiple scattered, discrete, vesicular lesions on the right leg for 5 days. There are golden-yellow, honey-colored, "stuck-on" crusts and erosions in some of those lesions. The culture yields *S. aureus*. The most likely diagnosis is

    (A) herpes simplex
    (B) varicella
    (C) herpes zoster
    (D) tinea corporis
    (E) impetigo   (Ref. 55)

96. A 6-year-old boy was found to have an eyelid rash for 2 months. The laboratory test is expected to show

    (A) leukopenia
    (B) elevated immunoglobulin E (IgE)
    (C) depressed immunoglobulin A (IgA)
    (D) depressed immunoglobulin G (IgG)
    (E) macrocytosis   (Ref. 55)

97. A 25-year-old male presents with multiple ulcers with raised borders at his right thigh for 2 weeks. Gram stain of an ulcer reveals group A streptococci. The most likely diagnosis is

    (A) varicella
    (B) ecthyma
    (C) herpes zoster
    (D) leishmaniasis
    (E) tinea corporis   (Ref. 2)

98. A 47-year-old female presents with increased hair shedding on the scalp during the past 3 months. She fears that this is hair thinning and is afraid that she may become bald. The patient is most likely suffering from

(A) alopecia areata

(B) premenopausal syndrome

(C) anxiety syndrome

(D) depression syndrome

(E) telogen effluvium   *(Ref. 55)*

DIRECTIONS (Questions 99 through 223): Each question consists of an introduction followed by some statements. Mark T (true) or F (false) after each statement.

99. Which of the following individuals are at a higher risk to develop malignant melanoma?

(A) persons with dysplastic nevi

(B) blood relatives of patients with malignant melanomas

(C) persons with dark skin pigmentation

(D) persons with a great number of moles

(E) indoor workers   *(Ref. 55)*

100. Managements for a patient with recurrent urinary tract infections (UTIs) include

(A) urine culture/sensitivity

(B) serum creatinine

(C) urethral dilatation

(D) voiding cystourethrogram for children

(E) radionuclide reflux studies   *(Ref. 3)*

101. Amblyopia is often associated with

(A) strabismus

(B) esotropia

(C) glaucoma

(D) blepharoptosis

(E) anisometropia   *(Ref. 56)*

102. The management of amblyopia involves

(A) correction of refractory errors

(B) calcium-channel blockers

(C) cycloplegic drugs

(D) occlusion of one eye

(E) in strabismus, surgical correction of the deviation prior to occlusive therapy   *(Ref. 56)*

103. Treatment of the common "cold sore" on the lips involves

(A) acyclovir (Zovirax)

(B) verapamil (Calan)

(C) cefazolin (Ancef)

(D) calcium gluconate

(E) riboflavin (vitamin B_2)   *(Ref. 55)*

104. Clinical features of acute sinusitis include

(A) pressure in the sinus region

(B) pain in the maxillary teeth

(C) nasal obstruction

(D) loss of the sense of smell

(E) sore throat   *(Ref. 10)*

105. Medical treatments of acute sinusitis include

(A) rifampin (Rifadin)

(B) nifedipine (Procardia)

(C) papain (Prevenzyme)

(D) melarsoprol (Mel B)

(E) amoxicillin   *(Ref. 10)*

106. Patients with which of the following conditions are advised to avoid air travel?

(A) acute low back strain

(B) acute otitis media

(C) acute sinusitis

(D) cardiothoracic surgery within the last 3 weeks

(E) myoma uteri   *(Ref. 9)*

107. Neurologic complications of herpes zoster include

(A) radiculitis

(B) Bell's palsy

(C) meningioma

(D) contralateral hemiplegia

(E) postherpetic neuralgia   *(Ref. 55)*

108. Nonorganic signs of low back pain include

    (A) camptocormic posture
    (B) use of a cane
    (C) sweating
    (D) increased muscle tension and tremor
    (E) stocking distribution of pain or numbness   (Ref. 63)

109. Common tenderness sites in fibrositis include the

    (A) fifth costochondral junction
    (B) sole of the right foot
    (C) midpoint of the left wrist
    (D) outer third of the forehead
    (E) interspinous ligaments of L4 to S1
    (Ref. 63)

110. Managements of fibrositis include

    (A) cimetidine (Tagamet)
    (B) cyclobenzaprine (Flexeril)
    (C) amitriptyline (Elavil)
    (D) propoxyphene (Darvon)
    (E) naproxen (Naprosyn)   (Ref. 63)

111. Symptoms of cutaneous larva migrans include

    (A) prickling, tingling discomfort in the skin
    (B) intense pruritus
    (C) threadlike burrows on the skin
    (D) bronchospasm
    (E) Löffler syndrome (pulmonary infiltrate with eosinophilia)   (Ref. 55)

112. Complications of contact lens use include

    (A) glaucoma
    (B) uveitis
    (C) infectious keratitis
    (D) *Acanthamoeba* infection
    (E) giant papillary conjunctivitis   (Ref. 56)

113. Ankylosing spondylitis is associated with

    (A) iridocyclitis
    (B) mitral stenosis
    (C) ulcerative colitis
    (D) urethritis
    (E) cardiac conduction defects   (Ref. 2)

114. Indications for a skin biopsy include

    (A) a skin lesion that cannot be diagnosed specifically through careful clinical examinations
    (B) recurrent urticarias
    (C) a small skin lesion measuring 0.2×0.3 mm that never heals
    (D) chronic bullous lesions
    (E) acute generalized erythematous lesions in the trunk and extremities   (Ref. 2)

115. In the management of UTIs

    (A) single-dose therapy is the treatment of choice for pregnant women
    (B) trimethoprim-sulfamethoxazole (Septra) is the drug of choice during pregnancy
    (C) in single-dose therapy, oral amoxicillin 3.0 g or trimethoprim-sulfamethoxazole 2 tablets are administered
    (D) when caused by *Chlamydia trachomatis*, the drug of choice is nitrofurantoin
    (E) the drug of choice for children with recurrent UTIs is doxycycline   (Ref. 3)

116. Initial treatments of acute low back strain include

    (A) surgical diskectomy
    (B) moist heat application
    (C) rest on a soft, comfortable mattress
    (D) avoidance of lifting objects
    (E) systemic corticosteroids   (Ref. 3)

117. In ankle sprain, when the foot is in plantar flexion, the forced inversion will most likely injure the

    (A) posterior talofibular ligament
    (B) calcaneofibular ligament
    (C) anterior talofibular ligament
    (D) superior deltoid ligament
    (E) deep deltoid ligament   (Ref. 63)

118. Over-the-counter nasal decongestant (eg, oxymetazoline) sprays are very effective to relieve the nasal obstruction of chronic rhinitis. However, prolonged use may induce

    (A) sedation
    (B) drowsiness
    (C) depression
    (D) rhinitis medicamentosa
    (E) impotence   *(Ref. 13)*

119. Treatments for an adult with acute otitis media include

    (A) oral penicillin
    (B) oral erythromycin
    (C) topical neomycin otic solution
    (D) topical corticosteroid otic solution
    (E) IV penicillin   *(Ref. 28)*

120. Managements of vertebral compression fractures include

    (A) medroxyprogesterone (Provera)
    (B) ibuprofen (Motrin)
    (C) reassurance
    (D) immobilization
    (E) calcium   *(Ref. 39)*

121. Complications of acute otitis media include

    (A) mastoiditis
    (B) chronic labyrinthitis
    (C) persistent otitis media
    (D) perforation of the tympanic membrane
    (E) bone-conduction hearing loss   *(Ref. 28)*

122. A 45-year-old female complains of heel pain aggravated by walking for 2 months. There is tenderness at the calcaneal origin of the plantar fascia. The most likely diagnosis is

    (A) heel arthritis
    (B) gout
    (C) Morton's neurinoma
    (D) plantar fascitis
    (E) hammertoe deformity   *(Ref. 84)*

123. A 35-year-old male is a long-distance runner. In the past 4 to 6 weeks, he has developed right knee pain, which worsens when he is walking down stairs. There is tenderness at the lower medial aspect of the patella. The most likely diagnosis is

    (A) meniscal tear of the right knee
    (B) prepatellar bursitis
    (C) patellar tracking syndrome
    (D) medial collateral ligament strain
    (E) osteoarthritis of the right knee   *(Ref. 3)*

124. A 30-year-old white male complains of fleeting arthralgia for 6 months, which has been followed in the last month by bilateral knee swelling, with heat and tenderness. Rheumatoid factor in a titer of 1:640 is present. Which of the following statements is/are correct?

    (A) The presence of a low synovial fluid complement is caused by deposition of immune complexes in synovium.
    (B) Rheumatoid factor is an isoantibody that can be safely transferred to another individual.
    (C) There is a family of rheumatoid factors which are of 19S or 7-11S species.
    (D) Chronic antigenic stimulation can lead to the development of rheumatoid factor.
    (E) Nonsteroidal anti-inflammatory drugs (NSAIDs) may be helpful.   *(Ref. 63)*

125. Which of the following drugs is the LEAST useful in the management of fibrositis?

    (A) cimetidine (Tagamet)
    (B) cyclobenzaprine (Flexeril)
    (C) amitriptyline (Elavil)
    (D) propoxyphene (Darvon)
    (E) antibiotics   *(Ref. 63)*

126. Adenoid hypertrophy may cause

    (A) nasal obstruction
    (B) serous otitis media
    (C) adenoid facies
    (D) fluctuating hearing loss
    (E) low-pitched voice   *(Ref. 28)*

127. To detect prostatic carcinoma in the early stage, you would

    (A) order a PSA test yearly
    (B) determine the serum alkaline phophatase level every 3 months
    (C) determine the serum acid phophatase level every 6 months
    (D) perform a urinalysis dipstick test yearly
    (E) perform digital rectal examinations to assess prostate condition regularly

    (Ref. 15)

128. Proliferative retinopathy may be seen in which of the following?

    (A) methemoglobinemia
    (B) macroglobulinemia
    (C) diabetes
    (D) central retinal vein occlusion
    (E) hemorrhage from hypertension   *(Ref. 56)*

129. A 2-year-old child comes in for a routine physical, and strabismus is noted. The parents should know which of the following?

    (A) A large number of children with strabismus have some degree of amblyopia.
    (B) Amblyopia should be prevented rather than treated.
    (C) In children with pure alternating strabismus, orthoptic treatment is usually unrewarding.
    (D) Practically all deviating eyes can be straightened by treatment.
    (E) The surgery should be carried out after age 10.   *(Ref. 56)*

130. Combined ulnar and median nerve injury at the level of the wrist is usually manifested by

    (A) ape hand
    (B) claw hand
    (C) the inability to approximate the small finger to the thumb
    (D) the inability to spread the fingers apart
    (E) wrist drop   *(Ref. 2)*

131. A 45-year-old woman presents with recent onset of inflammatory arthritis involving both hands. The differential diagnosis includes

    (A) rheumatoid arthritis
    (B) osteoarthritis
    (C) scleroderma
    (D) Reiter syndrome
    (E) systemic lupus erythematosus   *(Ref. 2)*

132. Necrotizing papillitis may be associated with

    (A) diabetes mellitus
    (B) sickle cell traits
    (C) vesicoureteral reflux
    (D) chronic use of analgesics
    (E) cirrhosis of the liver   *(Ref. 41)*

133. Uveitis is commonly associated with which of the following conditions?

    (A) diabetes mellitus
    (B) hypertension
    (C) rheumatoid arthritis
    (D) tuberculosis
    (E) sarcoidosis   *(Ref. 56)*

134. Which of the following conditions are precancerous?

    (A) senile keratosis
    (B) junctional nevus
    (C) blue nevus
    (D) arsenic hyperkeratosis
    (E) Bowen's disease   *(Ref. 27)*

135. Tuberous sclerosis is characterized by

    (A) mental deterioration
    (B) adenoma sebaceum
    (C) convulsions
    (D) retinal phacoma
    (E) pulmonary tuberculosis   *(Ref. 55)*

136. Ménière's disease in a middle-aged woman usually includes which of the following clinical features?

    (A) vertigo
    (B) nausea and vomiting

(C) deafness

(D) tinnitus

(E) blindness   *(Ref. 28)*

137. Nonunion of fractures is frequently associated with

(A) inadequate immobilization

(B) inappropriate reduction

(C) severe fracture

(D) extensive soft-tissue damage

(E) infection   *(Ref. 39)*

138. Which of the following features are part of Peutz–Jeghers syndrome?

(A) intestinal polyposis

(B) hematoma

(C) familial disease

(D) melanin pigmentation of the lips and oral mucosa

(E) recurrent colicky abdominal pain   *(Ref. 55)*

139. A 7-year-old boy complains of persistent severe pain and swelling at the left femoral region for 3 weeks. There was a history of injury. The most likely diagnosis is

(A) sprain

(B) osteosarcoma

(C) metastatic cancer of the lung

(D) relapse of prostatic cancer

(E) Osgood–Schlatter disease   *(Ref. 2)*

140. Chronic urethritis is characterized by

(A) urethral stenosis

(B) urethral discomfort

(C) burning on urination

(D) normal urinalysis

(E) nocturia   *(Ref. 2)*

141. Exophthalmos can be associated with

(A) high myopia

(B) macrophthalmia

(C) rhabdomyosarcoma

(D) fibroma

(E) hypothyroidism   *(Ref. 6)*

142. Osteoporosis may be caused by

(A) primary hyperparathyroidism

(B) Cushing syndrome

(C) hyperthyroidism

(D) rheumatoid arthritis

(E) Paget's disease   *(Ref. 2)*

143. Which of the following factors may increase the risk of perpetuating a UTI?

(A) vesicoureteral reflux

(B) vesical residual urine

(C) renal calculi

(D) vaginal colonization by pathogenic bacteria

(E) diabetes mellitus   *(Ref. 3)*

144. Kyphosis may be associated with

(A) neurofibromatosis

(B) poliomyelitis

(C) syringomyelia

(D) Frederick's ataxia

(E) Pott's disease   *(Ref. 1)*

145. Sialadenosis is associated with

(A) alcoholic cirrhosis

(B) diabetes mellitus

(C) pregnancy

(D) hypervitaminosis A

(E) hypothyroidism   *(Ref. 13)*

146. The differential diagnosis of fibromyalgia syndrome (FS) includes

(A) hypothyroidism

(B) malingering

(C) psychogenic rheumatism

(D) polymyalgia rheumatica

(E) flu syndromes   *(Ref. 3)*

147. Nephrotic syndrome is often associated with

(A) glomerulonephritis

(B) systemic lupus erythematosus (SLE)

(C) amyloidosis

(D) tinea versicolor

(E) diabetes mellitus   *(Ref. 41)*

148. Tuberculosis (TB) of the genital tract is characterized by which of the following clinical features?

(A) Painless swelling is usually presented in tuberculous epididymitis.

(B) It is often associated with extragenital tuberculosis.

(C) It may often cause persistent "sterile" pyuria.

(D) Intravenous pyelogram (IVP) may show a "moth-eaten" appearance of the involved ulcerated calyces.

(E) It may cause infertility.   *(Ref. 15)*

149. Tabes dorsalis may cause

(A) incontinence

(B) bladder distention

(C) Charcot's joint

(D) Argyll–Robertson pupils

(E) condyloma acuminatum   *(Ref. 6)*

150. Nephrocalcinosis is seen in which of the following conditions?

(A) primary nephrocalcinosis

(B) breast cancer with bone metastasis

(C) milk-alkali syndrome

(D) sarcoidosis

(E) hypoparathyroidism   *(Ref. 15)*

151. Acute prostatitis is characterized by

(A) insidious onset

(B) low back pain

(C) fever

(D) nocturia

(E) tender prostate   *(Ref. 2)*

152. Sporotrichosis is commonly seen in

(A) florists

(B) physicians

(C) gardeners

(D) fishermen

(E) paper manufacturers   *(Ref. 27)*

153. Xanthoma tendineum

(A) is associated with hypertension

(B) may produce hypoglycemia

(C) is an autosomal recessive disease

(D) is caused by too many hepatic hydroxymethylglutaryl coenzyme A (HMG CoA) reductase inhibitors

(E) is helpful with a high-cholesterol diet   *(Ref. 55)*

154. De Quervain's disease

(A) is a stenosing tenosynovitis

(B) produces positive Finkelstein test

(C) is located in the neck

(D) is treated with NSAIDs

(E) is often associated with infant care   *(Ref. 63)*

155. Still's disease is associated with

(A) uveitis

(B) retinal detachment

(C) keratitis

(D) hemianopsia

(E) eyelid edema   *(Ref. 6)*

156. Toxoplasmosis is characterized by

(A) retinal detachment

(B) chorioretinitis

(C) papillitis

(D) papilledema

(E) myalgia   *(Ref. 56)*

157. Trichinosis may produce

(A) nodular uveitis

(B) chorioretinitis

(C) eyelid edema

(D) keratomalacia

(E) subluxation of the lens   *(Ref. 54)*

158. Marfan syndrome may present with

(A) dissecting aneurysm

(B) subluxation of lens

(C) breast cancer

(D) mental deficiency

(E) erythema nodosum   (*Ref. 6*)

159. Glaucoma may result from the use of

(A) corticosteroids

(B) penicillin

(C) Donnatal (gastrointestinal anticholinergic sedative)

(D) amphetamines

(E) amitriptyline   (*Ref. 56*)

160. Clinical findings of hypertensive retinopathy include

(A) copper wire appearance

(B) arteriovenous (AV) crossing phenomena

(C) cotton-wool spots

(D) irregular hemorrhages

(E) papilledema   (*Ref. 56*)

161. Cataracts are associated with

(A) diabetes mellitus

(B) galactosemia

(C) corticosteroid use

(D) hypoparathyroidism

(E) rubella infection   (*Ref. 56*)

162. The common ocular manifestations of AIDS include

(A) hyphema

(B) strabismic amblyopia

(C) hyperopia

(D) cytomegalovirus (CMV) retinitis

(E) progressive exophthalmos   (*Ref. 2*)

163. Xanthopsia can be produced by

(A) chlorothiazide

(B) digoxin

(C) thiamine

(D) vitamin E

(E) penicillin   (*Ref. 29*)

164. Clinical presentations of retinitis pigmentosa include

(A) bitemporal hemianopsia

(B) ring scotoma

(C) night blindness

(D) chorioretinitis

(E) deafness   (*Ref. 56*)

165. Clinical presentations of optic neuritis include

(A) centrocecal scotoma

(B) visual acuity improved

(C) transient blurred vision

(D) eye pain

(E) mydriasis   (*Ref. 56*)

166. Glaucoma is characterized by

(A) an intraocular pressure of less than 10 mm Hg

(B) sharpening of central vision

(C) cup enlarging vertically

(D) arcuate scotoma

(E) severe eye pain   (*Ref. 56*)

167. The ocular findings in diabetes mellitus include

(A) microaneurysm

(B) rubeosis iridis

(C) blue sclerae

(D) chalazion

(E) cotton-wool spots   (*Ref. 56*)

168. Solar (eclipse) retinopathy is characterized by

(A) papilledema

(B) collapse of retinal arterioles

(C) engorgement of the retinal vein

(D) peripheral scotoma

(E) central scotoma   (*Ref. 6*)

169. Iritis is characterized by

(A) corneal opacity

(B) dilated pupils

(C) increased intraocular pressure

(D) phonophobia

(E) photophobia   (*Ref. 2*)

170. Pigmentary retinopathy can be produced by

    (A) hydroxychloroquine
    (B) thioridazine (Mellaril)
    (C) vitamin C
    (D) vitamin E
    (E) penicillin   *(Ref. 56)*

171. Ocular presentations of hypervitaminosis A include

    (A) band keratopathy
    (B) loss of eyebrows
    (C) retinal hemorrhage
    (D) nystagmus
    (E) ocular palsies   *(Ref. 6)*

172. Ocular findings in gout include

    (A) iridocyclitis
    (B) episcleritis
    (C) scleritis
    (D) conjunctivitis
    (E) glaucoma   *(Ref. 6)*

173. Retinal artery occlusion may be caused by

    (A) sickle cell disease
    (B) atheromas
    (C) temporal arteritis
    (D) retrobulbar hemorrhages
    (E) syphilis   *(Ref. 56)*

174. Which of the following conditions may arise from the meibomian glands?

    (A) chalazion
    (B) hordeolum
    (C) sebaceous cell carcinoma
    (D) uveitis
    (E) cataracts   *(Ref. 6)*

175. Myasthenia gravis may present with

    (A) ptosis
    (B) diplopia
    (C) difficulty in combing the hair
    (D) loss of facial expression
    (E) choking of food   *(Ref. 6)*

176. Osteogenesis imperfecta is characterized by

    (A) pink sclera
    (B) fragile bones
    (C) glaucoma
    (D) keratoconus
    (E) megalocornea   *(Ref. 75)*

177. The complications of central retinal vein occlusion include

    (A) retinal neovascularization
    (B) rubeosis iridis
    (C) glaucoma
    (D) cataracts
    (E) retinoblastoma   *(Ref. 56)*

178. Tay–Sachs disease is characterized by

    (A) a cherry-red spot in the disk
    (B) patients are all of Hispanic origin
    (C) dementia
    (D) deafness
    (E) blindness   *(Ref. 56)*

179. A 12-year-old boy is noted for asymmetry of the scapulae as he bends forward to touch his toes. You will now

    (A) order computed tomography (CT) of both scapulae
    (B) schedule magnetic resonance imaging (MRI) of the great toes
    (C) determine serum uric acid level
    (D) perform emergency surgical correction
    (E) evaluate similar conditions in all family members   *(Ref. 66)*

180. Osgood–Schlatter disease

    (A) mainly affects the elderly
    (B) occurs at the navicular bone
    (C) causes carpal tunnel syndrome
    (D) is treated by Flagyl (metronidazole)
    (E) patients should avoid kicking exercises
                                            (Ref. 4)

181. Morton's neuroma is

    (A) more prevalent in males than females
    (B) found between the third and fourth toes

(C) more prevalent in patients with short-ened first metatarsal and lengthened second toe

(D) characterized by pain in the forefoot

(E) characterized by patient's desire to take off the shoe and massage the foot

(Ref. 2)

182. Dermatomyositis is associated with

(A) Gottron's papules

(B) pulmonary fibrosis

(C) bronchogenic carcinoma

(D) myocarditis

(E) breast cancer   (Ref. 55)

183. "Growing pains"

(A) are caused by chlamydia

(B) are common in children

(C) usually occur at night

(D) commonly occur in the thighs

(E) can be severe   (Ref. 3)

184. A 45-year-old male presents with right knee pain for 2 years. The x-ray shows linear, stippled calcification of medial and lateral menisci. The disease may be associated with

(A) gout

(B) hemochromatosis–hemosiderosis

(C) hyperparathyroidism

(D) hypomagnesemia

(E) hereditary hypophosphatasia   (Ref. 63)

185. Tennis elbow is characterized by

(A) tenderness over the radial styloid

(B) pain at the glenohumeral joint

(C) pain exacerbated by extension of the wrist against resistance

(D) common occurrence in workers who swing a hammer

(E) improvement by rest   (Ref. 63)

186. Golfer's elbow is

(A) lateral epicondylitis

(B) patellar tendinitis

(C) carpal tunnel syndrome

(D) thoracic outlet syndrome

(E) medial epicondylitis   (Ref. 2)

187. Jumper's knee is due to

(A) patellar dislocation

(B) fracture of the femoral condyle

(C) fracture of the tibial condyle

(D) patellar fracture

(E) patellar tendinitis   (Ref. 2)

188. The iliotibial band syndrome is characterized by

(A) dislocation of the hip

(B) lateral knee pain

(C) scrotal pain

(D) improved by climbing up stairs

(E) femoral fractures   (Ref. 63)

189. Osteomalacia is often associated with

(A) intestinal malabsorption

(B) renal dialysis

(C) high intake of vitamin D

(D) anticonvulsants

(E) low intake of vitamin C   (Ref. 63)

190. A 53-year-old male presents with a painful left shoulder for 3 months after a vacation trip. He cannot abduct the arm more than 80 degrees away from the side. He is probably suffering from

(A) a dislocated left shoulder

(B) lateral epicondylitis

(C) frozen shoulder

(D) thoracic outlet syndrome

(E) cervical disk disease   (Ref. 2)

191. Nursemaid's elbow is

(A) usually seen in children less than 4 years old

(B) subluxation of the radial head

(C) diagnosed only by MRI

(D) treated by flexing the elbow to 90 degrees and rotating the forearm to supination

(E) suspected when the child refuses to use the affected arm   (Ref. 8)

192. Carpal tunnel syndrome is associated with

    (A) Colles' fracture
    (B) arthritic spurs
    (C) rheumatoid synovitis
    (D) pregnancy
    (E) hypertension   *(Ref. 63)*

193. Thoracic outlet syndrome is often presented

    (A) as hyperabduction of the arm that may decrease the radial pulse
    (B) as tenderness over the lateral epicondyle
    (C) as calcific bursitis
    (D) during the first trimester of pregnancy
    (E) as pain along the radial styloid   *(Ref. 1)*

194. Polyarteritis nodosa is manifested by

    (A) hypotension
    (B) fever
    (C) eosinophilia
    (D) cholecystitis
    (E) arthralgia   *(Ref. 55)*

195. Sinusitis may be a symptom of

    (A) Wegener's granulomatosis
    (B) orbital cellulitis
    (C) meningitis
    (D) osteomyelitis of facial bones
    (E) diabetes mellitus   *(Ref. 10)*

196. At a dinner party, a 53-year-old female suddenly experiences severe facial pain and she cannot close her mouth. The most likely problem is

    (A) herpes stomatitis
    (B) Bell's palsy
    (C) mandible dislocation
    (D) acute maxillar sinusitis
    (E) quinsy   *(Ref. 45)*

197. Reiter syndrome consists of

    (A) conjunctivitis
    (B) arthritis
    (C) urethritis

    (D) infectious diarrhea
    (E) chlamydial infection   *(Ref. 56)*

198. Peyronie's disease is characterized by

    (A) acute conjunctivitis
    (B) acute sinusitis
    (C) acute tonsillitis
    (D) scrotal swelling
    (E) penile induration   *(Ref. 15)*

199. The symptoms of pyelonephritis in adult patients may include

    (A) fever
    (B) flank pain
    (C) general malaise
    (D) vomiting
    (E) anorexia   *(Ref. 15)*

200. A 47-year-old male was found to have mild Paget's disease. To provide comprehensive and continuous total health care for him, you will be concerned with the early sign of malignant degeneration, which is most likely presented as

    (A) worsening of pain
    (B) hypomagnesemia
    (C) decreased urinary hydroxyproline
    (D) increased serum acid phosphatase level
    (E) prostatic hypertrophy   *(Ref. 2)*

201. Drugs that may cause hearing loss include

    (A) furosemide
    (B) quinidine
    (C) gentamycin
    (D) kanamycin
    (E) polymyxin B   *(Ref. 28)*

202. Ménière's disease is characterized by

    (A) vertigo
    (B) tinnitus
    (C) fluctuating hearing loss
    (D) nausea
    (E) nystagmus   *(Ref. 28)*

203. A 70-year-old Chinese woman complains of midback pain for 6 months. The examination shows a bump in the midback. No neurological signs are elicted. The most appropriate treatment plan is

(A) surgical resection of the back bump
(B) transcutaneous corticosteroid injection
(C) analgesics
(D) acupuncture
(E) immobilization   (Ref. 2)

204. Torsion of the testicle is characterized by

(A) sudden onset
(B) nausea
(C) fever
(D) pain alleviated by lifting up the testicle
(E) a posteriorly located epididymis
                                       (Ref. 15)

205. Acute epididymitis is usually characterized by

(A) sudden onset
(B) nausea
(C) anterior position of the epididymis
(D) pain increased by lifting up the testicle
(E) normal urinalysis   (Ref. 15)

206. A 70-year-old female has had osteoporosis for 2 years. After a fall at home, she now cannot stand and bear weight. Her right leg is shorter than her left leg. She is most likely suffering from

(A) poliomyelitis
(B) hip fracture
(C) Legg–Calvé–Perthes disease
(D) hip osteoarthritis
(E) metastatic breast cancer in the right leg
                                       (Ref. 2)

207. Cystinuria is characterized by

(A) flank pain
(B) hematuria
(C) renal colic

(D) the presence of cystine crystals in the urine
(E) renal insufficiency   (Ref. 15)

208. Which of the following occupations are at higher risk to develop noise-induced hearing loss?

(A) physicians
(B) pharmacists
(C) airport workers
(D) nurses
(E) gunfighters   (Ref. 28)

209. In otosclerosis

(A) most patients are in their infancy
(B) it may become worse during pregnancy
(C) it is often familial
(D) the hearing loss can be of sensorineural type
(E) tympanic membranes are usually normal
                                       (Ref. 28)

210. Low back pain may be produced by

(A) vertebral osteomyelitis
(B) pleural effusions
(C) abdominal aortic aneurysm
(D) multiple myeloma
(E) large bowel obstruction   (Ref. 63)

211. Sensorineural hearing loss is usually caused by

(A) hyperlipidemia
(B) head trauma
(C) hypothyroidism
(D) chronic renal disease
(E) acute otitis media   (Ref. 28)

212. Conductive hearing loss is usually produced by

(A) acute otitis media
(B) chronic otitis media
(C) serous otitis media
(D) impacted cerumen
(E) Paget's disease   (Ref. 28)

213. Complications of vasectomy include

(A) hematoma
(B) congestive epididymitis
(C) vasourinary fistula
(D) sperm granuloma
(E) hepatoma   *(Ref. 2)*

214. Acoustic neurinoma is characterized by

(A) conductive hearing loss
(B) dizziness
(C) tinnitus
(D) impaired speech discrimination
(E) angina pectoris   *(Ref. 28)*

215. A 45-year-old female complains of pain behind her right ankle that is aggravated by walking, particularly going up stairs. The range of motion of the ankle is normal, but there is tenderness behind the ankle. The most likely diagnosis is

(A) pre-Achilles bursitis
(B) Achilles tendinitis
(C) acute ankle sprain
(D) retrocalcaneal bursitis
(E) posterior tibialis tenosynovitis   *(Ref. 84)*

216. A pituitary tumor may produce

(A) central scotoma
(B) macular-sparing bitemporal hemianopsia
(C) macular-sparing homonymous hemianopsia
(D) bitemporal hemianopsia
(E) homonymous hemianopsia   *(Ref. 56)*

217. A tumor in the right visual cortex (occipital lobe) may produce

(A) right homonymous hemianopsia with macular sparing
(B) left homonymous hemianopsia
(C) right homonymous hemianopsia
(D) right homonymous hemianopsia with macular sparing
(E) bitemporal hemianopsia   *(Ref. 56)*

218. A cerebrovascular accident (CVA) lesion at the left optic tract may produce

(A) right total blindness
(B) right homonymous hemianopsia
(C) right homonymous hemianopsia with macular sparing
(D) bitemporal hemianopsia
(E) left homonymous hemianopsia   *(Ref. 56)*

219. Osteoarthritis is characterized by the enlargement of the proximal interphalangeal joint. The enlargement is

(A) a subcutaneous nodule
(B) a lymph node
(C) Bouchard's node
(D) a pseudocartilage
(E) Heberden's node   *(Ref. 63)*

220. Acute neurolabyrinthitis is characterized by

(A) sudden onset
(B) vertigo
(C) nystagmus
(D) nausea and vomiting
(E) hearing loss   *(Ref. 3)*

221. A tumor located at the left anterior temporal lobe may produce

(A) central scotoma
(B) bitemporal hemianopsia
(C) left congruous homonymous hemianopsia
(D) right upper quadrantanopsia
(E) left inferior quadrantanopsia   *(Ref. 56)*

222. Regarding corns and calluses

(A) corns are larger than calluses
(B) both are caused by pressure
(C) corns are malignant new growth
(D) calluses are premalignant lesions
(E) they occur most commonly in the upper back   *(Ref. 1)*

223. The side reactions of finasteride (Proscar) include

(A) headache
(B) impotency
(C) decreased libido
(D) decreased ejaculate volume
(E) increased prostatic volume   *(Ref. 35)*

DIRECTIONS (Questions 224 through 249): The following clinical set problem consists of clinical information presented in the format of questions or incomplete statements followed by a group of numbered options.

Indicate T if the option is true;
Indicate F if the option is false.

Questions 224 through 227

A female nurse caught you at the hospital cafeteria; she asked you to help her 9-month-old girl, who was irritable with a fever of 100.2°F. She was anorexic and vomited twice this morning. You would now

224. prescribe Prochlorperazine (campazine) 5 mg/teaspoonful qid

225. instruct her to use trimethobenzamide (Tigan) ½ suppository

226. tell her that you are fully occupied and run away from her

227. instruct her to try ice chips

Questions 228 through 232

The detailed history revealed that the baby also has had a slight cough, and the mother noticed that the baby has been pulling at her ears. The examination of both of the girl's eardrums revealed patchy, bright red spots on the tympanic membranes, which were not bulged. The throat was injected; the tonsils were enlarged, not red; and the lungs were clear to percussion and auscultation. The remaining parts of the examination were unremarkable. You would now

228. perform myringotomy

229. order a culture of the aspirate from tympanocentesis

230. perform a culture from nasopharyngeal secretions

231. perform an audiogram

232. order x-rays of both ears

Questions 233 through 236

A diagnosis of acute otitis media is considered. You would now prescribe which of the following antibiotics?

233. ampicillin PO 75 mg/kg/d for 10 days

234. isoniazid PO 10 mg/kg/d for 10 days

235. amoxicillin PO 75 mg/kg/d for 10 days

236. amphotericin B PO 1.0 mg/kg/d for 14 days

Questions 237 through 241

Complications of acute otitis media include

237. meningitis

238. recurrent infections

239. brain abscess

240. serous otitis media

241. facial nerve paralysis   *(Ref. 28)*

Questions 242 through 244

A 23-year-old female was married 4 days ago; she developed dysuria for 3 days. You will now

242. prescribe nitrofurantoin 100 mg 1 tablet qid for 10 days

243. give her 3 g oral amoxicillin stat

244. prescribe phenazopyridine (Pyridium) 200 mg 1 tablet tid for 3 days

Questions 245 through 249

A diagnosis of UTI is entertained; the high-risk groups of UTI include

245. patients taking cyclophosphamide

246. patients with diabetes mellitus

247. patients with pulmonary tuberculosis

248. patients receiving indwelling catheters

249. males with prostatic hypertrophy   *(Ref. 3)*

Answers and Explanations

1. **(C)** The most useful test in the diagnosis of lymphogranuloma venereum is the serologic (complement fixation) test. A serious complication is rectal stricture; tetracycline is effective.

2. **(A)** Acute neurolabyrinthitis is characterized by suden onset of vertigo, nausea, headache, and nystagmus. Neurologic examination is within normal limits.

3. **(E)** Presbycusis is mostly seen in the elderly. The hearing loss is bilateral, symmetric, and sensorineural. The onset is gradual, and the hearing loss is in the high-frequency area.

4. **(B)** Psoriasis is unusual at this age, and contact dermatitis from shoes is unlikely during the growing period due to frequent changes of shoes.

5. **(C)** *T. rubrum* infection (tinea pedis) is the most likely diagnosis.

6. **(E)** Screening efforts for prostate cancer include digital rectal exam, transrectal ultrasound, and serum tumor marker (PSA). Due to low sensitivity and low specificity of these three tests, a screening test for prostate cancer is yet to be developed. However, a few family physicians perform a rectal exam and a PSA determination yearly for male patients between 45 and 70.

7. **(C)** Acanthosis nigricans is a brownish, thickened papillomatous skin lesion that may be associated with obesity, hyperinsulinemia, stomach adenocarcinoma, lupus, scleroderma, Sjögren syndrome, Hashimoto, thyroiditis, ovarian hyperandrogenism, and uncontrolled diabetes. It can be induced by drugs such as nicotinic acid, estrogens, and corticosteroids.

8. **(D)** X-ray of the maxillary sinus will show opacity and sometimes a fluid level. If there is swelling of the cheek, either dental infection or antral tumor should be considered. The complications include spread to other sinuses (eg, frontal sinusitis), otitis media, laryngitis, pneumonia, or chronic paranasal sinusitis.

9. **(D)** In actinomycosis, pathognomonic "sulfur granules" are found in the pus. Treatment is with penicillin or clindamycin.

10. **(C)** Children often put foreign bodies in their noses. Paper wads, peas, pebbles, rubber erasers, and beans are the most common objects. The cardinal symptom is unilateral purulent nasal discharge.

11. **(B)** Actinic keratosis is a premalignant lesion, commonly seen on the dorsum of the hand. Farmers, fishermen, and sailors with actinic keratosis have an increased risk. The use of sunscreens is recommended. Rarely, keratoacanthoma may undergo malignant transformation to squamous cell carcinoma. Squamous cell carcinoma is also associated with leukoplakia, arsenic and tar exposures, lichen sclerosis et atrophicus (vulva), and radiation skin damages.

12. **(E)** The limited penetration in depth is a sign of good prognosis; frequent follow-ups for examination of the local site and regional lymph nodes are indicated. The follow-up continuity of care should be for life.

13. **(D)** Allergic rhinitis (hay fever) is best treated by eliminating the allergens or desensitization. Microscopically, the nasal secretions may reveal eosinophilia. Antihistamines are often used, and environmental control is needed.

14. **(C)** Quinsy is a collection of pus arising outside the capsule of the tonsil in close relationship to its upper pole. It is most frequently caused by *Streptococcus* as a complication of acute tonsillitis.

15. **(C)** The traumatic rupture of the tympanic membrane usually closes spontaneously in 3 months. All that is needed is to instruct the patient to protect the ear by using earplugs when the patient is shampooing and showering. The patient should avoid getting water in the ear canals.

16. **(C)** When the fourth cranial nerve is affected, a gross deviation is not often observed. The affected superior oblique muscle, however, will fail to intort the eye, and diplopia will result unless the patient tilts his head to the shoulder opposite the affected eye. This eliminates the need for intorsion, and fusion may be maintained.

17. **(B)** The most common causes of oculomotor paralysis (third cranial nerve) include trauma, carotid aneurysm, and diabetes. In diabetes, the pupillary responses are usually intact; in carotid aneurysm, they are almost never spared.

18. **(E)** In the common and benign form of subconjunctival hemorrhage, it should be noted that the gross hemorrhages that appear without cause are usually not related to hypertension or arteriosclerosis. However, when such hemorrhage is associated with extensive ecchymosis in the lids, one should consider an orbital neoplasm or a hemorrhagic dyscrasia. There is no treatment, and the hemorrhage is usually reabsorbed in about 2 to 3 weeks. The best treatment is reassurance.

19. **(A)** A symptom complex of headache, pain on chewing, malaise, or polymyalgia rheumatica in an elderly female with a high sedimentation rate may establish the diagnosis of temporal arteritis. One should look temporal to the eyes to find nodular, tortuous, or tender temporal arteries. Prompt treatment with high-dosage steroids appears to significantly prevent the irreversible blindness that occurs in 50% of cases.

20. **(B)** Werner syndrome is a rare hereditary disorder characterized ocularly by juvenile cataracts, glaucoma, and corneal opacities. It is probably transmitted as a recessive trait. The onset is usually between ages 20 and 30 years, with graying and thinning of the hair of the scalp, genital region, and axillas. Atrophic skin changes may also occur.

21. **(C)** Granuloma annulare occurs more frequently in diabetics and resembles a rheumatoid nodule. The eruptions are papules to nodules forming raised peripheral rings and central clearing.

22. **(E)** About one third of patients with central retinal vein occlusion have open-angle glaucoma in both eyes. This is considered to be a predisposing factor.

23. **(E)** Episodes of amaurosis fugax frequently occur as a result of atherosclerotic lesions of the ipsilateral internal carotid artery.

24. **(C)** Echothiophate iodide is an indirect-acting, irreversible anticholinesterase drug; thus, succinylcholine use should be avoided. Echothiophate iodide (phospholine iodide) is also believed to be cataractogenic in some patients.

25. **(D)** Sympathetic uveitis (ophthalmitis) is a bilateral granulomatous panuveitis that occurs after penetrating ocular trauma (may be associated with uveal prolapse) or following ocular surgery. The traumatized eye is the exciting eye and the other eye that develops uveitis later is called sympathizing eye. Sixty percent occur between 2 weeks and 3 months; 90% occur within a year.

26. **(B)** Thrombosis of the cavernous sinus is usually due to infection spreading along the venous channels, which drain the orbit, central face, throat, and nasal cavities.

27. **(B)** Acute glaucoma is an ophthalmologic emergency. The intraocular pressure is markedly increased, vision is severely decreased, the pupil is fixed and moderately dilated, and the cornea is edematous.

28. **(B)** Pellagra is due to niacin deficiency and low tryptophan intake. The sun-exposed areas of the body may develop erythematous vesiculation and hyperpigmentation. Depression and psychosis may also develop.

29. **(C)** Partial or complete obstruction of the sinus ostia causes secretion stagnation, decreased pH, and lowered oxygen tension to produce an environment favoring bacterial growth.

30. **(B)** The mongolian spot is a dusky blue pigmentation in the lumbosacral area of Oriental or black infants that usually disappears during childhood.

31. **(C)** The treatment plans for acute knee sprain include NSAIDs, immobilization, physical therapy, graded exercises, and the use of an assistive device. When a cane is used, it should be held on the contralateral side with a length of the distance between the foot and the greater trochanter to allow 20 to 30 degrees of elbow flexion.

32. **(B)** The medial meniscus is much more prone to laceration than the lateral. The typical cause of injury is a blow against the lateral aspect of the knee while it is flexed and the foot is fixed on the ground in an outwardly twisted position; thus, it is frequently incurred by young athletes and the elderly.

33. **(B)** The renal lesion of amyloidosis is usually not reversible and in time leads to progressive azotemia. The diagnosis is accurately made by renal biopsy.

34. **(A)** Treatment consists of resting the part and allowing the disorder to take its course.

35. **(A)** Hurler syndrome (gargoylism) is characterized by the excessive accumulation of intracellular mucopolysaccharides. X-ray often shows an enlarged skull with frontal and occipital hyperostosis; hypertelorism; a long, shallow sella turcica with anterior pocketing; and deformities of the facial bones.

36. **(D)** Colles' fracture of the wrist occurs in the elderly very frequently, possibly associated with osteoporosis. Although the bones are weak, they heal well. The median nerve is frequently injured.

37. **(A)** Ankylosing spondylitis (Marie–Strumpell's disease) is frequently seen in a young white man with chronic backache who develops progressive limitation of back motion, transient peripheral arthritis, uveitis, and aortic insufficiency. The late radiographic sign is "bamboo spine." Psoriatic arthritis may also cause backache and spondylitis but is a late manifestation, although it may occur as a primary disease. It is often associated with Reiter syndrome, psoriatic arthritis, and ulcerative colitis.

38. **(D)** Sjögren syndrome consists of dry eyes (keratoconjunctivitis sicca), dry mouth (xerostomia), and chronic arthritis. Lip biopsy specimens show infiltrates of plasma cells and lymphocytes in the minor salivary glands.

39. **(E)** Osteochondrosis of the femoral capital epiphysis (Legg–Calvé–Perthes disease) is most often unilateral. It is usually found in boys four to nine years of age and is characterized by hip joint irritation (protective limp and pain on forced motion) and referred knee joint pain.

40. **(C)** This is a classic history and description. Keratoacanthomas almost always respond to simple conservative surgical removal.

41. **(A)** Vitiligo has a strong familial tendency and is frequently associated with thyroid dis-

ease, adrenocortical insufficiency, scleroderma, alopecia areata, and pernicious anemia. The lesions are startlingly white, contain no pigment, and are frequently seen on periorbital areas, hands, axillas, perineum, and neck.

42. **(E)** Wine glass sign is usually seen in the calyces (spider crescent deformity). Sonography may reveal the association with polycystic liver. The treatment is usually symptomatic and supportive. In adults, the condition is transmitted by autosomal dominance, while in children, at least in some families, it is transmitted by autosomal recessive traits. Aneurysms of the arteries of the circle of Willis are frequently found. A normal hematocrit and renal failure may coexist.

43. **(A)** A normal young person can concentrate urine to 1.040. The urine-specific gravity increases as excessive water is lost. However, if the patient previously was unable to concentrate urine normally, the specific gravity may not rise even if severe water loss is present.

44. **(C)** Injury to the kidney usually can be revealed by a plain x-ray film. However, infusion urography should be done as soon as is practical. Retrograde urograms delineate the degree of injury quite clearly, but they are seldom needed. Infusion urography shows normal function and configuration if injury is minimal, delayed visualization if injury is present, and deformed renal pelvis or calyces if lacerations have occurred.

45. **(E)** The clinical findings of erythrasma are often difficult to differentiate from tinea cruris. The direct examination of scales with potassium hydroxide (KOH) will find hyphae in tinea cruris, as opposed to rods and filaments found in erythrasma. Erythrasma shows characteristic coral-red fluorescence by Wood's lamp examination.

46. **(B)** Prostatic secretion should be subjected to culture and sensitivity tests, though the cultures are usually negative. Three antimicrobials are usually active in prostatic tissue: erythromycin, oleandomycin, and trimethoprim. Since the bacteria are usually gram-negative rods, sulfonamide and trimethoprim may be administered.

47. **(B)** Nasal obstruction, yellowish nasal discharges, fever, headache, facial pain, and tenderness at the cheek and upper teeth characterize acute maxillary sinusitis. *Streptococcus pneumonia, Haemophilus influenzae,* and anaerobic bacteria are common organisms.

48. **(A)** Tinea versicolor is a superficial fungal infection of the skin, caused by *Pityrosporum orbiculare* and *Plasmodium ovale.* Involved areas are brown on untanned skin and pale on tanned skin. Loprox (ciclopirox olamine) 1% cream is very effective. Oral medications include ketoconazole, fluconazole, and itraconazole.

49. **(D)** Often, the differential diagnosis between pityriasis rosea and secondary syphilis is indicated clinically, and a VDRL (Veneral Disease Research Laboratory) test should be ordered. Pityriasis rosea is characterized by the herald patch and subsequent smaller eruptions in the trunk of "Christmas tree" distribution. This is a self-limited disease, which produces remission in 6 to 12 weeks.

50. **(B)** Nerve thickening and erythematous anesthetic lesion are characteristic of leprosy. Biopsy of the skin or nerve lesion usually confirms diagnosis. Dapsone and rifampin in combination are quite effective; however, they may cause "Lepra reaction" (fever, anemia, leukopenia, gastrointestinal symptoms, allergic dermatitis, hepatitis, mental disturbances), which can be treated with steroids.

51. **(D)** Nonallergic rhinitis with eosinophilia syndrome is characterized by sneezing attacks, profuse rhinorrhea, and itching in the nose or eyes. There is no seasonal preponderance, and congestion is not the major problem. Antihistamines and decongestants are not very effective, but nasal steroids produce dramatic improvement, with reduction of eosinophilia.

52. **(E)** Acute conjunctivitis, characterized by redness, chemosis, and mucopurulent discharge, is common in children, particularly in

newborn infants. Instillation into the eyes of prophylactic silver nitrate (for gonorrhea prophylaxis) frequently produces in the newborn a chemical irritation with a purulent discharge lasting 24 to 48 hours.

53. **(B)** Mycosis fungoides is T-cell lymphoma, and biopsy is indicated.

54. **(D)** Lichen planus is a chronic inflammatory disease associated with emotional stress in adults. There are gray lines on the flat surface of each papule (Wickham's striae). The eruptions are commonly seen along a linear scratch mark (Kobner's phenomenon). It can be caused by thiazide diuretics, gold, antimalarials, and phenothiazines. It is more commonly seen in diabetic patients.

55. **(C)** Salivary calculi usually present with a sharp pain and swelling at the area of salivary gland. X-rays reveal calcitic densities.

56. **(C)** In secondary syphilis, the skin lesions are often bright red vesicles with scaling. In gonococcemia, a few peripheral, raised, hemorrhagic necrotic pustules may be seen with arthralgias. In lymphogranuloma venereum, ulcers and papules are centered in the genitalia with fluctuant inguinal lymphadenopathy. In venereal warts, the lesions are commonly seen in the vulvar or perianal areas with pointed edges.

57. **(B)** Acute renal failure can be classified into prerenal causes, renal causes (proliferative glomerulopathies, contrast media, aminoglycosides, acute tubular necrosis, disseminated intravascular coagulation) and postrenal causes (obstructive uropathies). Prerenal causes are very common in the elderly and in children due to volume depletion. In volume depletion, urinalysis is normal (no proteinuria, no hematuria, no RBC casts, no eosinophils in the sediments), blood pressure is at normotension, and the ratio of BUN to creatinine is greater than 15.

58. **(C)** The glomus jugulare tumor arises from the glomus bodies located in the adventia of the dome of the jugular bulb. It may cause

tinnitus; hearing loss; throbbing, pulsating discomfort; and multiple cranial nerve paralyses (particularly nerve VII); profuse bleeding may follow manipulation. Surgical excision is indicated.

59. **(B)** Accutane (isotretinoin) decreases sebum production and is used 0.5 to 1 mg/day for 15 to 20 weeks. It may cause dry skin, dry mouth, nosebleed, irritated eyes, headaches, muscle pains, and fatigue. Accutane probably is harmful to unborn babies, so it should not be taken during pregnancy nor while nursing. Women taking the drug should use reliable birth control methods and should have at least one normal menstrual period after stopping therapy before becoming pregnant.

60. **(E)** Acute otitis externa is often associated with swimming ("swimmer's ear"), seborrheic dermatitis, or diabetes. It is characterized by pain, itching, and discharges. The ear canal shows crusting, scaling, erythema, and swelling. Topical antibiotics such as polymyxin B or neomycin can be used; corticosteroid ear drops are useful for underlying dermatitis.

61. **(A)** The diagnosis of gout is strongly suggested in a male by acute arthritis in the great toe following heavy alcohol ingestion. The presence of urate crystal in the synovial fluid is diagnostic. However, in clinical practice, the diagnosis of gouty arthritis is usually made through a detailed history and characteristic physicals with minimal laboratory test findings, including leukocytosis, elevated erythrocyte sedimentation rate (ESR), hyperuricemia, and dramatic therapeutic response to colchicine. However, in equivocal cases, synovial analysis and biopsy of a soft tissue mass or synovial membrane are required.

62. **(D)** In viral conjunctivitis, the discharge is serous, the conjunctiva is injected, and periauricular adenopathy is present. Usually, a history of precedent upper respiratory infection with pharyngitis (sore throat) can be elicited. Itching is usually not present in viral conjunctivitis but is a prominent symptom of

allergic conjunctivitis. In iritis, a small pupil and keratic precipitates are present; blurred vision with vomiting is present in glaucoma. In viral conjunctivitis, lymphocytes are found in scrapings from the infected eye. There is no specific treatment available. Antibiotics and corticosteroids are not indicated. The disease is contagious, and the patient should avoid spreading the disease.

63. **(E)** Ramsay–Hunt syndrome is herpes zoster oticus, characterized by facial paralysis, otalgia, and vesicles in the external auditory canal. Treatment includes topical anesthetic (dibucaine), analgesics, steroids, and acyclovir.

64. **(D)** Calculi of the salivary glands are most commonly found in the submaxillary glands, followed by the parotid glands and the sublingual glands. The presence of a stone in the submaxillary gland can be determined by bimanual palpation of the floor of the mouth, probing of the duct, and x-ray examination.

65. **(D)** Penis size varies in a range fairly constant in the normal male. However, the concern over the size of the penis is practically universal among men. The size of the penis is in the range of 7 to 11 cm in the flaccid state and 14 to 18 cm in the erect state. The size of penis bears no direct relationship to the body size, and the flaccid dimension bears little relation to the erect dimension. The female genitalia have a wide adaptability to penis size.

66. **(B)** Psychologic factors are the greatest cause of impotence. In over 90% of cases, impotence can be traced to conflict between the sexual impulse and its expression because of fear, anxiety, anger, or moral prohibition. The common causes of impotence due to organic factors include diabetes, castration, and multiple sclerosis.

67. **(E)** Lice infestation occurs in epidemics among children and is often passed to adults in their families. Pyrethrin (A-200) is the drug of choice for lice. Lindane (Kwell) is also helpful.

68. **(E)** All answers may be correct; however, the presentation is characteristic for quinsy (peritonsillar abscess), which may necessitate incision and drainage.

69. **(B)** Stevens–Johnson syndrome is a variation of erythema multiforme. It begins with a sudden febrile onset and involves subepidermal vesiculations which become ulcerated in the mucous membranes of the lips, buccal cavity, eyes, and genitalia. Pneumonia and arthritis may also be present. It is commonly caused by phenytoin and sulfa drugs.

70. **(A)** Hidradenitis suppurativa is a chronic, suppurative, and cicatricial disease of apocrine gland-bearing skin, mainly in the axilla (female) and perianal (male) areas. Dense fibrosis ("bridge" scar) and sinus tracts may develop. Etiology is from apocrine duct obstruction with infections. Microorganisms responsible include staphylococci, streptococci, *Proteus, Pseudomonas, E. coli*, and anaerobes. Obese patients are at a higher risk.

71. **(C)** Lichen simplex chronicus, also called neurodermatitis, is a circumscribed, itching area of lichenification. It is worsened by emotional stresses and results from repeated rubbing or scratching due to itching. It occurs mostly in the nuchal areas, feet, and anogenital areas.

72. **(C)** Sarcoidosis is a noncaseating granulomatous disease of unknown etiology that involves the reticuloendothelial system and can affect all organs. The Kveim test is positive in 70% of cases. Erythema nodosum, bilateral hilar lymphadenopathy, anemia, elevated serum calcium, increased gamma globulins, and ocular involvement are usually present (chronic bilateral uveitis).

73. **(E)** Presbycusis is characterized by bilateral, gradual, and progressive sensorineural hearing loss, initially occurring at high frequencies. Otologic examinations are usually normal; there is no history of systemic disease, inner ear toxicity, or ear diseases.

74. **(D)** Seborrheic keratoses are often associated with autosomal dominance. It is more common in males after 30 years of age.

75. **(E)** Most cases of otitis media with effusion resolve spontaneously, and observation is all that is necessary. However, the use of antibiotics for 10 days may increase the resolution rate with possible risk of untoward reactions.

76. **(B)** Tinea capitis is treated with oral griseofulvin (15 mg/kg/d for 4 to 12 weeks), fluconazole (50 mg/kg/d for 3 weeks), itraconazole (3 to 5 mg/kg/d for 4 to 6 weeks) or terbinafine (3 to 6 mg/kg/d for 4 weeks).

77. **(A)** Mild cases of dyshidrotic eczematous dermatitis usually revolve spontaneously in 1 to 2 weeks, and continuous care with regular follow-up is recommended. For moderate cases, steroids and antibiotics may be needed. Secondary infections with group A β-hemolytic streptococcus are common, and the large blisters are best to be burst. For severe cases, hospital care may be needed.

78. **(D)** Pemphigus is characterized by bullae that may start in the mouth. Nikolsky's signs are often positive, and corticosteroids often helpful. Pemphigus may be associated with D-penicillamine and captopril administration.

79. **(C)** Erysipelas is caused by group A streptococcus or, less likely, by group G streptococcus. It is a red, warm, raised, brawny, sharply bordered cellulitis. It often occurs on a preexisting skin wound and is most likely to happen on the face and leg.

80. **(A)** Erythrasma is caused by the diphtheroid organism *Corynebacterium minutissimum.* Treatment is by oral erythromycin 250 mg qid for 14 days.

81. **(E)** Ludwig's angina is the cellulitis at the deep facial submandibular space. It results from dental abscess, which is commonly caused by anaerobic bacteroids. Prophylactic tracheostomy may be needed to prevent glottic or hypopharyngeal edema.

82. **(D)** Herpes zoster is characterized by unilateral pain and a group of vesicles. It is associated with immunosuppression and human immunodeficiency virus (HIV) infection. Treatment is acyclovir 800 mg five times daily for 7 days.

83. **(B)** Epidemic Kaposi's sarcoma is characterized by violaceous nodules and edema secondary to lymphatic obstruction. It is more likely to occur in homosexuals, and AIDS is a real possibility. Immediate biopsy is needed to establish the diagnosis.

84. **(E)** At birth, the cremasteric reflex is weak or absent and the testicle is in the scrotum. In response to the exaggerated or strong cremasteric reflex, the retractile testicle is withdrawn into the inguinal canal. Repeated examinations may establish the diagnosis since the retractile testicle can be brought down into the scrotum by a warm, relaxed environment. The condition usually resolves by puberty without problems of cryptorchidism.

85. **(C)** A communicating hydrocele is an infant's scrotal mass that fills and empties with time or with changes in position. The hydrocele usually communicates with the peritoneal cavity and should be treated as an indirect inguinal hernia.

86. **(C)** Acrochordon is common polyps on the skin surface, also called skin tags. Treatment is electrodesiccation. It usually occurs in the eyelid, neck, axilla, inframammary, and groin areas.

87. **(D)** Systemic lupus erythematosus is frequently precipitated by hydralazine hydrochloride (Apresoline), phenylbutazone, phenytoin (Dilantin), reserpine, trimethadione (Tridione), and mephenytoin (Mesantoin). Antinuclear antibody (ANA), peripheral rim pattern of nuclear fluorescence, and antidouble-stranded deoxyribonucleic acid (DNA) antibodies are useful in diagnosis.

88. **(B)** Sturge–Weber syndrome is characterized by a port wine hemangioma on one side of the face following the distribution of the

trigeminal nerve. Unilateral infantile glaucoma with chorioid hemangioma may develop. Laser therapy is used.

89. **(C)** Rosacea is associated with marginal corneal ulcers and blepharoconjunctivitis. Alcohol should be avoided. Oral antibiotics (erythromycin or tetracyclines) are effective, and 0.75% topical metronidazole can be used.

90. **(E)** Oncolysis is often the prominent sign of pustular psoriasis. Psoriasis is characterized by silvery-white scaling plaques. HIV is the risk factor, and lithium, steroids, alcohol, and chloroquine can aggravate the condition.

91. **(A)** Neurofibromatosis is an autosomal dominant trait manifested by hypertensive headache (pheochromocytomas), pathologic fractures (bone cysts), mental retardation, brain tumor (astrocytoma), short stature, precocious puberty (early menses, clitoral hypertrophy). Sarcomas may arise within plexiform neuromas.

92. **(C)** Dermatitis herpetiformis is associated with gluten-sensitive enteropathy, IgA skin deposits, human lymphocyte antigen (HLA) B8, and HLA DR3, and is dramatically responsive to sulfones (Dapsone) and sulfonamides. Erythematous vesicles are often seen symmetrically in the elbows, knees, and buttocks in adults, with intense itching.

93. **(C)** Solar lentigo is a flat, dark brown macule of 1- to 3-cm size, usually present at the exposed areas such as cheeks, forearms, dorsal side of the hand, upper back, and chest.

94. **(D)** It is commonly seen in outdoor workers (farmers, ranchers, sailors) and outdoor sports persons (tennis players, golfers, deep-sea fishers, mountain climbers). Old age, blue eyes, childhood freckling, renal transplant recipients, and immunocompromised patients are at increased risk.

95. **(E)** Impetigo contagiosa frequently occurs in children in hot, humid climates. However, it can also occur in adults, often caused by infected children in the household. It is due to

S. aureus and/or group A β-hemolytic streptococci. Mupirocin topical ointment is useful, and oral dicloxacillin is effective.

96. **(B)** This patient is very likely suffering from atopic dermatitis, which usually shows an elevated IgE level.

97. **(B)** Ecthyma (ulcerative impetigo) is caused by group A streptococci and staphylococci. It is to be treated with oral antibiotics, especially erythromycin.

98. **(E)** Alopecia areata is the single- or multiple-patched hair loss resulting in localized balding. Telogen effluvium is a diffuse hair loss following stressful events by 2 to 4 months. These events include pregnancy, abortion, high fever, crash dieting, surgical procedures, and injuries. In time, complete regrowth of hair is usually the case. Reassurance is all that is necessary.

99. **(A)-T, (B)-T, (C)-F, (D)-T, (E)-T.** The following individuals are at a higher risk of developing malignant melanoma: persons with dysplastic nevi and their blood relatives; the blood relatives of patients with malignant melanomas; persons with light skin pigmentation; persons with a great number of moles; affluent indoor workers; individuals receiving intermittent, intense ultraviolet radiation in adolescence; persons with congenital nevi or with giant hairy nevi; and individuals receiving excessive sun exposure.

100. **(A)-T, (B)-T, (C)-F, (D)-T, (E)-F.** For patients with recurrent UTIs, liberal use of urine cultures and sensitivity studies to characterize the causal organisms will control the problems. Routine excretory urography, cystoscopy, serum creatinine, and BUN are needed for recurrent and prolonged UTIs. For young men and children, voiding cystourethrogram is needed to detect vesicoureteral reflux.

101. **(A)-T, (B)-T, (C)-F, (D)-T, (E)-T.** Amblyopia is reduced vision without organic causes; it affects 5% of the population. It is often associated with congenital cataracts, blepharopto-

sis, anisometropia, spherophakia, aphakia, strabismus, esotropia, and exotropia.

102. **(A)-T, (B)-F, (C)-T, (D)-T, (E)-F.** The management of amblyopia is to encourage use of the amblyopic eye by limiting use of the non-amblyopic eye. Occlusive therapy or cycloplegic drugs (such as atropine) are instituted as soon as amblyopia are identified in early infancy. Refractory errors are to be corrected by glasses or by continuous-wear contact lenses. In strabismus, occlusive therapy is attempted before surgical correction of the deviation.

103. **(A)-T, (B)-F, (C)-F, (D)-F, (E)-F.** For the initial episode, treat with acyclovir 200 mg PO five times a day for 7 to 10 days. For recurrent episodes, acyclovir 200 mg PO five times a day for 5 days may be tried but is less effective.

104. **(A)-T, (B)-T, (C)-T, (D)-T, (E)-T.** Clinical features of acute sinusitis include facial pain and pressure, dental pain, nasal congestion, purulent nasal discharge and postnasal drip, headache, fever, foul odor, nasal bleeding, sinus tenderness, swelling of the face or periorbital area, and middle-ear effusion.

105. **(A)-F, (B)-F, (C)-F, (D)-F, (E)-T.** Medical treatments of acute sinusitis include antibiotics; amoxicillin (children: 50 to 100 mg/kg/d orally; adults: 250 to 500 mg orally three times daily); alternatives for patients who are allergic to penicillin (erythromycin: 250 to 500 mg orally four times daily; tetracycline: 250 to 500 mg orally four times daily); systemic decongestants: Drixoral (dexbrompheniramine, pseudoephedrine; one tablet twice daily); and Dimetapp (brompheniramine, phenylephrine, phenylpropanolamine, one teaspoonful three times daily).

106. **(A)-F, (B)-T, (C)-T, (D)-T, (E)-F.** Contraindications to air travel include (1) absolute contraindications (unlikelihood of surviving flight, active contagious disease, complete immobility); (2) relative contraindications (cardiopulmonary condition,and recent myocardial infarction [until patient resumes normal activity], uncontrolled hypertension, severe congestive heart failure, symptomatic valvular disease, uncontrolled arrhythmia, unstable angina, room-air hypoxia, severe restrictive lung disease, congenital pulmonary cysts, pneumothorax, recent cardiothoracic surgery [3 weeks]); (3) neurologic and psychiatric conditions (recent cerebrovascular accident [3 weeks], uncontrolled epilepsy, recent skull fracture, brain tumors [primary or metastatic], uncontrolled violent behavior, claustrophobia, or aerophobia); (4) eye, ear, nose, and throat conditions (recent ophthalmologic surgery [2 weeks], sinusitis and otitis, mandibular fracture); and (5) other conditions (late pregnancy, anemia [hemoglobin < 7.5 g/dL], sickle cell disease, uncontrolled diabetes mellitus, recent cast placement, diverticulitis and/or peptic ulcer disease, recent abdominal surgery with anastomosis or fistula).

107. **(A)-T, (B)-T, (C)-F, (D)-T, (E)-T.** Neurologic complications of herpes zoster include isolated muscle weakness in the involved dermatome, anesthesia in the involved dermatome, encephalitis, meningitis, contralateral hemiplegia, post-herpetic neuralgia, myelitis, Bell's palsy, Ramsay–Hunt syndrome, Guillain–Barré syndrome, neurogenic bladder, ipsilateral deafness, diaphragmatic paralysis, optic neuropathy, and Brown–Séquard syndrome.

108. **(A)-T, (B)-T, (C)-T, (D)-T, (E)-T.** The following signs are common in nonorganic causes of low back pain: tenderness at light touch in nonanatomic distribution; exacerbation of pain with light pressure on the head while the patient stands; exacerbation of pain with passive rotation of the shoulders and pelvis in the same plane while the patient stands; muscle weakness or rigidity of nonanatomic distribution; disproportionate verbalization or facial expression; collapsing; and pain decreased by distraction.

109. **(A)-F, (B)-F, (C)-F, (D)-F, (E)-T.** Common tenderness sites in fibrositis are the midpoint of the upper fold of the trapezius muscle; second costochondral junction; site 2 cm distal to the lateral epicondyle; origin of the supraspinatus muscle above the scapular

spine near the medial border; anterior aspects of the intertransverse ligaments of C4–6; interspinous ligaments of L4 to S1; upper outer quadrants of the buttocks in the gluteus medius muscle; and medial fat pad of the knee.

110. **(A)-F, (B)-T, (C)-T, (D)-T, (E)-T.** Fibrositis should be managed with (1) patient education and counseling—definition of the syndrome, natural history of the syndrome, exacerbating factors (stress, biomechanical factors, sleep disturbance), and continuing follow-up; (2) physical modalities (particularly lower back and neck)—physical therapy; (3) exercise—low-level aerobic exercise; and (4) drug therapy—analgesics, NSAIDs, tricyclics and other antidepressants, and muscle relaxants.

111. **(A)-T, (B)-T, (C)-T, (D)-T, (E)-T.** Cutaneous larva migrans is mainly caused by *Ancylostoma braziliense*. The therapy is by oral thiabendazole, 20 mg/kg/d for 2 days. Side reactions include dizziness, headache, nausea, vomiting, and diarrhea. Topical application of 10% thiabendazole suspension qid is effective. The localized allergic reactions can be treated by topical steroids or systemic antihistamines.

112. **(A)-F, (B)-F, (C)-T, (D)-T, (E)-T.** To prevent contact lens-related infections, thermal disinfection is recommended for soft lenses with a low water content; chemical decontamination is preferred for soft contact lenses with a high water content. Patients with giant papillary conjunctivitis can change to rigid gas-permeable lenses.

113. **(A)-T, (B)-F, (C)-F, (D)-F, (E)-T.** Ankylosing spondylitis is often associated with uveitis, iridocyclitis, cardiac conduction defects, aortic insufficiency, aortitis, and restrictive lung diseases.

114. **(A)-T, (B)-F, (C)-T, (D)-T, (E)-F.** The following lesions should be biopsied: chronic ulcers; chronic bullous lesions; rapidly growing lesions (especially nevi); lesions with irregularly notched borders; congenital, raised, pig-mented lesions; and lesions that are difficult to diagnose.

115. **(A)-F, (B)-F, (C)-T, (D)-F, (E)-F.** Single-dose therapy is recommended for nonpregnant young women with symptoms lasting for less than 5 days. During pregnancy, trimethoprim-sulfamethoxazole is not recommended. Tetracyclines and erythromycin are effective against *C. trachomatis*. Doxycycline is not recommended for use in children.

116. **(A)-F, (B)-T, (C)-F, (D)-T, (E)-F.** Initial treatments of acute low back strain include bedrest on hard mattress, lying flat on the back without pillows with knees flexed, analgesics such as NSAIDs, and a low back support. An extension/flexion-graded exercise for the low back can be started after pain relief; the patient needs to avoid lifting heavy objects, and sudden back motion is to be avoided. Weight reduction is recommended for obese patients.

117. **(A)-F, (B)-F, (C)-T, (D)-F, (E)-F.** The anterior talofibular ligament is located in the lateral ankle. It crosses anteriorly from the fibula to attach to the talus. It prevents the anterior translation of the talus on the tibia. This ligament is tight in plantar flexion and is most frequently torn with plantar flexion and inversion.

118. **(A)-F, (B)-F, (C)-F, (D)-T, (E)-F.** Rhinitis medicamentosa is rebound rhinitis, which is the result of abuse of nose drops and/or nasal spray. The sympathomimetic decongestants cause vasoconstriction which accumulate vasodilatation substances. A rebound vasodilatation produces nasal congestion again.

119. **(A)-T, (B)-T, (C)-F, (D)-F, (E)-F.** After 7 years of age the most common microorganism for acute otitis media is *S. pneumoniae*, followed by group A streptococcus. The treatment of choice is oral penicillin; erythromycin is the alternative drug. Parenteral penicillin may increase the risk of anaphylaxis. The topical antibiotics are used for otitis externa.

120. **(A)-F, (B)-T, (C)-T, (D)-F, (E)-T.** Vertebral compression fractures are stable fractures; immobilizations or surgical interventions are not necessary; counseling and supports are provided along with analgesics to relieve the pain. Once the pain subsides, graded exercises are begun to enhance muscular support. Estrogens, calcium, fluoride, vitamin D, and calcitonin are often used to prevent osteoporosis, which results in vertebral compression fractures. Long-term use of estrogen may be associated with an increased risk of endometrial carcinomas.

121. **(A)-T, (B)-F, (C)-T, (D)-T, (E)-F.** Complications include persistent otitis media, recurrences of otitis media, chronic serous otitis media, air conduction hearing loss, mastoiditis, brain abscess, and meningitis.

122. **(A)-F, (B)-F, (C)-F, (D)-T, (E)-F.** Plantar fasciitis is the tenderness in the sole of the foot about the midarch area. The most common tender point is the tendon of the flexor hallucis longus. It is more common in long-distance runners.

123. **(A)-F, (B)-F, (C)-T, (D)-F, (E)-F.** Patellar tracking syndrome (chondromalacia) presents as knee pain with tenderness around the lower medial aspect of the patella or the adjacent tibial plateau. The pain is worst when walking down stairs and can be reproduced by firm compression of the patella into the medial femoral groove while the knee is in slight flexion. It is called runner's knee if runners do not exercise to strengthen the quadriceps and stretch the hamstring.

124. **(A)-T, (B)-T, (C)-T, (D)-T, (E)-T.** Rheumatoid arthritis (RA) is frequently seen in women. Painful, swollen, small joints with morning stiffness are frequently experienced. Rheumatoid nodules in the lung may cavitate to resemble malignant lesions roentgenographically. Synovial fluid analysis may show inflammatory reactions with lymphocytosis. Aspirin remains the best drug for RA. The dosage for anti-inflammatory effects is higher than that for analgesic effects, and the doses tolerated by individuals tend to vary inversely with their ages. Gold salt therapy is useful but often must be discontinued due to unwanted side effects, which include the involvement of oral mucosa, bone marrow, kidney, and skin.

125. **(A)-F, (B)-F, (C)-T, (D)-F, (E)-F.** The treatment of fibromyalgia (fibrositis) is symptomatic. Trigger points can be injected with local anesthetics and steroids; give analgesics (acetaminophen, NSAIDs) and psychotropic drugs (such as amitriptyline in low doses) to patients as needed. The patient may benefit from comprehensive and continuous total health care.

126. **(A)-T, (B)-T, (C)-T, (D)-T, (E)-F.** Adenoid hypertrophy may cause nasal obstruction, leading to mouth breathing, poor rest at night, and a slight nasality of the voice. Chronic mouth breathing during the age when facial bones are changing toward the adult configuration often produces a high arch to the hard palate, pinching in of the nose, shortening of the upper lip, malocclusion of the teeth, and a dull facial expression (adenoid facies). Partial blocking of the eustachian tube may cause recurrent suppurative otitis media, serous otitis media, tinnitus, and fluctuating hearing loss.

127. **(A)-F, (B)-F, (C)-F, (D)-F, (E)-T.** Prostatic cancer is the most prevalent cancer in the male. There is no acceptable screening method at the present time. A family physician should perform prostatic examinations for all male patients beyond age 50 and should initiate appropriate work-ups for high-risk patients. A hard, fixed prostatic nodule is suspicious for malignancy.

128. **(A)-F, (B)-T, (C)-T, (D)-T, (E)-T.** Proliferative retinopathy (often referred to as retinitis proliferans) consists of the growth of retinal vessels into the vitreous, usually at the disk. They proliferate in a network pattern, may bleed and cause massive hemorrhage into the vitreous, or contract in scar formation that will detach the retina. Patients with any significant degree of retinopathy should be evaluated by fluorescent angiography.

129. **(A)-T, (B)-T, (C)-T, (D)-T, (E)-F.** Parents should know that practically all deviating eyes can be straightened by corrective lenses, miotic therapy, orthoptics, surgery, or some combination thereof, and that the straightening should be accomplished at the earliest possible time.

130. **(A)-T, (B)-T, (C)-T, (D)-T, (E)-F.**

Peripheral Nerve	Involvement
Median	Thumb and thenar eminence
Ulnar	Little finger and hypothenar eminence
Radial	Wrist drop
Femoral	Absent knee jerk
Peroneal	Foot drop
Sciatic	Pain down lateral thigh, absent ankle jerk

131. **(A)-T, (B)-T, (C)-T, (D)-F, (E)-T.** Reiter syndrome is characterized by nonspecific urethritis, conjunctivitis, keratoderma blennorrhagia, and arthritis. It is commonly seen in young men, and the arthritis is commonly asymmetric, with involvement of knees, ankles, and sacroiliac joints. The HLA B27 test is frequently positive. The other four types of arthritis all may involve both hands in a middle-aged woman with inflammatory reactions.

132. **(A)-T, (B)-T, (C)-T, (D)-T, (E)-T.** Necrotizing papillitis (papillary necrosis) is often due to the complications of pyelonephritis; however, it is also often associated with vesicoureteral reflux, diabetes, cirrhosis, sickle cell traits, and prolonged use of analgesics, such as aspirin or phenacetin. There may be fever, oliguria, renal tenderness, pyuria, bacteriuria, azotemia, and shock. Appropriate antibiotics may be used and underlying diseases controlled.

133. **(A)-T, (B)-F, (C)-T, (D)-T, (E)-T.** Uveitis is characterized by acute painful red eye with photophobia and blurred vision. It is often associated with diabetes mellitus, rheumatoid arthritis, gout, ankylosing spondylitis (HLA B27), Behçet's disease (relapsing iritis, aphthous and genital ulceration, HLA B5), Crohn's disease, ulcerative colitis, Reiter's disease (urethritis, conjunctivitis, arthritis, HLA B27), tuberculosis, sarcoidosis, toxoplasmosis, sympathetic ophthalmia, histoplasmosis, and nematode endophthalmitis; hypertension mainly causes retinopathy.

134. **(A)-T, (B)-T, (C)-F, (D)-T, (E)-T.** The blue nevus is rarely the source of melanoma, while junctional nevus is frequently implicated as the source of malignant melanoma. Senile keratosis is potentially a precancerous lesion. Arsenic hyperkeratosis frequently becomes malignant. Bowen's disease is usually a precancerous lesion of basal cell carcinoma.

135. **(A)-T, (B)-T, (C)-T, (D)-T, (E)-F.** The characteristic cerebral lesions are sclerotic patches (tubers) scattered throughout the cortical gray matter. Convulsions, mental defect, rhabdomyoma of the heart, and renal tumors are often associated. Adenoma sebaceum is the most characteristic skin lesion. It consists of small, bright red or brownish nodules in a butterfly configuration on the nose and cheeks. Hypopigmented skin macules on the arms, legs, and trunk are usually present from birth. The patient's risk of contracting tuberculosis does not increase.

136. **(A)-T, (B)-T, (C)-T, (D)-T, (E)-F.** Vertigo is intermittent, with attacks lasting between several minutes and several hours, taking the form of a definite feeling of rotation. It is preceded by pressure in the ear and is followed by malaise for several days. Deafness is perceptive and is more marked before and during an attack. The audiogram shows a perceptive deafness. The curve is fairly flat (the losses for high tones and low tones are similar). A calorigram may show nystagmus. Blindness usually does not occur.

137. **(A)-T, (B)-T, (C)-T, (D)-T, (E)-T.** In nonunion, the fracture is not united and will remain so indefinitely. The actual causes for this are not clear. Radiologically, there is a definite gap at the fracture site, the ends of the bone are sclerotic and smooth, and occasionally one end of the fragment has a cupped appearance.

138. **(A)-T, (B)-F, (C)-T, (D)-T, (E)-T.** Peutz–Jeghers syndrome is an uncommon familial disease manifested by intestinal polyposis (the colon and rectum are also involved in one third of the cases and the stomach in about one fourth) and brown pigmentation of the skin and mucous membranes. The hamartomas are of low malignancy potential, but ovarian and duodenal carcinomas are at increased risk of development. Recurrent colicky abdominal pain caused by transient intussusception is frequent. Surgical treatment is polypectomy.

139. **(A)-F, (B)-T, (C)-F, (D)-F, (E)-F.** Osteosarcoma of the femur usually presents with persistent pain at rest with swelling. There is often history of trauma. It is associated with bilateral retroblastoma. Ten to 20% of cases are due to metastases of cancers of the lung, but it is more common below the knee or elbow. Relapses are most likely from lung, cancers. Prostatic cancer is not common in children.

140. **(A)-T, (B)-T, (C)-T, (D)-T, (E)-T.** Chronic urethritis is a very common problem and is often called the urethral syndrome of the female. The patient may complain of burning on urination, frequency, nocturia, and urethral discomfort and stenosis. The urine examination may show no abnormalities, although it is often caused by *Ureaplasma ureolyticus* (sensitive to tetracyclines) or *Chlamydia* (sensitive to erythromycin or tetracyclines).

141. **(A)-T, (B)-T, (C)-T, (D)-T, (E)-F.** The most common cause of exophthalmos is Graves' disease (hyperthyroidism). Other causes include trauma, orbital cellulitis, cavernous sinus thrombosis, aneurysms, dermoid cysts, rhabdomyosarcoma, fibroma, paralysis of the rectus muscles, macrophthalmia, lymphoma, leukemia, and high myopia.

142. **(A)-T, (B)-T, (C)-T, (D)-T, (E)-T.** The etiology of osteoporosis includes (1) failure to develop normal skeletal mass during growth and development due to poor nutrition or inadequate exercise; (2) endocrine deficiency or excess—estrogen deficiency or testosterone deficiency, Cushing syndrome, hyperthyroidism or hyperparathyroidism; (3) immobilization or weightlessness; (4) hematologic malignancies; (5) inherited defects of collagen synthesis; (6) systemic mastocytosis; (7) heparin therapy; (8) rheumatoid arthritis; and (9) idiopathic juvenile osteoporosis.

143. **(A)-T, (B)-T, (C)-T, (D)-T, (E)-T.** UTIs are often associated with urinary tract anomalies, urinary stasis and obstruction or stenosis of the urinary tract, instrumentations, diabetes mellitus, pregnancy, renal calculi, initial sexual activities ("honeymoon cystitis"), and neurogenic bladders. Chronic UTIs can be suppressed by daily ingestion of trimethoprim-sulfamethoxazole (Bactrim) for 6 to 12 months.

144. **(A)-T, (B)-T, (C)-T, (D)-T, (E)-T.** Most causes of kyphosis are unknown. The onset is usually insidious and is more common in girls than in boys. There appears to be familial incidence. The condition may cause psychological problems, and empathetic support is necessary.

145. **(A)-T, (B)-T, (C)-T, (D)-F, (E)-T.** Noninflammatory, nonneoplastic enlargement of salivary glands, usually the parotid, is termed sialadenosis. Other conditions include ovarian or testicular atrophy, menopause, hypoproteinemia, malabsorption, obesity, pellagra, generalized malnutrition, beriberi, and hypovitaminosis A.

146. **(A)-T, (B)-T, (C)-T, (D)-T, (E)-T.** The conditions of FS are similar to the following conditions: metabolic problems (bone disease [eg, osteomalacia], hypothyroidism); inflammatory conditions (early rheumatoid arthritis, polymyalgia rheumatica, systemic lupus erythematosus [SLE], polyarteritis nodosa, seronegative spondyloarthropathy); infections (viral prodromes, subacute bacterial endocarditis, sequelae of viral infections or vaccinations, brucellosis and other unusual infections, acute leukemias); anatomic problems (hypermobility syndromes, idiopathic edema, muscle overuse syndromes, Paget's

disease); and neurologic conditions (early multiple sclerosis, early Parkinson's disease).

147. **(A)-T, (B)-T, (C)-T, (D)-F, (E)-T.** Nephrotic syndrome is associated with infections from syphilis, tuberculosis, and bacterial endocarditis, but there is no known association with tineas. Children with nephrotic syndrome usually run a fairly benign course. Adults with nephrosis fare less well, particularly when disease is associated with glomerulonephritis, SLE, amyloidosis, renal vein thrombosis, or diabetic nephropathy.

148. **(A)-T, (B)-T, (C)-T, (D)-T, (E)-T.** TB of the prostate and seminal vesicles usually causes no symptoms. The first clue is tuberculous epididymitis characterized by painless swelling and chronic draining scrotal sinus. Diagnosis is by chest x-ray, showing pulmonary tuberculosis and observation of tuberculous bacilli in urine. Infertility may be caused by TB salpingitis and TB orchitis.

149. **(A)-T, (B)-T, (C)-T, (D)-T, (E)-F.** Tabes dorsalis is a type of neurosyphilis that causes progressive degeneration of the parenchyma of the posterior columns of the spinal cord and of the posterior sensory ganglia and nerve roots. Signs of neurogenic bladder (painful bladder spasm, distention of bladder, and incontinence) may develop. Crises are common, including abdominal pain and dyspnea. Argyll–Robertson pupils are poorly reactive to light but well reactive to accommodation. Charcot's joint is joint damage as a result of lack of sensory innervation. Condyloma acuminatum is caused by human papillomavirus (HPV).

150. **(A)-T, (B)-T, (C)-T, (D)-T, (E)-F.** Chronic hypercalciuria and hyperphosphaturia may result in precipitation of calcium salts in the renal parenchyma. The most common causes are hyperparathyroidism, hypervitaminosis D, high intake of calcium and alkali, osteoporosis following immobilization, sarcoidosis, De Toni–Fanconi's syndrome, destruction of bone by metastatic carcinoma, and chronic pyelonephritis.

151. **(A)-F, (B)-T, (C)-T, (D)-T, (E)-T.** Acute prostatitis produces symptoms of urinary tract infection (frequency, urgency, dysuria), abrupt onset, fever, chills, low back pain, and nocturia. The prostate is tender, warm, swollen, boggy, or indurated. Common organisms include *E. coli*, *Pseudomonas*, and *Proteus*. Treatment with trimethoprim-sulfamethoxazole, ciprofloxacin, or ofloxacin is effective.

152. **(A)-T, (B)-F, (C)-T, (D)-F, (E)-T.** Sporotrichosis is caused by *Sporothrix schenckii* and characterized by a subcutaneous, indurated nodule with central ulceration in linear lymphatic distributions. It is common in farmers, lawn laborers, forestry workers, and rosebush cultivators. It is associated with patients with diabetes, HIV, alcoholism, carcinoma, and immunosuppressive therapy.

153. **(A)-F, (B)-F, (C)-T, (D)-F, (E)-F.** Xanthoma tendineum is a yellow subcutaneous tumor moving with the extensor tendon. It is a symptom of familial hypercholesterolemia caused by a defect in the low-density lipoprotein (LDL) receptors. A diet low in cholesterol and saturated fat is necessary. Cholestyramine and mevacor (Lovastatin) are helpful.

154. **(A)-T, (B)-T, (C)-F, (D)-T, (E)-T.** De Quervain's disease is a stenosing tenosynovitis involving the abductor pollicis longus and the extensor pollicis brevis tendons. In the Finkelstein test, the patient is instructed to make a fist with the thumb tucked inside the other fingers. Sharp pain develops when the wrist deviates to the ulnar side. It often occurs in postpartum women holding babies.

155. **(A)-T, (B)-F, (C)-T, (D)-F, (E)-F.** Still's disease is associated with uveitis, bilateral iridocyclitis, and band keratitis.

156. **(A)-F, (B)-T, (C)-T, (D)-T, (E)-T.** Chorioretinitis is most commonly caused by *Toxoplasma gondii*. Acquired toxoplasmosis is associated with fever, myalgia, and lymphadenopathy. All pregnant women need serology tests; if negative, infection of the fetus should be avoided (the probability is

1:10,000). Congenital toxoplasmosis may present with convulsions, scattered intracranial calcifications, chorioretinitis, papillitis, and papilledema.

157. **(A)-F, (B)-F, (C)-T, (D)-F, (E)-F.** *Trichinella spiralis* occasionally localizes in the extraocular muscles to produce conjunctivitis, lid edema, eosinophilia, fever, and muscle pain.

158. **(A)-T, (B)-T, (C)-F, (D)-F, (E)-F.** Marfan syndrome is autosomal dominant inheritance. The patient may present with arachnodactyly, laxity of joints, tall stature, ectopia lentis, retinal detachment, blue sclerae, glaucoma, and dissecting aortic and thoracic aneurysms. Intelligence is normal.

159. **(A)-T, (B)-F, (C)-T, (D)-T, (E)-T.** Glaucoma may be induced by the use of steroids, anticholinergics (atropine, belladonna), amphetamines, and hexamethonium. Periodic monitoring of intraocular pressure is advised.

160. **(A)-T, (B)-T, (C)-T, (D)-T, (E)-T.** Funduscopic changes in hypertension include vessel spasm, retinal edema, hemorrhages, cotton-wool spots, and papilledema; these are relatively reversible.

161. **(A)-T, (B)-T, (C)-T, (D)-T, (E)-T.** Cataracts are associated with diabetes mellitus, galactosemia, Down syndrome, myotonic dystrophy, hypophosphatemia, hypocalcemia, atopic dermatitis, gargoylism, hypothyroidism, and hypoparathyroidism. Cataracts can also be caused by the long-term use of drugs, including steroids, ethanol, phenothiazines, busulfan, and echothiophate iodide (a strong miotic used for the treatment of glaucoma).

162. **(A)-F, (B)-F, (C)-F, (D)-T, (E)-F.** Common ocular lesions associated with AIDS are cotton-wool spots, CMV retinitis, retinal hemorrhages, Kaposi's sarcoma of the conjunctiva, keratitis sicca, cranial nerve paralysis, and papilledema. CMV retinitis occurs in around one half of AIDS patients. Patients present with sudden, painless vision loss. The ocular manifestations include hemorrhage, cotton wool-spots, necrosis along the vasculature, and intense whitening of the retina.

163. **(A)-T, (B)-T, (C)-F, (D)-F, (E)-F.** Xanthopsia (yellow vision) can be caused by the use of digitalis or chlorothiazide.

164. **(A)-F, (B)-T, (C)-T, (D)-F, (E)-F.** Retinitis pigmentosa causes night blindness, gun barrel vision, and ring scotoma (loss of the peripheral visual field) and may be associated with abetalipoproteinemia, cataract, and glaucoma.

165. **(A)-T, (B)-F, (C)-T, (D)-T, (E)-F.** Central scotoma may be associated with optic neuritis and macular degeneration. Optic neuritis is associated with diabetes mellitus, multiple sclerosis, pernicious anemia, methanol, tobacco, quinine, lead, and salicylate. It is characterized by loss of vision, eye pain, transient blurred vision, and equal and normal size of both pupils.

166. **(A)-F, (B)-F, (C)-T, (D)-T, (E)-T.** It is estimated that one million Americans have undetected glaucoma, and the detection of glaucoma by the measurement of intraocular pressure becomes an important procedure in family practice. Any asymptomatic patients beyond 35 years of age with eye pressure beyond 22 mm Hg are suspicious. Acute symptoms include red eye, eye pain, nauseousness, and vomiting. Central vision may diminish; cup may enlarge to exceed 1:3 normal cup-to-disk ratio. It may cause arcuate scotoma in the early stage and progress to peripheral constriction later.

167. **(A)-T, (B)-T, (C)-F, (D)-F, (E)-T.** Diabetes causes formation of new vessels on the surface of the iris (rubeosis iridis), microaneurysm, hemorrhage, retinal detachment and cataract, and refractive error.

168. **(A)-F, (B)-F, (C)-F, (D)-F, (E)-T.** Direct observation of the sun during a solar eclipse may result in solar retinopathy, which presents with a macular hole resulting in central scotoma. The patient complains of painless loss of central vision.

169. **(A)-F, (B)-F, (C)-F, (D)-F, (E)-T.** Iritis is inflammation of the iris, presented with red eyes. There are no conjunctival injections or discharges. There is photophobia and constricted pupils. The cornea is not edematous, and the intracranial pressure is normal. Iritis should be differentiated with conjunctivitis and glaucoma.

170. **(A)-T, (B)-T, (C)-F, (D)-F, (E)-F.** Dilated pupils and pigmentary retinopathy may occur with the administration of phenothiazines, particularly chlorpromazine (Thorazine) and thioridazine (Mellaril).

171. **(A)-F, (B)-T, (C)-T, (D)-T, (E)-T.** Hypervitaminosis A may produce ocular palsies, retinal hemorrhages, exophthalmos, nystagmus, diplopia, strabismus, loss of eyebrows and eyelashes, blepharoconjunctivitis, and papilledema (pseudotumor cerebri). Band keratopathy is caused by hypervitaminosis D.

172. **(A)-T, (B)-T, (C)-T, (D)-F, (E)-F.** Gout may cause uveitis, iridocyclitis, scleritis, and episcleritis. Often, uric acid crystals may deposit at the cornea, resulting in urate band keratopathy.

173. **(A)-T, (B)-T, (C)-T, (D)-T, (E)-T.** Retinal artery occlusion appears as a cherry-red spot with pallor of the retina. It is most commonly caused by embolization. Retinal artery embolism may be caused by cholesterol, calcific, or platelet emboli due to valvular heart disease, polycythemia, sickle cell disease, or carotid artery stenosis.

174. **(A)-T, (B)-T, (C)-T, (D)-F, (E)-F.** Hordeolum is staphylococcal infection of the meibomian gland; warm, moist compression with topical antibiotics will resolve the infection. Chalazion is a chronic inflammation of the meibomian gland, probably resulting from a resolved hordeolum. Recurrent chalazion raises the possibility of sebaceous cell carcinoma.

175. **(A)-T, (B)-T, (C)-T, (D)-T, (E)-T.** Myasthenia gravis is characterized by easy fatigability of striated muscles, with unilateral ptosis and diplopia.

176. **(A)-F, (B)-T, (C)-T, (D)-T, (E)-T.** Osteogenesis imperfecta is characterized by multiple fractures, blue sclera, and deafness.

177. **(A)-T, (B)-T, (C)-T, (D)-F, (E)-F.** The central retinal vein occlusion may show vein dilatation, cotton-wool spots, hemorrhages, and swollen disk.

178. **(A)-F, (B)-F, (C)-T, (D)-T, (E)-T.** Tay–Sachs disease is the deficiency of hexosaminidase A with accumulation of GM$_2$ ganglioside in the ganglion cells of the retina. Mostly patients are of Ashkenazic Jewish ancestry. It is characterized by a cherry-red spot in the macula, dementia, spasticity, blindness, and deafness.

179. **(A)-F, (B)-F, (C)-F, (D)-F, (E)-T.** To provide comprehensive and continuous total health care for him, you will be concerned with the early sign of degeneration, which is scoliosis in the lateral curvature of the spine. A standing posterior–anterior (PA) spine x-ray is evaluated to determine the degree of curvature. A curvature less than 15 degrees needs continuous follow-up care, and a curvature greater than 40 degrees may need surgery. A curvature between 20 and 40 degrees may be corrected by a brace or with electrical stimulation. Eighty percent of scolioses are idiopathic; however, 5% of scolioses are congenital, and all family members should be screened.

180. **(A)-F, (B)-F, (C)-F, (D)-F, (E)-T.** Osgood–Schlatter disease is frequently seen in children 12 to 15 years of age, and x-ray shows irregular fragmentation of the tibial tuberosity. It is a common cause of knee pain in adolescents. The patient needs to avoid resisted knee extension, including running, climbing, and kicking.

181. **(A)-F, (B)-T, (C)-T, (D)-T, (E)-T.** Morton's neuroma is more prevalent in females between the ages of 15 and 55. It occurs between the third and the fourth toes, and neuroma can be palpated. Direct compression of the space reproduces the pain.

182. **(A)-T, (B)-T, (C)-T, (D)-T, (E)-T.** Dermatomyositis is often associated with scaling eczematoid dermatitis; Gottron's papules (flat-topped violaceous papules); telangiectasia; elevated creatine phosphokinase (CPK), aldolase, glutamic oxaloacetic transaminase (GOT), and lactic dehydrogenase (LDH); pulmonary fibrosis; and malignancy of breast, ovary, lung, and gastrointestinal tract.

183. **(A)-F, (B)-T, (C)-T, (D)-T, (E)-T.** Growing pains are common in children. The pain is poorly localized; is usually mild but can be severe; is mostly in the thighs, calves, back, and arms; and occurs at night.

184. **(A)-T, (B)-T, (C)-T, (D)-T, (E)-T.** In addition, chondrocalcinosis is also associated with hypothyroidism and neurogenic arthropathy. The synovial fluid shows leukocytosis and characteristic crystals of calcium pyrophosphate dihydrate.

185. **(A)-F, (B)-F, (C)-T, (D)-T, (E)-T.** Lateral epicondylitis (tennis elbow) is a tear in the extensor tendon, resulting in pain upon extending the wrist against resistance. It is associated with tennis players, throwing athletes, and workers who swing a hammer or heavy weight. There is tenderness over the lateral epicondyle of one humerus. It is an overuse syndrome, and rest and NSAIDs may be helpful.

186. **(A)-F, (B)-F, (C)-F, (D)-F, (E)-T.** Golfer's elbow is a result from the overuse of the wrist flexors, and it shows tenderness over the medial epicondyle of the humerus. Although golfers may also suffer from lateral epicondylitis (tennis elbow), they are more likely to suffer from medial epicondylitis. Rest and NSAIDs may be helpful.

187. **(A)-F, (B)-F, (C)-F, (D)-F, (E)-T.** Jumper's knee is the result of patellar tendinitis, which causes pain at the patellar tendon. Rest and NSAIDs are helpful. Quadriceps and hamstring muscle exercises are useful.

188. **(A)-F, (B)-T, (C)-F, (D)-F, (E)-F.** The iliotibial band syndrome is characterized by lateral knee pain distal to the joint line. It is aggravated by going up or down stairs.

189. **(A)-T, (B)-T, (C)-F, (D)-T, (E)-F.** Osteomalacia is due to intestinal malabsorption, renal diseases, renal dialysis, anticonvulsants, and inadequate intake of vitamin D. It causes generalized bone tenderness, and alkaline phosphatase is usually elevated. Serum calcium and phosphate are low or normal.

190. **(A)-F, (B)-F, (C)-T, (D)-F, (E)-F.** Frozen shoulder (adhesive capsulitis) characteristically occurs in middle-aged patients. The shoulder capsule shrinks and becomes a "check-rein" that restricts shoulder motion. Rest, NSAIDs, and gradual exercises may be helpful.

191. **(A)-T, (B)-T, (C)-F, (D)-T, (E)-T.** Nursemaid's elbow is the subluxation of the radial head caused by sudden traction of force on the child's forearm. It is common in children between 18 months and 3 years of age. Diagnosis is usually established by clinical findings.

192. **(A)-T, (B)-T, (C)-T, (D)-T, (E)-F.** Carpal tunnel syndrome is characterized by pain starting at the wrist and radiating into the fingers, innervated by median nerves. It is associated with pregnancy, gout, rheumatoid arthritis, and tenosynovitis—often associated with trauma.

193. **(A)-T, (B)-F, (C)-F, (D)-F, (E)-F.** Thoracic outlet syndrome is caused by the compression of brachial plexus nerve roots by a cervical rib, scalenus muscle, or the clavicle, causing a burning pain radiating from the neck through the shoulder and down the arm.

194. **(A)-F, (B)-T, (C)-T, (D)-T, (E)-T.** Polyarteritis nodosa may cause fever, weakness, anorexia, myalgia, arthralgia, hypertension, and glomerulosclerosis. Periarteritis of the gallbladder may cause cholecystitis and perforation. Arthritis of the hip, knee, ankle, and elbow without improvement by NSAIDs is common.

195. **(A)-T, (B)-T, (C)-T, (D)-T, (E)-F.** Complications of sinusitis may include osteomyelitis of facial bones, orbital cellulitis, intracranial infections, and meningitis. Wegener's granulomatosis causes nonbacterial rhinorrhea, sinusitis, myalgias, arthralgias, purpura, and glomerulonephritis, often leading to terminal uremia.

196. **(A)-F, (B)-F, (C)-T, (D)-F, (E)-F.** Acute dislocation of the mandible can be unilateral or bilateral and usually occurs due to overopening of the mouth while eating or yawning. The condyle becomes located anterior to the articular eminence.

197. **(A)-T, (B)-T, (C)-T, (D)-T, (E)-T.** Reiter syndrome is characterized by conjunctivitis (or iritis), arthritis, and urethritis. The discharge is usually free of bacteria; the agent is possibly *Chlamydia*, and tetracycline is useful. HLA B27 is often positive; ESR may be elevated and is associated with infectious diarrhea.

198. **(A)-F, (B)-F, (C)-F, (D)-F, (E)-T.** Peyronie's disease is fibrosis of the covering sheaths of the corpora cavernosa, which usually occurs in men over 45 years of age.

199. **(A)-T, (B)-T, (C)-T, (D)-T, (E)-T.** The differentiation of pyelonephritis with cystitis is often difficult. In pyelonephritis, the urine is usually cloudy, shows a little protein, and contains large amounts of pus and bacteria, with systemic symptoms.

200. **(A)-T, (B)-F, (C)-F, (D)-F, (E)-F.** Paget's disease of the bone commonly involves the spine, skull, pelvis, femur, and tibia. Initially, the pain is intermittent and mild. The urinary hydroxyproline will be increased, along with elevated serum alkaline phosphatase with normal serum calcium level. Following osteolytic and osteoblastic processes, the affected bone may result in deformity and fractures. It can also develop nerve compression, head enlargement, warmth of overlying skin, and high-output heart failure. Rapidly worsening pain is an early sign of malignant degeneration.

201. **(A)-T, (B)-T, (C)-T, (D)-T, (E)-T.** Ototoxicity often occurs in aminoglycoside and diuretics. It often is dose/duration-related but can occur even in the therapeutic range.

202. **(A)-T, (B)-T, (C)-T, (D)-T, (E)-T.** Ménière's disease causes tinnitus, whirling vertigo, and sensorineural hearing loss. Hearing loss is in the low tones, with fairly good high-tone hearing.

203. **(A)-F, (B)-F, (C)-T, (D)-F, (E)-F.** During the acute stage of vertebral compression fracture due to osteoporosis, bedrest is recommended. Analgesics (acetaminophen or NSAIDs) are used to relieve the pain. Gradually, a supervised exercise program is arranged for the patient. Cigarette smoking should be stopped, but alcohol is allowed in moderation. Calcium supplementation and estrogen (hormone replacement) therapy are recommended to prevent further progression of osteoporosis. The use of vitamin D, calcitonin, bisphosphonates, fluoride, parathyroid hormone, insulin-like growth factor I, growth hormone, and androgens should be used according to individual needs.

204. **(A)-T, (B)-T, (C)-T, (D)-F, (E)-F.** Torsion of the testicle is a condition almost exclusively seen in prepubertal boys, although it may happen in newborn males. Patients with cryptorchid testis are at higher risk to develop torsion of the testicle. Many patients may develop this condition during sleep, and many may develop it following or during vigorous activities (including sexual activity). Testes that are apt to develop torsion lie horizontal when the patient is standing. The examination of the genitalia reveals a swollen, tender right testicle that is retracted upward. Pain is increased by lifting the testicle up over the symphysis. The epididymis is felt in the anterior position. The lower portion of the spermatic cord appears to be thickened.

205. **(A)-F, (B)-F, (C)-F, (D)-F, (E)-F.** The typical epididymitis occurs in patients over 25 years of age. There is usually a history of infection with gradual onset. There are no systemic symptoms, including nausea and vomiting. How-

ever, fever may develop, with pyuria in the urinalysis. The epididymis is in the posterior position, with alleviation of pain by lifting up the testicle. The scrotum is red and swollen.

206. **(A)-F, (B)-T, (C)-F, (D)-F, (E)-F.** Osteoporosis increases the risk of fractures of the vertebral bodies (most commonly in the thoracic and lumbar spines), wrists, humerus, and tibia. The most catastrophic fracture is hip fracture, which may cause disability or even death (possibly from fat embolism).

207. **(A)-T, (B)-T, (C)-T, (D)-T, (E)-T.** The hexagonal crystals in the urine are pathognomonic for cystinuria. Cystine stones account for 1% to 2% of all urinary tract calculi. Hematuria, flank pain, renal colic, and UTI may be complicated by renal insufficiency.

208. **(A)-F, (B)-F, (C)-T, (D)-F, (E)-T.** Any services of intense noise, such as woodworking equipment, chain saws, internal combustion engines, heavy machinery, gunfire, or aircraft, may damage the hair cells in the organ of Corti. Any noise greater than 85 db is damaging. Noise exposure causes hearing loss in the high-frequency range, beginning at 1000 Hz, with a characteristic 4000-Hz notch. At 8000 Hz, the hearing loss is less.

209. **(A)-F, (B)-T, (C)-T, (D)-T, (E)-T.** Otosclerosis is the most common cause of progressive conductive hearing loss in adults (mostly in later teenage years and early adulthood) with a normal tympanic membrane. However, the hearing loss can also be of sensorineural type. It may progress rapidly in pregnancy. Carhart's notch is seen in the bone conduction curve (at 2000 Hz) of otosclerosis.

210. **(A)-T, (B)-T, (C)-T, (D)-T, (E)-T.** Low back pain can be produced by degenerative, inflammatory, metabolic, neoplastic, traumatic, congenital, and infectious causes. In addition, the back has always been a particularly susceptible "target organ" for patients with psychogenic disease. Low back pain is a very common problem in family practice. Eighty percent of adults will experience at least one incapacitating episode of low back pain dur-

ing their lifetime. It is the number one cause of restricted activity in patients under 45 and the number three cause in patients over 45 (after heart disease and arthritis).

211. **(A)-T, (B)-T, (C)-T, (D)-T, (E)-F.** Sensorineural hearing loss results from damage of the cochlea and/or eighth nerve. The common causes include drug toxicity (furosemide), abnormal glucose tolerance, hyperlipidemia, head trauma, neurosyphilis, and chronic renal disease.

212. **(A)-T, (B)-T, (C)-T, (D)-T, (E)-F.** Conductive hearing loss occurs when sound cannot reach the cochlea. The blockage may be due to abnormality of the canal, eardrum, or ossicles, including the footplate of the stapes. Lesions central to the footplate produce sensorineural hearing loss. Otitis externa, otitis media, and most cases of otosclerosis may produce conductive hearing loss.

213. **(A)-T, (B)-T, (C)-T, (D)-T, (E)-F.** About 500,000 vasectomies are performed in the United States each year. The complications include persistent sperm, spontaneous recanalization, occasional ejaculated sperm, hematoma, incisional infection, sperm granuloma, congestive epididymitis, and vasourinary fistula.

214. **(A)-F, (B)-T, (C)-T, (D)-T, (E)-F.** Acoustic neurinoma is derived from Schwann cells. The eighth, fifth, and seventh cranial nerves can be involved. Hearing loss and tinnitus are characteristic. Hearing loss is of the sensorineural type, with impaired speech discrimination. The patient may present with dizziness and unsteadiness, but true vertigo is rare.

215. **(A)-F, (B)-F, (C)-F, (D)-T, (E)-F.** Between the anterior border of the Achilles tendon and the posterior margin of the superior calcaneal tuberosity lies the retrocalcaneal bursa, which is frequently inflamed, resulting in posterior heel pain. It more commonly occurs in young women and may be associated with rubbing of the shoe against the back of the heel.

216. **(A)-F, (B)-F, (C)-F, (D)-T, (E)-F.** The site of damage along the visual pathway brings about the visual field changes. A pituitary tumor sits just above or below the chiasm. It often destroys nerve fibers supplying the inner (nasal) half of both retinas with defects of bilateral temporal visual fields.

217. **(A)-T, (B)-F, (C)-F, (D)-F, (E)-F.** A tumor in the right occipital lobe usually will result in loss of function of the left (opposite to the side affected) halves of both visual fields, to produce left homonymous hemianopsia with macular sparing.

218. **(A)-F, (B)-T, (C)-F, (D)-F, (E)-F.** A CVA lesion at the left optic tract may produce loss of function in the right (opposite to the affected side) halves of both visual fields, resulting in right homonymous hemianopsia. Occasionally, the hemianopsia is incongruous.

219. **(A)-F, (B)-F, (C)-T, (D)-F, (E)-F.** Heberden's nodes are bony hypertrophic or osteophytic articular nodules on the distal interphalangeal joints. Bouchart's nodes are the nodules on the proximal interphalangeal joints.

220. **(A)-T, (B)-T, (C)-T, (D)-T, (E)-T.** Acute neurolabyrinthitis is characterized by sudden onset of vertigo, nystagmus, and nausea and vomiting. There may be hearing loss and tinnitus. Symptoms usually resolve in a few days to a few weeks.

221. **(A)-F, (B)-F, (C)-F, (D)-T, (E)-F.** A lesion in the optic radiation usually produces congruous homonymous hemianopsia without macular sparing, resulting in poor central vision; a lesion in the temporal lobe produces upper quadrantanopsia in the opposite side; a lesion in the parietal lobe produces lower quadrantanopsia in the opposite side.

222. **(A)-F, (B)-T, (C)-F, (D)-F, (E)-F.** Corns are sharply delineated, smooth hyperkeratoses; calluses are large, diffuse, thickened skin. Both are the skin's physiologic responses to friction and pressure. Most commonly in the feet, corns tend to be round and measure from 3 to 10 mm in diameter. Calluses are usually much larger. Both are benign, and soft shoes with soft padding are helpful. The following are causes for corns and calluses: high-heel shoes, shoes too small, and faulty weight distribution.

223. **(A)-T, (B)-T, (C)-T, (D)-T, (E)-F.** Finasteride is the first-line treatment for mild to moderate benign prostatic hyperplasia. It reduces 5-α-dihydrotestosterone (DHT) with decreased prostatic volume. However, following discontinuation, DHT returns to baseline.

224. **(F)**

225. **(F)**

226. **(F)**

227. **(F)**

228. **(F)**

229. **(F)**

230. **(F)**

231. **(F)**

232. **(F)**

233. **(T)**

234. **(F)**

235. **(T)**

236. **(F)**

237. **(T)**

238. **(T)**

239. **(T)**

240. **(T)**

241. **(T)**

Although the curbstone consultation is often unavoidable, you should insist that the mother bring the baby to your office to form a professional relationship and to provide needed comprehensive and continuous total health care for the entire family. Acute otitis media is often diagnosed upon clinical findings, and the selection of antibiotics is usually based upon epidemiologic experiences. *S. pneumoniae* is often the most common pathogen, followed by *H. influenzae.* Thus, oral ampicillin 50 to 100 mg/kg/d in four divided doses or amoxicillin 20 to 40 mg/kg/d in three divided doses is usually initiated for 10 days. No response in patients may be caused by β-lactamase producing ampicillin-resistant strains of *H. influenzae,* and cefaclor (Ceclor), or trimethoprim-sulfamethoxazole (Septra or Bactrim) can be used. Oral decongestants, antihistamines, analgesics, and antipyretics are tried by some clinicians with variable results.

242. **(F)**

243. **(F)**

244. **(F)**

245. **(T)**

246. **(T)**

247. **(T)**

248. **(T)**

249. **(T)**

Although this patient is probably suffering from "honeymoon cystitis," detailed history taking and physicals are in order to differentiate among many conditions, including irritation of genitalia, vaginitis (this patient was in fact also found to harbor trichomonads), cervicitis, emotional stresses, and pyelonephritis. When acute cystitis is the probable cause of the presenting genitourinary symptoms, urinalysis is mandatory to identify the causal microorganisms in selecting appropriate antibiotics. *E. coli* is by far the most common pathogen, and single-dose therapy with amoxicillin or trimethoprim-sulfamethoxazole (Septra DS 2 tablets) is often effective. Urine culture and antimicrobial drug sensitivity test should be ordered. If bacteriuria (10^5 or more colonies) persists in 3 to 4 days, a 10-day course of ampicillin (250 mg qid) or Septra (1 DS tablet bid) may be continued. For those patients with pyuria and sterile culture, *C. trachomatis* is the likely pathogen, and doxycycline (Vibramycin) 100 mg bid for 10 days can be prescribed. Persistent bacteriuria and recurrent UTIs require thorough work-ups to identify structural or functional abnormalities of urinary organs and to determine current pathogens (such as candidiasis or schistosomiasis) or other etiologic factors (including sexual activities) for provision of continuity of care.

CHAPTER 6

Community Medicine and Geriatrics
Questions

DIRECTIONS (Questions 1 through 81): Each of the numbered items or incomplete statements in this section is followed by answers or by completions of the statement. Select the ONE lettered answer or completion that is BEST in each case.

1. The important characteristic of urban family medicine research is that it emphasizes

   (A) cross-sectional studies
   (B) inpatient care
   (C) a laboratory-based perspective
   (D) physiologic correlates of psychosocial variables in the inner-city environment
   (E) teaching hospital orientation   *(Ref. 5)*

2. According to the American Cancer Society, to detect lung cancer in an asymptomatic female, you would perform

   (A) chest x-rays
   (B) pelvic examination
   (C) sputum cytology
   (D) bronchoscopy
   (E) none of the above   *(Ref. 2)*

3. According to the American Cancer Society, for an asymptomatic woman following two normal examinations one year apart, a Pap smear is recommended

   (A) every month
   (B) every 2 months
   (C) every 3 years

   (D) every 10 years
   (E) no more required   *(Ref. 5)*

4. If a community is to double its population size in 23 years, the expected annual rate of increase is approximately

   (A) 1%
   (B) 3%
   (C) 5%
   (D) 10%
   (E) 25%   *(Ref. 54)*

5. When a disease lasts 2 to 3 weeks with a fatality rate of 80%, then its incidence

   (A) is higher than its prevalence
   (B) is equal to its prevalence
   (C) is lower than its prevalence
   (D) has no relationship to its prevalence
   (E) is one half of its prevalence   *(Ref. 3)*

6. Primary prevention programs

   (A) work to lower the incidence of psychiatric disorders
   (B) are planned for early identification of schizophrenics
   (C) minimize the handicapping effect of mental illness
   (D) operate for adolescents in jail
   (E) intend to build more mental hospitals   *(Ref. 3)*

7. In the 1990 U.S. census, it was found that

   (A) one-person households represented 25% of all households
   (B) all households were nuclear families
   (C) female-headed households comprised less than 5% of all households
   (D) most minority groups were settled in the suburban areas
   (E) almost all family households were headed by male adults   *(Ref. 3)*

8. Routine health screenings for an asymptomatic 55-year-old male include

   (A) complete blood count (CBC)
   (B) serologic test for syphilis
   (C) serum electrolytes
   (D) erythrocyte sedimentation rate (ESR)
   (E) stool for parasitic ova   *(Ref. 3)*

9. In a family practice center, there are 100 diabetic patients; through reviews of medical records, you found that 70 of them drink more than 32 glasses of milk a day. You will now

   (A) conclude that diabetes is caused by milk consumption
   (B) conclude that milk consumption is a risk factor for diabetes
   (C) advise all diabetic patients to stop drinking milk
   (D) advise all healthy individuals to stop drinking milk
   (E) conduct a study in the matched controls   *(Ref. 51)*

10. Patients/families visiting urban family practice centers frequently request help from family physicians in finding resources to meet their basic needs. The most likely reason is

   (A) family practice patients are sicker than patients visiting other specialists
   (B) family physicians are personally concerned with patients' welfare
   (C) patients find it easier to manipulate family practice team members

   (D) social services agencies rarely exist in the urban area
   (E) 90% of urban family practice centers are housed inside of social services agencies   *(Ref. 5)*

11. In the 1990 U.S. census, it was found that

   (A) all households in the rural areas were family households
   (B) all households in the urban areas were nuclear families
   (C) 90% of family households in the urban areas were headed by male adults
   (D) there were an average of 6.5 members in the family
   (E) 25% of all children under 18 were living with one parent   *(Ref. 3)*

12. The family physician is one who

   (A) serves as the physician of first contact and provides the patient a means of entry into the health-care system
   (B) evaluates the patient's total health needs and provides medical care within the sphere of his or her own competency
   (C) assumes the responsibility of total health care of the patient and his family within the medical community
   (D) accepts responsibility for the patient's total health care, including the use of consultants, within the context of their environment, including the community, the family, or the comparable social unit
   (E) all of the above   *(Ref. 2)*

13. In urban areas, there are often more physicians seeking jobs than there are jobs available. The most likely reason is

   (A) employment opportunities for spouses
   (B) most medical students are committed to urban underserved communities
   (C) most family practice residencies are located in the urban areas
   (D) most family practice residency graduates are interested in practicing in urban areas
   (E) less costly to live in the urban cities   *(Ref. 5)*

14. In 1990, most graduates of family practice residencies were practicing in

(A) inner cities
(B) suburbs
(C) large metropolitan areas
(D) midsize cities
(E) small towns   *(Ref. 4)*

15. In 1992, the leading cause of death in the United States was

(A) chronic obstructive pulmonary disease (COPD)
(B) suicide
(C) diabetes mellitus
(D) homicide
(E) heart diseases   *(Ref. 54)*

16. Concerning physician manpower

(A) the national average physician/population ratio is about 1:1000
(B) "overabundance" of physicians has been seen in other countries
(C) the number of osteopathic physicians is drastically declining in recent years
(D) 90% of physicians are engaged in primary care
(E) there is no shortage of family physicians in the United States   *(Ref. 2)*

17. In 1993, the number of homeless in the United States was estimated to be

(A) 0
(B) 0 to 1000
(C) 1000 to 10,000
(D) 10,000 to 100,000
(E) 250,000 to 3,000,000   *(Ref. 5)*

18. In 1989, the life expectancy of blacks was

(A) 10 years longer than whites
(B) the same as whites
(C) the same as Hispanics
(D) 10 years longer than Hispanics
(E) 6 years shorter than whites   *(Ref. 5)*

19. Qualitative data are often tested for significance by the

(A) t-test
(B) chi-square test
(C) analysis of variance
(D) product–moment correlation
(E) relative risk   *(Ref. 50)*

20. Concerning residences of blacks in the United States

(A) 90% of blacks live in the rural South
(B) 75% of blacks live in the inner cities
(C) 75% of blacks live in the rural Midwest
(D) 95% of blacks live in the suburbs of the large metropolitan areas
(E) 90% of blacks live in the small towns of the Northwestern states   *(Ref. 5)*

21. Two groups of 100 infants are compared for the effect on weight change of two different family counseling methods. You would use the

(A) chi-square test
(B) t-test
(C) product–moment correlation
(D) nonparametric test
(E) incidence rate   *(Ref. 50)*

22. The standard deviation is

(A) a measure of location
(B) equivalent to the range
(C) a measure of normality of the data
(D) a measure of the variability
(E) a measure of central tendency   *(Ref. 50)*

23. Three groups of 100 patients are randomly assigned to three treatment plans to measure the changes in blood glucose. The method of statistical analysis to employ is the

(A) chi-square test
(B) t-test
(C) analysis of variance
(D) product–moment correlation
(E) Spearman's correlation coefficient

(Ref. 50)

24. Concerning urban community resources
    (A) there are no agencies that provide emergency services
    (B) all agencies provide continuous long-term services
    (C) they provide services according to geographic boundaries; therefore, all areas are well covered without duplicating services
    (D) there are "working poor" who have problems in accessing needed services because their incomes are above the assistance level
    (E) when the urban poor are in crisis there are no agencies available to provide basic survival needs   *(Ref. 5)*

25. To grasp a central tendency, the best information is represented by
    (A) median
    (B) mode
    (C) mean
    (D) range
    (E) standard error   *(Ref. 50)*

26. The most powerful epidemiologic study is
    (A) prospective cohort studies
    (B) retrospective case control studies
    (C) cross-sectional studies
    (D) histolic time analyses
    (E) secondary data analyses   *(Ref. 49)*

27. Hallux valgus
    (A) is the medial displacement of the third metatarsal
    (B) is more likely to occur in boys aged 2 to 4
    (C) may cause lateral displacement of the fourth metatarsal
    (D) may cause pain
    (E) is the pathologic fracture of the thumb   *(Ref. 44)*

28. It is often difficult for a family physician to find satisfactory employment in an inner city. The most likely reason is
    (A) oversupply of physicians in the inner city
    (B) intense competition among family physicians in the inner-city area
    (C) difficulty obtaining specialist consultation in inner-city community hospitals
    (D) inadequate financial resources in the inner city to support a new family physician
    (E) inadequate continuing medical education programs in the urban areas   *(Ref. 5)*

29. At present, which of the following family practice settings is most attractive to the medical student?
    (A) inner city
    (B) underserved areas
    (C) large metropolitan areas
    (D) urban communities
    (E) rural communities   *(Ref. 5)*

30. A "typical" urban primary-care physician is most likely to be
    (A) one with a rural background
    (B) one who receives clinical training at urban clinics
    (C) one who prefers a suburban lifestyle
    (D) one whose significant others value rural living
    (E) one who takes a rural family practice residency   *(Ref. 5)*

31. The best appointment schedule in the urban family practice office is
    (A) 10-minute increments
    (B) prohibition of walk-ins
    (C) the stream system of 10 minutes per visit
    (D) the modified wave
    (E) avoidance of the long visit (eg, new patients)   *(Ref. 5)*

32. Strength of association between two variables can be tested by the

    (A) chi-square test
    (B) *t*-test
    (C) standard deviation
    (D) product–moment correlation
    (E) standard error   *(Ref. 50)*

33. Concerning family physicians' urban hospital privileges, which of the following is the most correct statement?

    (A) The intensive care unit (ICU) privilege is the easiest privilege to obtain.
    (B) Limited privileges for family physicians are usually related to their inadequate training.
    (C) As a general rule, the larger the city the easier for a family physician to obtain comprehensive, unrestricted privileges.
    (D) There are absolutely no problems for a family physician to obtain unrestricted obstetric privileges (including cesarean sections) at any urban hospital.
    (E) There tends to be a direct correlation between limited privileges for family physicians and the number of specialists practicing in that area at the urban hospitals.   *(Ref. 5)*

34. Urban "Medicaid mills" serve only Medicaid patients. Medicaid is

    (A) administered by the family practice residencies
    (B) exclusively for the person aged beyond 65 years
    (C) need-based entitlement
    (D) available only in urban settings
    (E) a cash-benefit program for the enrollee   *(Ref. 5)*

35. Which of the following is the most useful health screening procedure for an asymptomatic individual aged 50 years?

    (A) CBC
    (B) stool guaiac slide test

    (C) electrocardiogram (ECG)
    (D) chest x-rays
    (E) urinalysis   *(Ref. 5)*

36. Specificity is calculated by

    (A) true positive and false positive
    (B) true negative and false positive
    (C) false positive and false negative
    (D) true negative and false negative
    (E) true positive and true negative   *(Ref. 5)*

37. Sensitivity is calculated by

    (A) true positive and false positive
    (B) true positive and true negative
    (C) false positive and false negative
    (D) false negative and true negative
    (E) false negative and true positive   *(Ref. 5)*

38. The positive predictive value of a test is calculated by

    (A) true positive and false positive
    (B) true negative and false positive
    (C) true negative and false negative
    (D) false negative and true positive
    (E) false positive and false negative   *(Ref. 5)*

39. The prevalence of a disease entity can be estimated by the grand total (ie, the test population) and which of the following test results?

    (A) true positive and false positive
    (B) true negative and false positive
    (C) true positive and true negative
    (D) true positive and false negative
    (E) false negative and false positive   *(Ref. 5)*

40. An alternative hypothesis is

    (A) the null hypothesis
    (B) the correct hypothesis
    (C) to be accepted if the null hypothesis is rejected
    (D) to be accepted if the null hypothesis is accepted
    (E) the wrong assumption   *(Ref. 50)*

41. The most common skin problem in the elderly is

    (A) pityriasis rosea
    (B) varicella
    (C) basal cell carcinoma
    (D) pruritus
    (E) condyloma acuminata   *(Ref. 44)*

42. A discipline that studies the distribution of disease and its determinants in population groups is called

    (A) statistics
    (B) psychosomatic medicine
    (C) demography
    (D) epidemiology
    (E) operations research   *(Ref. 5)*

43. Which of the following is most commonly used in assessing community health?

    (A) infant mortality rate
    (B) prevalence of cigarette smokers
    (C) breast self-examination rate
    (D) median housing value
    (E) diptheria–pertussis–tetanus (DPT) immunization completion rate   *(Ref. 5)*

44. An example of secondary prevention is

    (A) detection of asymptomatic diabetes mellitus
    (B) use of seat belts
    (C) coronary bypass surgery
    (D) influenza vaccines for the elderly
    (E) DPT immunizations for infants   *(Ref. 5)*

45. An elderly patient newly admitted to a nursing home is negative for the purified protein derivative (PPD) test. You will

    (A) order an upper gastrointestinal (GI) series
    (B) order a chest x-ray
    (C) retest PPD
    (D) prescribe vitamin B$_6$
    (E) prescribe isoniazid (INAH)   *(Ref. 44)*

46. During an average month, 750 out of 1000 adults will experience one (or more) illness or injury. Of these 750 patients

    (A) all will be admitted to a hospital
    (B) all will be seen by a physician
    (C) one third will be seen by a physician
    (D) one third will be admitted to community hospitals
    (E) one third will be admitted to university medical centers   *(Ref. 4)*

47. Incidence is calculated by the number of

    (A) old cases during the study period
    (B) new cases during the study period
    (C) new cases at a point in time
    (D) old cases at a point in time
    (E) existing cases at a study period   *(Ref. 52)*

48. In epidemiologic studies

    (A) controls are not needed in retrospective studies
    (B) cases are not needed in determining frequency distribution of a disease
    (C) denominators are not needed to derive prevalence
    (D) characteristics of time, place, and person are usually described
    (E) population instead of samples is to be used for data collection at all times

    (Ref. 52)

49. In normal distribution

    (A) median equals mean divided by mode
    (B) 68% of observations lie within one standard deviation from the mean
    (C) 95% of observed values lie outside of mean ± 1.96 standard deviations
    (D) 5% of observed values are greater than 5.96 standard deviations from the mean
    (E) standard error is derived by the square root of the mean   *(Ref. 50)*

50. Recurrent cases are to be included in the calculation of

    (A) incidence
    (B) prevalence

(C) infant mortality rate

(D) crude death rate

(E) fatality rate   *(Ref. 52)*

51. Infant mortality rate is

(A) newborn deaths within one month per 1000 live births

(B) infant deaths under one year of age per 1000 live births

(C) total deaths per 1000 population

(D) one-year deaths with pneumonia

(E) infant deaths under one year of age per 1000 population   *(Ref. 52)*

52. In 1997, the number of deaths that occurred in a city of 10,000 was 98. The conventional expression of the crude death rate for this city is

(A) 9.8 per 1000 population

(B) 0.98%

(C) 98

(D) 980 per 100,000 population

(E) 980   *(Ref. 51)*

53. If the sensitivity of a screening test for a defined disease is 95%, then it may be expected that

(A) the test will be positive in 95% of individuals with the disease

(B) the test will be negative in 95% of individuals without the disease

(C) of the positive individuals, 95% will have the disease

(D) of the negative individuals, only 5% will have the disease

(E) 5% of the patients actually have no disease   *(Ref. 5)*

54. When measles virus is introduced into an isolated community that has had no known cases for 50 years, which of the following might be expected?

(A) sporadic cases largely limited to children

(B) sporadic cases involving both children and adults

(C) an epidemic largely involving children, sparing adults

(D) an epidemic involving children and adults under 50 years of age

(E) a completely unpredictable situation
                                               (Ref. 53)

55. Diseases are usually developed by

(A) the agent only

(B) the evil spirit

(C) the interaction of agent, host, and environmental factors

(D) the yin-yang forces

(E) random chance   *(Ref. 52)*

56. The advantages of the retrospective study as compared to the prospective study include

(A) relatively lower costs

(B) relatively small sample requirements

(C) easy-to-select matched controls

(D) extremely accurate data collected

(E) exceptionally reliable exposure information   *(Ref. 52)*

57. The characteristic triangular, broad-based pattern of the population pyramid in developing countries indicates

(A) low birth rate

(B) low death rate

(C) young median age

(D) high proportion of older people

(E) low proportion of children   *(Ref. 51)*

58. In a hospital, 72% of patients with a first myocardial infarction (MI) were smokers; this was the most common factor observed. What, if any, conclusions can be drawn?

(A) Smoking is a risk factor for MI.

(B) One needs to know the periods and intensity of smoking for these patients.

(C) One needs to know the age–sex–race composition of these patients.

(D) One needs a control group from the same hospital.

(E) This hospital provides excellent care for cardiac patients.   *(Ref. 50)*

59. Causality in the etiology of disease

    (A) requires a specific single agent
    (B) can be explained as due to multiple factors
    (C) cannot be determined by observational studies
    (D) can be determined by clinical impression only
    (E) must be determined before the disease can be controlled   *(Ref. 50)*

60. Health Maintenance Organizations (HMOs)

    (A) evolved from prepaid group practices
    (B) are limited to prepaid group practices
    (C) provide only preventive services
    (D) provide only multiphasic screening services
    (E) provide only inpatient services   *(Ref. 2)*

61. The neonatal death rate is

    (A) newborn deaths within one month per 1000 live births
    (B) infant deaths under one year of age per 1000 live births
    (C) total deaths per 1000 population
    (D) one-year deaths with pneumonia
    (E) newborn deaths within one month per infant deaths under one year of age
                                           (Ref. 51)

62. In your study, five blocks are selected randomly from 50 homogeneous blocks; 20 households are then selected randomly from each of these five blocks for household interviews to determine the health needs of the family members. This sampling design is called

    (A) area-cluster sampling
    (B) systematic sampling
    (C) simple random sampling
    (D) biased sampling
    (E) stratified sampling   *(Ref. 49)*

63. One hundred families are drawn from the problem-oriented records of a family physician's office on the basis of a randomly selected last digit of the family number. These 100 families are selected according to

    (A) area-cluster sampling
    (B) systematic sampling
    (C) simple random sampling
    (D) stratified sampling
    (E) purposive sampling   *(Ref. 49)*

64. One hundred households are selected from the entire 2500 households in the area on the basis of a table of random numbers. This sampling method is

    (A) area-cluster sampling
    (B) systematic sampling
    (C) simple random sampling
    (D) stratified sampling
    (E) purposive sampling   *(Ref. 49)*

65. Managed competition

    (A) is intended to escalate cost
    (B) is intended to limit access
    (C) is based on the fee-for-service payment mechanism
    (D) will greatly lower the quality of health services
    (E) offers independent providers to compete for consumers   *(Ref. 2)*

66. Most elderly Americans are

    (A) ambulatory and functional
    (B) bedbound
    (C) institutionalized
    (D) alone and isolated
    (E) without families   *(Ref. 2)*

67. The administration of aminoglycosides and cephalosporins to a 75-year-old female who is currently on furosemide may increase the risk of developing

    (A) necrotizing enteropathy
    (B) acute renal failure
    (C) hypocalcemic tetany
    (D) pulmonary fibrosis
    (E) thrombocytopenic purpura   *(Ref. 44)*

68. Falls among the elderly most commonly occur in

(A) the home
(B) the workplace
(C) public institutions
(D) streets
(E) motor vehicles   *(Ref. 44)*

69. Most elderly in the urban setting

(A) are alone
(B) are isolated
(C) have no family ties
(D) are independent
(E) are without friends   *(Ref. 2)*

70. A 70-year-old male living alone was brought to your office by his neighbor for irritability and confusion. He appears emaciated, and his tongue is reddish and swollen, with atrophy of papillae and ulcerations. His skin is dry, scaly, and hyperpigmented. The treatment of choice is

(A) mycostatin
(B) amphotericin B
(C) ascorbic acid
(D) nicotinamide
(E) tetracyclines   *(Ref. 9)*

71. In 1991, the elderly population accounted for

(A) 2% of the population
(B) 5% of the population
(C) 8% of the population
(D) 10% of the population
(E) 13% of the population   *(Ref. 2)*

72. A 65-year-old female with chronic osteoarthritis of the right hip develops intractable pain for 3 months. You will

(A) schedule for right hip total replacement surgery
(B) start intensive psychotherapy
(C) inject vitamin B_{12} IM

(D) prescribe Premarin 1.25 mg daily for 28 days
(E) consult an alternative medicine specialist
          (Ref. 2)

73. Your nursing home patient requires chronic indwelling bladder catheterization. You will

(A) use a closed drainage system
(B) prescribe campicillin 250 mg PO daily
(C) start imipramine 25 mg PO hs
(D) perform urethral dilation twice a week for 6 weeks
(E) irrigate the catheter twice a week with normal saline   *(Ref. 15)*

74. To provide long-term care for the elderly, the caregiver should

(A) avoid telling the patient the unfavorable prognosis
(B) perform all daily tasks for the patient
(C) restrict the patient's contact with friends
(D) leave the patient to perform daily tasks he or she can accomplish
(E) train the patient to follow only the caregiver's orders   *(Ref. 7)*

75. The sleep pattern in the elderly shows

(A) decreased nocturnal awakenings
(B) increased deep sleep
(C) increased rapid eye movement (REM)
(D) "lark" sleep patterns
(E) increased sleep latency   *(Ref. 44)*

76. For nursing home patients, the most important role of the family is

(A) to maintain the patient's outside contact
(B) to seal the negative feelings toward the patient
(C) to trust the judgment of the health professionals in the nursing home
(D) to relieve the heavy burden of caring for the patient
(E) to serve as the liaison between the attending physician and the nursing home staff   *(Ref. 7)*

77. The most common cause of tooth loss in the elderly is

    (A) osteoporosis
    (B) vitamin C deficiency
    (C) acute paranasal sinusitis
    (D) chronic periodontal disease
    (E) herpes labialis   *(Ref. 44)*

78. In a healthy, asymptomatic elderly female (over age 65), you would NOT provide which of the following health maintenance services?

    (A) influenza immunization
    (B) pneumococcal vaccination
    (C) mammogram
    (D) tetanus toxoid (Td)
    (E) bacille Calmette–Guérin (BCG)   *(Ref. 2)*

79. The best treatment for urge incontinence is

    (A) phenylpropanolamine 25 mg PO bid
    (B) a bladder training program
    (C) Premarin 0.625 mg PO qd
    (D) doxazosin (Cardura) 2 mg qd
    (E) amylodipine (Norvasc) 5 mg qd   *(Ref. 22)*

80. A 70-year-old female complained of urine loss during lifting of furniture for 4 months. She is most likely suffering from

    (A) urge incontinence
    (B) stress incontinence
    (C) overflow incontinence
    (D) reflex incontinence
    (E) functional incontinence   *(Ref. 15)*

81. In the elderly

    (A) platelet counts decrease
    (B) blood volume decreases
    (C) hematocrit is unchanged
    (D) white blood cells decrease
    (E) hemoglobin concentration decreases
                                           (Ref. 44)

DIRECTIONS (Questions 82 through 103): Each question consists of an introduction followed by some statements. Mark T (true) or F (false) after each statement.

82. Concerning DRG, which of the following statements is/are correct?

    (A) It is a retrospective payment system.
    (B) All physicians are employed by a fixed salary under this system.
    (C) It stands for Diagnosis Related Groups.
    (D) It considers only principal procedures for its classification.
    (E) It adopts ICD-9-CM for coding.   *(Ref. 44)*

83. In urban family practice, home visits are commonly made for

    (A) patient education
    (B) routine check-ups for chronic illness
    (C) administration of medications
    (D) acute illness evaluation
    (E) performing an appendectomy   *(Ref. 5)*

84. An 82-year-old healthy female traveled overseas, where she received cholesterol testing. She was told that her cholesterol was "high." You would prescribe

    (A) fluvostatin (Lescol) 20 mg PO qd
    (B) fluvostatin (Lescol) 40 mg PO qd
    (C) gemfibrozil (Lopid) 300 mg PO bid
    (D) cholestyramine (Questran) 4 mg PO qd
    (E) no medications   *(Ref. 2)*

85. Common eye changes in an elderly person include

    (A) presbyopia
    (B) reduced tear secretion
    (C) ectropion
    (D) entropion
    (E) arcus senilis   *(Ref. 47)*

86. Fecal incontinence in the elderly is most likely caused by

    (A) encopresis
    (B) depression

(C) dementia

(D) fecal impaction

(E) hemorrhoid   *(Ref. 22)*

87. Alzheimer's disease is characterized by which of the following presentations?

(A) a lack of voluntary movement

(B) poor immediate recall

(C) prior history of stroke

(D) progressive intellectual impairment

(E) inability of self-care   *(Ref. 7)*

88. Pressure sores mostly develop in the

(A) sacrum

(B) ischial tuberosity

(C) greater trochanter

(D) lateral malleolus

(E) tuberosity of the calcaneus   *(Ref. 44)*

89. Common causes of contact dermatitis in the elderly include

(A) neomycin

(B) nitrofurazone (Furacin)

(C) parabens

(D) vitamin E

(E) lanolin   *(Ref. 44)*

90. Cervical spondylosis is characterized by

(A) numbness and tingling of fingers

(B) clumsiness in buttoning shirts

(C) increased tone in the lower extremities

(D) impaired vibration perceptions in the legs

(E) postural instability   *(Ref. 44)*

91. Constipation in the elderly is often associated with

(A) lack of motility

(B) decreased fluid intake

(C) laxative abuse

(D) depression

(E) poor nutrition   *(Ref. 44)*

92. Halitosis in the elderly may be associated with

(A) leukemia

(B) ketoacidosis

(C) uremia

(D) depression

(E) hepatic failure   *(Ref. 47)*

93. The components of community-oriented primary care (COPC) include

(A) primary-care practice

(B) defined population to be served by the practice in the community

(C) systematically addressing major health problems of the population

(D) utilization of epidemiologic principles

(E) establishment of a primary-care practice in the community   *(Ref. 2)*

94. The crude death rate of community A is 6.8/1000; that of community B is 8.6/1000. The likely explanations include

(A) the death data may be more complete in community B

(B) the population of community A may be much younger than the population of community B

(C) the population size of community B may be smaller

(D) community A enjoys a higher health status than community B

(E) age-specific death rates may be lower in community A than in community B
     (Ref. 51)

95. An urban family practice center is open 24 hours a day, 7 days a week, 365 days a year. This will

(A) improve accessibility

(B) improve continuity

(C) improve availability

(D) increase the chance of robbery

(E) increase the possibility of assault   *(Ref. 5)*

96. The use of computers in the urban family practice office includes

    (A) scheduling of appointments
    (B) processing insurance claims
    (C) summarizing patient information
    (D) billing service statements
    (E) facilitating managed care   *(Ref. 5)*

97. Accessibility of care in the urban setting is improved by

    (A) adequate transportation system
    (B) establishment of urban family practice residencies
    (C) house calls
    (D) provision of free care
    (E) implementation of COPC   *(Ref. 5)*

98. The problem-oriented medical record (POMR) is simply a convenient way of displaying the patient's problems. This record is implemented when

    (A) a defined database is completed
    (B) a numbered and titled problem list is kept
    (C) a problem list is placed at the front of the record and regularly updated
    (D) progress notes are numbered and titled for each problem
    (E) the subjective, objective assessment, and plan (SOAP) system is adopted   *(Ref. 2)*

99. In Los Angeles, California, a city with heavy air pollution, it is found that

    (A) the incidence of lung cancer in the residents is 10 times higher than that of national average
    (B) 90% of the elderly are sick at all times due to air pollution
    (C) the children have had 10 times the incidence of upper respiratory infections (URIs) per year than children in the rural Midwest

    (D) 80% of the adults have had COPD due to continuous exposure to air pollution
    (E) the prevalence of allergic rhinitis is 200 times higher than the prevalence in Rhode Island   *(Ref. 54)*

100. A problem is

    (A) a symptom complex
    (B) a specific diagnosis
    (C) a working impression
    (D) an abnormal physical sign
    (E) an abnormal lab result   *(Ref. 2)*

101. Which of the following diseases may show a family predisposition?

    (A) epilepsy
    (B) schizophrenia
    (C) febrile seizures
    (D) alcoholism
    (E) varicose veins   *(Ref. 3)*

102. A positive family history is often present in the patient with

    (A) atherosclerosis
    (B) peptic ulcer
    (C) polycystic kidney disease
    (D) diabetes mellitus
    (E) breast cancer   *(Ref. 3)*

103. Multiple screening programs are effective and justified when

    (A) the screening test is simple, specific, reasonably cheap, and sensitive
    (B) methods and facilities are available to confirm the diagnosis and to manage the disease
    (C) incidence of the disease is sufficiently high
    (D) the screening test uncovers an appreciable number of new cases
    (E) the yield is high and the cost of resources expended is affordable   *(Ref. 2)*

DIRECTIONS (Questions 104 through 123): The following clinical set problem consists of clinical information presented in the format of questions or incomplete statements followed by a group of numbered options.

Indicate T if the option is true;
Indicate F if the option is false.

Sixty people attended a picnic at which the following foods were served: fried chicken, fruit salad, rolls, butter, coffee with cream and sugar, ice cream, and custard-filled pastry. Drinking water came from a spring adjacent to a river. Between 2 and 5 hours after the meal, 45 individuals became ill with nausea, vomiting, abdominal cramps, diarrhea, or a combination of these symptoms. Stools were watery, with some containing mucus but no blood. Temperatures ranged from 37.0°C (98.6°F) to 38.0°C (100°F). Attacks lasted for 24 to 72 hours. Recovery was uneventful in all cases.

Which of the following was the most likely cause of the epidemic?

104.   sewage pollution of the water

105.   *Staphylococcus* enterotoxin

106.   arsenic poisoning

107.   *Salmonella*

108.   *Shigella*

Which of the following laboratory examinations would be most likely to determine the causative agent?

109.   chemical analysis of the food

110.   bacteriologic examination of the drinking water

111.   bacteriologic culture of the leftover foods

112.   stool cultures of the people who became ill

113.   stool cultures of the people who prepared the food

Which of the following was the most likely source of the epidemic?

114.   an intestinal carrier of a pathogenic organism

115.   contamination of the spring by sewage

116.   an insecticide

117.   an attendant's common cold

118.   a pustular lesion on the hand of the baker

Which of the following was most likely infected?

119.   drinking water

120.   ice cream

121.   fried chicken

122.   custard-filled pastries

123.   rolls

(*Ref. 4*)

Answers and Explanations

1. **(D)** Important characteristics of urban family medicine research are (1) emphasis of ambulatory rather than inpatient care; (2) examination of clinical problem from an applied (eg, office-based) rather than basic (eg, laboratory-based) research perspective; (3) emphasis on longitudinal (over time) rather than cross-sectional studies; (4) a need for data that is not routinely collected as part of the clinical record; (5) examination of the role that psychosocial and other nondisease-specific factors play in response to disease; and (6) a need to conduct educational research to evaluate family medicine outcome.

2. **(E)** Chest x-rays and sputum cytology in an asymptomatic adult are not useful.

3. **(C)** A Pap smear is recommended every 3 years after two normal examinations 1 year apart; initial examination is recommended at age 20 or when sexually active. More frequent examinations are recommended for high-risk groups, including multiple partners (more than three) and early intercourse (before age 17).

4. **(B)** Neglecting migration (population growth is determined by the difference between immigration and emigration), the rate of population growth is expressed as the difference between the crude birth and death rates. A useful approximation is: years to double equals 70 divided by annual percentage increase.

5. **(A)** The prevalence (P) is related to both incidence (I) and duration (d) of disease: $P \approx I \times$ d. When d is short (acute) or there is a high fatality rate, then prevalence is low as compared to incidence. In chronic diseases, the duration is long and the prevalence will be relatively large in relation to incidence. If the incidence and duration have both been stable over a long period of time and the population is also stable, then $P = I \times d$, where d is the mean duration.

6. **(A)** Primary prevention programs exist to prevent maladaptation or malfunctioning from ever occurring. Programs for early detection and treatment of the diseases are programs for secondary prevention, while tertiary prevention limits or reduces the handicapping effect of the disease process.

7. **(A)** In the 1990 census, 25% of all households were adults living alone, a 75% increase in numbers from 1970.

8. **(B)** The most important health screening is a detailed history and physical examination. Serum cholesterol and serologic test for syphilis are ordered and stool for occult blood is performed. Other tests are to be ordered for high-risk individuals.

9. **(E)** The milk-drinking behavior of the healthy individuals should be compared with the diabetic patients' to determine the association of milk consumption and diabetes.

10. **(B)** Common reasons why patients/families request help from family physicians include (1) access to family practice centers is easier than in other community agencies; (2) family

physicians know the patients well and are truly concerned with their welfare; and (3) access to resources has been medicalized.

11. **(E)** By 1990, 16.6 million children were living with only one parent, a 5% increase from 1980. There were 3 million households that had cohabiting couples, an increase of 2.5 million since 1970. In 1991, only 26% of all households in the United States consisted of a married couple living together with children.

12. **(E)** The family physician is oriented to care for the whole family and the whole patient. He or she guides rehabilitation, practices preventive medicine, and is a medical advocate for his or her families. He or she assumes continuing responsibility for the health care needs of the family and provides comprehensive health care and disease management for all of the family members. Family practice is a useful way to meet community health needs.

13. **(A)** Many young physicians, both men and women, are married to people with their own careers. Large cities generally offer more employment possibilities for spouses, particularly those in the professions, than do small towns.

14. **(E)** Percentages of graduates by area settled are as follows: (1) small towns—63%; (2) suburbs—12%; (3) cities (100,000–500,000 population)—13%; (4) large cities—10%; (5) inner city—2%. With the expansion of urban family practice residencies, it is expected that many more graduates will settle in the large metropolitan areas and the inner cities.

15. **(E)** The 10 leading causes of death are: heart disease, cancer, stroke, COPD, accidents, pneumonia and influenza, diabetes, human immunodeficiency virus (HIV), suicide, and homicide.

16. **(B)** In 1992, the physician/population ratio was 1:392, and 4% of physicians were osteopathic physicians who have showed a steady growth in number during recent years. There were 72,000 family and general practitioners,

representing 11% of the total physician force. There is an acute "shortage" of family physicians. "Overabundance" of physicians has been seen in other countries; many physicians engage in nonmedical activities (such as taxi drivers), and many migrate to other countries.

17. **(E)** In 1993, the number of homeless in the United States was estimated to be 250,000 to 3,000,000, around 0.5% of the total population.

18. **(E)** In 1989, the life expectancy for whites was 75.9 years and that of blacks was 69.7 years.

19. **(B)** The chi-square test is used to test the null hypothesis of "independence" for the two classifications of a contingency table:

$$X^2 = \frac{\sum (\text{Observed number} - \text{Expected number})^2}{\text{Expected number}}$$

20. **(B)** Seventy-five percent of blacks live in inner cities, 34% of them in seven cities: New York; Chicago; Detroit; Philadelphia; Washington DC; Los Angeles; and Baltimore.

21. **(B)** The *t*-test is used to compare group means in two independent samples. It is particularly suitable to use in small samples (sample size less than 25).

22. **(D)** The standard deviation is the square root of the variance, which is the average squared deviation around the mean:

$$SD = \sqrt{\frac{\sum (\chi - M)^2}{N}}$$

However, the sample standard deviation is

$$S = \sqrt{\frac{\sum (\chi - \bar{\chi})^2}{n - 1}}$$

23. **(C)** The analysis of variance is used for comparing two or more sample means.

24. **(D)** There is an abundance of agencies that may create duplication and fragmentation of

services. Strict adherence to geographic boundaries often means that some areas are left without needed services. Many agencies provide basic survival needs for the urban poor on an emergency or crisis basis, but they need long-term solutions.

25. **(C)** The mean (average value) measures the central tendency. The mean is the sum of total value from all items divided by the number of items:

$$M = \frac{\Sigma x}{N}$$

26. **(A)** The prospective cohort study is that in which a group of people (cohorts) who are free of disease are classified by exposure (control and experimental groups) to a factor and followed prospectively (forwardly) for the development of disease.

	Exposure to the Specific Factor	
	+	−
Disease State	Experimental Group	Control Group
+ (with disease)	a	b
− (without disease)	c	d
Total	a + c	b + d

Relative risk = (a/a+c) / (b/b+d)
Absolute risk = (a/a+c) − (b/b+d)

27. **(D)** Hallux valgus is the lateral displacement and subluxation of the first metatarsal of the foot, commonly seen in the elderly female who may complain of pain and irritation. The second metatarsal may sublux or dislocate, forming a hammertoe. It is a bunion, and the shoe should be wide enough to relieve the pressure. Pads can be placed for cushioning.

28. **(D)** The retirement of many community family physicians and the lack of qualified replacements has produced a tremendous deficit of urban family physicians. However, the poor, inner-city communities most in need of physicians are also the least able to support financially the practice that may employ a new physician.

29. **(E)** With the promotion of the urban family-medicine model in predoctoral training and with the awareness that there still exists a shortage of family physicians in urban America, despite an overall "surplus" of physicians in years to come, many medical students will be attracted to the urban family practice.

30. **(B)** Common characteristics of a typical urban primary-care physician include (1) urban background; (2) spouse with urban background; (3) preference for urban living; (4) urban training; (5) valuing short, flexible hours; (6) valuing clinical support facilities and personnel; and (7) contacts with colleagues or academic settings.

31. **(D)** The modified wave scheduling may accommodate the family physician's "art style." It provides for walk-in or emergency patients. It schedules patients in groups or clusters to ensure that there will always be a patient to be seen by the physician. In addition, the delay of an appointment by a patient does not disrupt the entire appointment schedule.

32. **(D)** The correlation coefficient is used for studying the degree of linear relationship between two variables.

33. **(E)** The overabundance of specialists and subspecialists practicing in the urban hospitals has created difficulties for family physicians to obtain privileges, particularly in obstetrics, intensive-care medicine, and pediatrics, particularly in eastern large cities.

34. **(C)** Medicaid's need-based entitlements include Medicaid (Medi-cal in California), food stamps, Aid to Families with Dependent Children (AFDC), Supplemental Security Income (SSI), Social Security Disability (SSD), and workers' compensation. Medicaid's age-based entitlements include Social Security and Medicare.

35. **(B)** After the age of 50 years, an annual guaiac slide test is recommended. After two negative examinations 1 year apart, sigmoid-

oscopy should be done every 3 to 5 years. Annual mammography is recommended for women until age 65. A Pap smear is recommended every 3 years after two negative examinations 1 year apart.

36. **(B)**

$$\text{Specificity} = \frac{\text{True negative}}{\text{True negative} + \text{False positive}}$$

37. **(E)**

$$\text{Sensitivity} = \frac{\text{True positive}}{\text{True positive} + \text{False negative}}$$

38. **(A)**

$$\text{Positive predictive value} = \frac{\text{True positive}}{\text{True positive} + \text{False positive}}$$

39. **(D)** Prevalence is the percentage of the population in which the condition exists.

40. **(C)** If it is very unlikely that the observed outcome could occur if the null hypothesis (that no true difference exists) were true, then the null hypothesis is rejected and the alternative hypothesis (that a true difference exists) is accepted.

41. **(D)** Pruritus is the most common skin problem for which the elderly seek care. Alkaline soaps, overbathing, low humidity, rough clothing, alcohol use, and poor nutrition may aggravate pruritus. Pruritus is associated with scabies, dermatitis herpetiformis, chronic renal failure, iron deficiency anemia, diabetes, thyrotoxicosis, and xerosis.

42. **(D)** Epidemiology also is concerned with the planning process of health services, including the assessment of needs, the choice of alternative policies, the formulation of objectives, and evaluation of the results of implementation.

43. **(A)** The following considerations are often used to assess community health: (1) dependency ratio = (population <20 + >65/population 20–64); (2) median family income; (3) percent of poor families, per capita income, percent with public assistance; (4) infant mortality rate = (infant death <1 yr/live births) × 1000; (5) fetal mortality rate = (stillbirths/live births) × 1000; (6) crude death rate = (deaths/population) × 1000; (7) education level; and (8) percent of overcrowding (>1.01 persons/ room).

44. **(A)** Other examples of secondary prevention include treatment of hypertension, education of adults to stop alcohol drinking or cigarette smoking, and a weight-reduction program.

45. **(C)** Screening for tuberculosis is recommended for all elderly persons admitted to the nursing home. Shallow and slow administration of PPD is recommended to produce the best wheal reaction. If the test is negative, a second "booster" test is applied 7 to 10 days later to detect an infected person whose cell-mediated immunity to the tuberculin test has waned.

46. **(C)** Most of these 750 people (so-called "patients") are managed by themselves while only 250 patients (one third) will consult a physician. Of these, only five patients will be referred to a specialist, and nine will be admitted to the hospital—eight to the community hospitals and only one to the university medical center. Thus, a patient seen in the university medical center does not represent having a typical disease pattern in the community; and medical education received at the university medical center needs community orientation to be relevant to the community health needs.

47. **(B)** Incidence rate is the number of new cases divided by the population at risk during a specific period of time (ie, the study period) as shown by the formula:

$$\text{Incidence} = \frac{\text{No. of new cases occurring during a specific time period}}{\text{Midperiod population}}$$

48. (D) The following characteristics are usually examined in relation to disease occurrence: (1) time—seasonal variation, secular trends; (2) place—residence, urban/rural differentials, geographic areas; and (3) person—including age, sex, ethnic group, marital status, education, socioeconomic status, occupation, and behavior (including health-care behavior).

49. (B) A normal curve is the symmetric bell-shaped curve in which the distribution centers symmetrically about the mean (which is the midpoint of the curve) with a clustering of the data in the vicinity of the mean and tapers off gradually with asymptotic tails. The further an observation is from the mean, the less likely the observation is to exist. The proportion of observations that lie within the standard deviation from the mean ($X \pm 1$ SD) is 68.26% of all the values; 95.44% of all observations lie between the two standard deviations from the mean ($X \pm 2$ SD); 99.72% of all values lie between three standard deviations from the mean ($X \pm 3$ SD); 95% of all values lie between 1.96 standard deviations from the mean ($X \pm 1.96$ SD). It follows that the percentage of observed values that are more than plus and less 1.96 standard deviations from the mean is 5% (100% − 95% = 5%) which is often stated as probability at 5% level.

50. (B) The prevalence rate (point prevalence) is the number of existing cases divided by the population at risk at a point in time. The existing cases include new and chronic cases, as well as recurrent cases. The formula is:

$$\text{Prevalence} = \frac{\text{No. of existing cases at a point in time}}{\text{Total population at risk at a point in time}}$$

51. (B) The most commonly used ratio is the infant mortality, which is derived by:

$$\text{Infant mortality} = \frac{\text{No. of deaths} <1 \text{ yr. of age in a year}}{\text{No. of live births in the same year}} \times 1000$$

52. (A) The crude death rate is the number of deaths reported in a calendar year per 1000 population (estimated as of the middle of the year).

53. (A)

Result of Screening Test	Disease State	
	Disease	No disease
Positive	True positive (TP)	False positive (FP)
Negative	False negative (FN)	True negative (TN)

$$\text{Sensitivity} = \frac{TP}{TP + FN} \qquad \text{Specificity} = \frac{TN}{TN + FP}$$

Sensitivity is the percentage of people with the disease who are detected by the test; specificity is the percentage of people without the disease who are correctly labeled by the test as having no disease.

54. (D) The organism and the level of immunity of the population are crucial for the development of illness. The introduction of measles (or mumps) into a virgin population (ie, one in which an organism has not been present for many years, if ever) will affect adults as well as children. The upper age limit is determined by the number of years since the virus last circulated in the community.

55. (C) When a factor must be present for a disease to occur, it is called the agent of that disease (eg, influenza virus is the agent of influenza). However, an agent is considered to be a necessary but not sufficient cause of disease, because suitable conditions of the host (intrinsic factors) and environment (extrinsic factors) must also be present for disease to develop. Host factors affect susceptibility to disease, and factors in the environment influence exposure and often indirectly affect susceptibility. The interactions of these two factors determine whether disease develops.

56. (A) In a retrospective study, people diagnosed as having a disease (cases) are compared with persons who do not have the disease (controls). Relative risk is then calculated by dividing the incidence rate among the exposed (cases) by the incidence rate among the nonexposed (controls). In a prospective study, a group of people (cohort) who are free of disease are classified by exposure or lack of exposure to a factor and followed for the development of disease. In addition to relative risk, the attributable risk is also calculated by the absolute difference in incidence rates between an exposed group and a nonexposed group.

57. **(C)** The determinants of population dynamics—births, deaths, and migration—can be shown pictorially by a population pyramid, which presents the population of an area or country in terms of its composition by age and sex at a point in time. The shape of the pyramid reflects the major influences on births and deaths, plus any changes due to migration, over the three to four generations preceding the date of the pyramid. The population pyramids of developing countries frequently show triangular, broad-based patterns reflecting high birth and death rates. Only a small proportion of persons have survived into the older age groups, so the median age is relatively young.

58. **(D)** In an investigation of etiological factors in disease, it is necessary to study not only the cases of the disease, but healthy individuals (controls) from the same environment as well. This is termed the denominator principle in epidemiology.

59. **(B)** The generally accepted concept of the etiology of disease is multiple causation of illness. The concept maintains that illness is the result of a basic imbalance in a person's adaptation to the multiple short- and long-term physical and emotional stresses within the environment. A more precise terminology for multiple causation might be a "chain of causation" or a "web of causation." Epidemiologic studies (descriptive, analytic, and experimental) are conducted to determine the causal factors of the disease. Control of the disease is often successfully achieved long before the etiology of the disease is found. For example, although the exact cause of lung cancer is still unknown, the control of

cigarette smoking will possibly lower the risk of developing lung cancer.

60. **(A)** HMOs carry full responsibility for health services to individuals for a fixed annual payment. The emphasis is frequently on ambulatory care (both curative and preventive) instead of hospital services to lower the cost of medical care.

61. **(A)**

$$\text{Neonatal death rate} = \frac{\text{Newborn deaths within one month of age}}{\text{Live births in a year}} \times 1000$$

62. **(A)** The area-cluster sampling is frequently employed in the household health needs survey in a large homogeneous area due to less traveling expense.

63. **(B)** Systematic sampling is the most frequently used sampling procedure in record analysis. If the last digit of the family number is assigned on the basis of a selective factor (eg, income level, ethnicity, or residence), then there will be a bias.

64. **(C)** Simple random sampling usually will result in a fairly representative sample; however, the required traveling to the scattered sample households makes it expensive.

65. **(E)** There are almost 35 million Americans without health insurance; to provide universal access to all Americans (citizens and legal aliens), President Clinton proposed an employer-based system (companies paying 80% of premiums, workers 20%). Regional health alliances will be established to pool people together and bargain for the best prices for "womb-to-tomb" coverage of care. To hold down the health-care cost of $1 trillion (14% of gross domestic product), a global budget may be set, and independent providers will compete for consumer markets with capitation coverage (ie, "managed competition"). Managed competition is intended to hold down the cost and to improve the quality. Family physicians will be gatekeepers of the system.

66. **(A)** In regard to American elderly, 4.5% live in an institutionalized setting (an extended-care facility or skilled nursing home); 5% are bedbound or homebound; and 90% are ambulatory and function well in the community.

67. **(B)** In the elderly with dehydration or pre-existing renal insufficiency or who are using furosemide, the administration of aminoglycosides (gentamicin) and cephalosporins may cause acute renal failure (tubulointerstitial injury). The kidney's ability to concentrate urine may decrease, the glomerular filtration rate may decrease, proteinuria may develop, and blood urea nitrogen (BUN) and creatinine may be increased.

68. **(A)** Falls are a major medical problem in the elderly that lead to fractures, dependency, and often death. The home remains the most common site of fatal accidents in the elderly, followed by highways, hospitals, and nursing homes.

69. **(D)** Most elderly in the urban setting are not alone and isolated; they are ambulatory, functional, and independent. Markets, banks, churches, clinics, social agencies, and shops are often within walking distance. Most of them establish satisfactory relationships with neighbors and friends.

70. **(D)** The risk of pellagra is increased in patients with alcoholism, liver cirrhosis, chronic diarrhea, diabetes mellitus, tuberculosis, thyrotoxicosis, malignant carcinoid, and neoplasia.

71. **(E)** In 1991, there were 35 million Americans beyond the age of 65 years, accounting for 13% of the total population. In 1900, only 4% of the population was elderly, and in 2050 it is expected to be 23%.

72. **(A)** The main indication for the joint replacement surgery is the intractable pain, commonly arising from chronic osteoarthritis. The pain is often relieved following joint replacement. The functional ability of the patient with rheumatoid arthritis may improve following replacement surgery. Younger patients (less than 55 years) should try medical therapy as far as possible. Antibiotic prophylaxis improves the result of the total hip replacement. The most common complication is thromboembolism. The long-term durability of hip replacement may be compromised by bone resorption (osteolysis).

73. **(A)** Many nursing home patients may require long-term indwelling bladder catheterization (such as patients with traumatic cord injury). These patients are at increased risk for urinary tract infections (UTIs) with subsequent septicemia and even mortality. With open drainage system, urinary tract infections usually develop in the patient with an indwelling catheter; the use of sterile closed system may delay the occurrence of infection.

74. **(D)** In long-term care for the elderly, the caregiver should bolster the elderly patient's self-esteem and let the elderly patient exert control and maintain confidence. The caregiver should assess the patient's functional ability of daily living (such as ambulation, eating, bathing, dressing, toileting, and communication). The caregiver should perform for the patient only those daily tasks he or she cannot accomplish and let the patient perform those tasks he or she can accomplish.

75. **(D)** The elderly spend more time in bed, but sleep time is often decreased (or unchanged); thus, the sleep efficiency is decreased. The elderly experience increased nocturnal awakening, decreased REM, and deep sleep with a "lark" pattern (fall asleep earlier and awaken earlier).

76. **(E)** Many nursing home patients are lonely and often feel isolated. Family members serve as the patient's social support system and should maintain social relationships for the patient to maintain contact with the outside world.

77. **(D)** Periodontal disease may cause gingivitis, bleeding gums, gingival abscesses, and tooth loss. It is prevalent in 90% of the elderly and is more common to cause tooth loss than are dental caries.

78. (E) BCG is not recommended for the elderly. It may reduce the usefulness of the tuberculin test in detecting the tuberculous infection early.

79. (B) Urge incontinence is the most common cause of urinary incontinence due to involuntary detrusor contractions. The patient feels a strong urge to void, yet experiences loss of urine on the way to the bathroom. The bladder retraining program is to be instituted. Anticholinergic agents (oxybutymin [Ditropan] 2.5 mg tid), and tricyclic antidepressants (imipramine [Tofranil] 25 mg qd) are also useful.

80. (B) In stress incontinence, the urine leaks when the patient coughs, sneezes, laughs, or engages in physical activities. The leakage is usually in the daytime and not at night. It is far more common in females than males.

81. (C) The hematopoietic system is basically unchanged. Hemoglobin concentration and hematocrit are essentially unchanged. Blood volume is maintained, and platelets are the same. Leukocytes remain the same, but periphery T cells are decreased.

82. (A)-F, (B)-F, (C)-T, (D)-F, (E)-T. The type of hospitalized patients (called "case mix") can be grouped into 467 categories, diagnoses, or procedures (including an additional three DRGs of ungroupable records, a total of 470 DRGs) according to principal diagnosis and procedure, secondary diagnosis and procedure, age, sex, complications, and discharge status.

There are 23 major diagnostic categories in DRGs, and ICD-9-CM (International Classification of Disease, 9th Revision, Clinical Modification) is adopted for its reporting upon which a predetermined (ie, prospective) payment schedule is reimbursed for an average length of hospital stay.

83. (A)-T, (B)-T, (C)-T, (D)-T, (E)-F. In urban family practice, the following types of home visits are frequently made: (1) acute illness evaluation; (2) routine health-maintenance check-ups for chronic illness; (3) posthospitalization follow-ups; (4) death and dying counseling and care; (5) home evaluation for social and family counseling; (6) medication and laboratory (blood and ECG); and (7) patient education.

84. (A)-F, (B)-F, (C)-F, (D)-F, (E)-T. Cholesterol screening for healthy elderly patients is not necessary. All that is needed is counseling the patient on the risk of coronary heart disease and healthy life styles.

85. (A)-T, (B)-T, (C)-T, (D)-T, (E)-T. Presbyopia, a phenomenon that occurs with aging, is due to the elastic tissue of the lens showing a diminished activity to increase in thickness and curvature. Due to this change, the eye becomes less able to focus on near objects. There is a yellowing of the lens, sclera, and, occasionally, vitreous humor, as well as a reduction in the size of the pupil. Entropion (inversion of the eyelids) and ectropion (eversion of the eyelids) are aging processes. There is generally a decrease in tear production. Cataracts and macular degeneration occur very often in the elderly.

86. (A)-F, (B)-F, (C)-F, (D)-T, (E)-F. Fecal impaction not only causes fecal incontinence but also develops urinary incontinence. Disimpaction of stool restores fecal and urinary continence. Fecal incontinence also can be caused by diarrhea, decreased anal sphincter tone, dementia, and lack of toilet facility.

87. (A)-F, (B)-F, (C)-T, (D)-F, (E)-F. Alzheimer's disease is the most common cause of dementia. The patient suffers from progressive intellectual and cognitive deterioration. Recent memory and immediate recall are poor, but remote memory is well preserved. The patient is unable to perform self-care. Physical and neurological examinations are unremarkable. There is no history of stroke.

88. (A)-T, (B)-T, (C)-T, (D)-T, (E)-T. Ninety-five percent of pressure sores develop in sacrum, ischial tuberosity, greater trochanter, tuberosity of the calcaneus, and lateral malleolus. The scapula is also a common site. Hypoalbuminemia, fecal incontinence, immobility, weight loss, hypotension, fractures, anemia, diabetes, and dementia are at high risk to develop pressure sores.

89. **(A)-T, (B)-T, (C)-T, (D)-T, (E)-T.** Contact dermatitis is usually present with erythematous macules, papules, and vesicles, with hot and warm inflammatory reactions. In the elderly, there may be little vesiculation or inflammation, and instead there will be scaling, lichenification, and itching.

90. **(A)-T, (B)-T, (C)-T, (D)-T, (E)-T.** Cervical spondylosis may cause hand clumsiness, tingling and numbness of fingers, increased tone and impaired vibration perception in legs, and postural instability. This is a common cause of falls in the elderly.

91. **(A)-T, (B)-T, (C)-T, (D)-T, (E)-T.** Irritable bowel syndrome is often common in the elderly. Complications include fecal impaction, intestinal obstruction, megacolon, and fecal incontinence. Regular mealtime, adequate fluid intake, high-fiber diet, adequate nutrition, and elimination of motility-inhibiting drugs (anticholinergics) as well as laxatives will be helpful.

92. **(A)-T, (B)-T, (C)-T, (D)-T, (E)-T.** Halitosis (bad breath) is often due to gingivitis, periodontitis, oral candidiasis, xerostomia (may be caused by antidepressants and antihypertensives), oral cancer, leukemia, hepatic failure, renal failure, ketoacidosis, depression, schizophrenia, and temporal lobe epilepsy.

93. **(A)-T, (B)-T, (C)-T, (D)-T, (E)-F.** The characteristic feature of COPC is that the health care of the community and the health care of individuals are brought together in a single integrated practice that endeavors to identify the community's main health problems and implement defined programs to deal with these in a systematic manner, while at the same time providing clinical care for individuals. Epidemiology provides the basis for the development and evaluation of these programs. Establishment of a primary-care practice cannot guarantee community-oriented service to manage systematically major

health problems of the community, although it does provide personal care for community members who request it.

94. **(A)-T, (B)-T, (C)-T, (D)-T, (E)-T.** All the explanations may be true. Age-adjusted death rates should be calculated to compare the two communities prior to reaching the conclusion. Although the crude death rate is a readily obtainable health statistic, it is not a sensitive measurement of the health status of a community due to its influence by the age composition of the population. The elderly have a relatively higher risk for death, and a community comprised of a higher proportion of the elderly may show a higher crude death rate.

95. **(A)-T, (B)-T, (C)-T, (D)-T, (E)-T.** An urban clinic with evening hours may increase the chance of robbery, rape, and assault.

96. **(A)-T, (B)-T, (C)-T, (D)-T, (E)-T.** Although the manual system is still prevalent, in many inner-city family practice offices, computer systems are now in progress. However, the cost of instituting the computerized system should justify the returns in the inner-city family practice office, where many patients and families are poor.

97. **(A)-T, (B)-T, (C)-T, (D)-T, (E)-T.** The need to bring new family physicians practicing the biopsychosocial model into inner-city communities to practice was obvious in the 1970s. Urban family practice residencies appeared in Chicago, Cleveland, New York, Philadelphia, San Francisco, Los Angeles, and elsewhere in the mid-1970s. Since the 1980s, COPC has been implemented to improve accessibility.

98. **(A)-T, (B)-T, (C)-T, (D)-T, (E)-T.** POMRs are very useful in recordkeeping for ambulatory patient care services; thus, many family practice centers are adopting POMR as their recordkeeping system. Progress notes frequently include the SOAP system. Plans should include diagnoses to be ruled out. The format of a flow sheet is frequently used for the progress notes.

99. **(A)-F, (B)-F, (C)-F, (D)-F, (E)-F.** There is no clear-cut evidence that air pollution increases urban health risk. Air pollution does not increase mortality, morbidity, or respiratory illness of urban residents, even in Los Angeles. The role of SO_2 in the development of lung cancer is not clear.

100. **(A)-T, (B)-T, (C)-T, (D)-T, (E)-T.** Problems are selected and identified from the analysis of the currently available database. Thus, sometimes a general term such as headache will appear on the problem list. The objective evidence obtained from subsequent studies may change the problem into a specific diagnosis, such as migraine headache, or the problem may remain on the problem list until resolved.

101. **(A)-T, (B)-T, (C)-T, (D)-T, (E)-T.** Epilepsy is not a hereditary disease, but it does show a familial predisposition. Schizophrenia has a hereditary predisposition. Febrile seizures show a familial disposition. Alcoholism is not hereditary; however, family members of alcoholics are at increased risk of becoming alcoholics. Almost one half of patients with varicose veins may show a family predisposition.

102. **(A)-T, (B)-T, (C)-T, (D)-T, (E)-T.** Many illnesses and diseases are clustered in certain families—some are genetically determined through inheritance (hereditary illnesses), and some show familial aggregation without a definite inheritance pattern. In these instances, the family should be the unit of care to provide preventive and counseling services for other members of the family who are not ill (but who are at risk of developing similar diseases). A detailed family history of these diseases with familial predisposition should be recorded.

103. **(A)-T, (B)-T, (C)-T, (D)-T, (E)-T.** Multiple screening programs are designed for the community-wide testing of individuals for several diseases at the same visit. Such programs are expensive, and evaluation of the cost/benefit ratio is in order.

104. (F)
105. (T)
106. (F)
107. (F)
108. (F)
109. (F)
110. (F)
111. (T)
112. (F)
113. (F)
114. (F)
115. (F)
116. (F)
117. (F)
118. (T)
119. (F)
120. (F)
121. (F)
122. (T)
123. (F)

The most common food poisoning in the United States is by enterotoxin of the *Staphylococcus* organism. This disease is characterized by acute nausea, vomiting, and diarrhea, which occur 2 to 4 hours after ingestion of contaminated food. The patient usually recovers after 24 hours. It is usually due to contamination of food from infections existing on the body of the food handler, typically boils on the hands or other body surfaces. The food implicated includes milk, milk products, and custard- or cream-filled pastries.

CHAPTER 7

Internal Medicine
Questions

DIRECTIONS (Questions 1 through 205): Each of the numbered items or incomplete statements in this section is followed by answers or by completions of the statement. Select the ONE lettered answer or completion that is BEST in each case.

1. *Treponema pallidum* is the causative organism of

   (A) granuloma inguinale
   (B) condyloma latum
   (C) condyloma acuminatum
   (D) herpes progenitalis
   (E) fibrocystic disease   *(Ref. 2)*

2. Ciguatera poisoning

   (A) is prevented by cooking fish in a microwave oven
   (B) may cause the reversal of cold to hot sensation in touch and taste
   (C) can be treated with an antidote
   (D) is caused by the action of histamine
   (E) is caused by the toxins concentrated in the gonads (ichthyotoxic)   *(Ref. 2)*

3. In the elderly, which atypical presentation is frequently the first clue of sepsis?

   (A) pain
   (B) fever
   (C) tachycardia
   (D) confusion
   (E) leukocytosis   *(Ref. 2)*

4. Tinnitus is most likely associated with

   (A) retinal detachment
   (B) hyperthyroidism
   (C) hypertension
   (D) acute otitis media
   (E) acute rhinitis   *(Ref. 2)*

5. Good recordkeeping includes documentation that is

   (A) complete
   (B) consistent
   (C) accurate
   (D) timely recorded
   (E) all of the above   *(Ref. 2)*

6. Decline of which of the following physiologic functions in the elderly places them at risk of falling?

   (A) sexual drive
   (B) sense of smell
   (C) vision
   (D) hearing
   (E) thinking process   *(Ref. 2)*

7. Neurosyphilis is characterized by all of the following presentations EXCEPT

   (A) apathetic behavior
   (B) forgetfulness
   (C) chancre
   (D) Argyll–Robertson pupils
   (E) ataxic gait   *(Ref. 7)*

8. A 17-year-old high school student notes the onset of severe sore throat, malaise, and fever of 102°F of 1 day's duration. On physical examination, he has bilateral enlarged tonsils with several white plaques and diffuse erythema. There are several 1-cm submandibular nodes and postcervical nodes. As a child, he developed wheezing and urticaria following penicillin therapy. When you see him, you do a throat culture, and strep screen is positive. You would treat him with

(A) clindamycin 300 mg PO qid for 10 days
(B) tetracycline 250 mg PO qid for 10 days
(C) tetracycline 500 mg PO qid for 10 days
(D) erythromycin 250 mg PO qid for 10 days
(E) oral cephalexin 500 mg PO qid for 4 days
(Ref. 2)

9. A 50-year-old nurse with chronic bronchitis develops influenza and then develops an acute patchy bronchopneumonia. Gram stain of the sputum grows gram-positive cocci in clusters. Antibiotic therapy should be

(A) oral phenoxymethyl penicillin
(B) adequate penicillin, 2,000,000 units every 6 hours
(C) benzathine penicillin G 2,400,000 units IM
(D) oxacillin 2 g IV every 6 hours
(E) chloramphenicol 0.5 g IV every 6 hours
(Ref. 2)

10. Which of the following will most likely increase high-density lipoprotein (HDL)?

(A) cigarette smoking
(B) high-magnesium diet
(C) an executive position
(D) exercise
(E) vitamin A 10,000 IU for 10 days   *(Ref. 2)*

11. Which of the following conditions is most likely to occur in elderly hypertensives?

(A) increased peripheral resistance
(B) increased plasma renin level
(C) increased stroke volume
(D) increased intravascular volume
(E) increased renal blood flow   *(Ref. 2)*

12. The most common reason for antibiotic failure is

(A) gross overuse for viral or nonbacterial illnesses
(B) inappropriate route of administration
(C) prolonged time intervals between administered doses
(D) inadequate dosage
(E) patient noncompliance   *(Ref. 43)*

13. Thiazide diuretics may produce which of the following biochemical changes?

(A) hyperuricemia
(B) hyperkalemia
(C) hypoglycemia
(D) hypouricemia
(E) hypermagnesemia   *(Ref. 2)*

14. Beta blockers are recommended for a hypertensive patient with which of the following conditions?

(A) bronchial asthma
(B) depression
(C) Raynaud's phenomenon
(D) impotence
(E) mitral prolapse   *(Ref. 43)*

15. An executive has had a 3-day history of upper respiratory infection (URI) prior to his air travel from Los Angeles to Honolulu for a scuba diving activity. Upon his return, he complains of frontal aching and pressure sensations. The patient most likely has

(A) depression
(B) leprosy
(C) cocaine use
(D) barosinusitis
(E) acquired immune deficiency syndrome (AIDS)   *(Ref. 10)*

16. Cigarette smoking increases the risk of developing all of the following conditions EXCEPT

   (A) chronic hepatitis
   (B) coronary artery disease
   (C) lung cancer
   (D) respiratory illness in smoker's children
   (E) bladder cancer   *(Ref. 2)*

17. A 25-year-old man develops onset of fever and hacking cough of 5 days' duration. His cough comes in uncontrolled paroxysms. He has a fever of 101°F. Chest examination reveals minimal scattered rales at the left lower lung. Chest x-ray shows bilateral alveolar and interstitial infiltrates in the left lower end and right middle lung fields. After culturing his sputum, you would

   (A) treat him with 1,200,000 units per day of aqueous or procaine penicillin in appropriately divided doses for 10 days
   (B) administer erythromycin 500 mg qid for 1 week
   (C) administer clindamycin 300 mg qid if he is penicillin allergic
   (D) administer erythromycin 500 mg qid for 3 weeks
   (E) none of the above   *(Ref. 2)*

18. Proper empiric therapy for a community-acquired pneumonia for a 27-year-old woman would be

   (A) Augmentin (amoxicillin plus clavulinic acid)
   (B) erythromycin
   (C) Septra (trimethoprim-sulfamethoxazole)
   (D) clindamycin
   (E) dicloxacillin   *(Ref. 2)*

19. A 52-year-old asymptomatic woman is found to have hepatomegaly on a routine physical examination. The liver measures 11 cm in total span and is firm and palpable 2 cm below the right costal margin. Laboratory evaluation reveals a normal complete blood count, normal renal function, and normal hepatic function. A radionuclide liver scan shows multiple filling defects within the right lobe and one within the left lobe of the liver. A directed-needle biopsy of the liver demonstrates metastatic carcinoid tumor. A 24-hour urine specimen for 5-hydroxyindoleacetic acid reveals a value of 58 mg/24 h. Which of the following is the best approach to further management?

   (A) systemic chemotherapy with 5-fluorouracil plus streptozocin
   (B) exploratory laparotomy and placement of a hepatic artery catheter for subsequent chemotherapy
   (C) therapy with serotonin antagonists and antihistamines
   (D) hepatic irradiation to a total dose of 2,200 rad
   (E) continuity of care with careful observation and regular follow-ups   *(Ref. 22)*

20. The principal cause of death of patients with Kaposi's sarcoma associated with AIDS is

   (A) hepatic metastases
   (B) pulmonary metastases
   (C) opportunistic infections
   (D) complications of chemotherapy
   (E) progressive cutaneous ulceration *(Ref. 2)*

21. Which of the following symptoms is most likely to occur in heart failure?

   (A) rectal bleeding
   (B) micturition pain
   (C) fever
   (D) hemoptysis
   (E) weight loss   *(Ref. 2)*

22. Which of the following tests is most useful in distinguishing thalassemia minor from pure iron deficiency anemia?

    (A) peripheral blood smear
    (B) osmotic fragility test
    (C) Ham test
    (D) hemoglobin electrophoresis on paper
    (E) serum iron determination   (Ref. 73)

23. In prescribing nitrofurantoin (Macrodantin) to treat urinary tract infections (UTIs), which of the following statements is correct?

    (A) It should be taken with food.
    (B) It is the drug of choice for pregnant women with UTIs at term.
    (C) Its absorption is increased in an empty stomach.
    (D) It is the first-line medication for neonatal UTIs.
    (E) It is the only drug to be used in renal insufficiency.   (Ref. 15)

24. Vestibular causes of dizziness are characterized by:

    (A) aphasia
    (B) dyspraxia
    (C) dysphagia
    (D) hearing loss
    (E) weight loss   (Ref. 3)

25. A 70-year-old female has long-standing osteoarthritis of her left knee, which is well controlled by a nonsteroidal anti-inflammatory drug (NSAID). Now she complains of occasional tarry stool. The most likely reason is

    (A) Alzheimer's disease
    (B) peptic ulcer disease (PUD)
    (C) hemorrhoid
    (D) depression
    (E) colon cancer   (Ref. 2)

26. Which of the following conditions is the most common cause of chronic cough?

    (A) gastroesophageal reflux
    (B) duodenal ulcer
    (C) pneumothorax
    (D) allergic rhinitis
    (E) smoking withdrawal   (Ref. 77)

27. Silo-filler's disease is characterized by

    (A) calcified pleura
    (B) bronchiolitis fibrosa obliterans
    (C) miliary tuberculosis
    (D) laryngeal edema
    (E) intestinal obstruction   (Ref. 22)

28. Lactic acidosis is often caused by

    (A) dimethylbiguanide (DBI) phenformin
    (B) tetracycline
    (C) insulin
    (D) antacids
    (E) vitamin B   (Ref. 2)

29. Which of the following microorganisms is frequently found in AIDS patients?

    (A) *Giardia lamblia*
    (B) *Mycobacterium avium intracellulare*
    (C) *Pseudomonas maltophilia*
    (D) *Mycobacterium marinum*
    (E) *T. pallidum*   (Ref. 2)

30. According to current concepts, which of the following individuals are at a higher risk to develop AIDS?

    (A) classmates of school children with AIDS
    (B) nonsexual partners of AIDS patients' family members
    (C) family physicians providing continuity of care for AIDS patients at their offices
    (D) infants of mothers with AIDS
    (E) nurses who take care of AIDS patients at hospital wards   (Ref. 2)

31. Which of the following dietary regimens is recommended in chronic renal failure?

    (A) low potassium
    (B) low sodium
    (C) high phosphorus
    (D) high protein
    (E) high purines   (Ref. 48)

32. The most likely eletrocardiographic (ECG) finding in the early stage of acute viral pericarditis is

   (A) T inversion
   (B) ST elevation with upward concavity
   (C) ST depression
   (D) ST elevation with downward convexity
   (E) P pulmonale   (Ref. 2)

33. Vitamin D deficiency may be associated with

   (A) acute hepatitis
   (B) biliary cirrhosis
   (C) angina pectoris
   (D) lactose intolerance
   (E) hypertension   (Ref. 2)

34. The most common vitamin deficiency in the alcoholic is

   (A) riboflavin deficiency
   (B) folic acid deficiency
   (C) pyridoxine deficiency
   (D) niacin deficiency
   (E) thiamine deficiency   (Ref. 2)

35. The most common side reaction of isoniazid (INH) is

   (A) gynecomastia
   (B) convulsions
   (C) peripheral neuropathy
   (D) agranulocytosis
   (E) optic neuritis   (Ref. 43)

36. Pseudomembranous enterocolitis is most likely to be caused by

   (A) nitroglycerin
   (B) verapamil
   (C) sucralfate
   (D) clindamycin
   (E) morphine   (Ref. 72)

37. Transient ischemic attacks (TIAs) most often

   (A) are microembolic
   (B) are small clots blocking carotids
   (C) are related to blood pressure fluctuations
   (D) occur with syncope
   (E) are due to occlusion of the intracranial arteries   (Ref. 2)

38. The most common site of occlusion of blood vessels to the head is

   (A) carotid
   (B) middle cerebral artery
   (C) anterior cerebral
   (D) anterior choroidal
   (E) postcerebral   (Ref. 22)

39. Thrombocytosis is commonly detected in patients with

   (A) PUD
   (B) diabetes mellitus
   (C) hypertension
   (D) myeloproliferative disorders
   (E) pneumonia   (Ref. 73)

40. In the management of the elderly patient with stroke sequelae at home, you would

   (A) start medications for diastolic hypertension and stop medication for systolic hypertension
   (B) stop aspirin if stroke is from thromboembolic disease
   (C) order a high-protein, high-cholesterol, high-fat diet to speed recovery
   (D) instruct the family to let the patient participate in as many family affairs as he or she can
   (E) prescribe fen-phen (fenfluramine/phentermine) to prevent poststroke depression   (Ref. 7)

41. A 52-year-old man is admitted to the hospital with an acute myocardial infarction of the anterior wall. On the third hospital day, he suddenly experiences severe dyspnea, diaphoresis, and hypotension. A new systolic murmur is heard at the left sternal border and a thrill is palpated in the same region. A chest x-ray discloses pulmonary edema. The most likely cause of these findings is

   (A) rupture of a papillary muscle
   (B) acute aortic dissection
   (C) rupture of the ventricular septum
   (D) rupture of a mitral chordae tendineae
   (E) pulmonary embolism   (Ref. 75)

42. When an acyanotic middle-aged adult has roentgenographic evidence of enlarged pulmonary arteries and increased lung markings, the most likely diagnosis is

   (A) ventricular septal defect
   (B) coarctation of the aorta
   (C) pulmonary valvular stenosis
   (D) atrial septal defect (ASD)
   (E) truncus arteriosus   (Ref. 22)

43. A 70-year-old female has had a history of progressive memory and intellectual slowness for 2 years. There is urinary incontinence and ataxic gait disturbance. The most likely diagnosis is

   (A) Alzheimer's disease
   (B) metastatic breast cancer of the brain
   (C) Pick's disease
   (D) normal pressure hydrocephalus
   (E) multiple sclerosis   (Ref. 7)

44. Each of the following statements concerning vitamin B_{12} deficiency is true EXCEPT

   (A) Howell–Jolly bodies are present in circulating erythrocytes
   (B) blood transfusions correct the megaloblastic maturation of erythroid precursors in the bone marrow
   (C) serum folate levels are usually normal or elevated

   (D) pancreatic insufficiency causes malabsorption of vitamin B_{12}
   (E) the Schilling test is useful for confirming vitamin B_{12} malabsorption in patients treated with vitamin B_{12} (Ref. 73)

45. Which of the following abnormal hemoglobins characteristically produces targeting in the peripheral blood?

   (A) hemoglobin M
   (B) hemoglobin S
   (C) hemoglobin Zurich
   (D) hemoglobin C
   (E) hemoglobin Barts   (Ref. 73)

46. Chloracne is associated with long-term exposure to

   (A) zinc
   (B) arsenic
   (C) organophosphate
   (D) trichloroethane
   (E) polychlorinated biphenyls (PCBs)   (Ref. 27)

47. Long-term use of which of the following over-the-counter (OTC) medications is often associated with dyspepsia?

   (A) ibuprofen (Motrin)
   (B) cimetidine (Tagamet)
   (C) ranitidine (Zantac)
   (D) Tavist D
   (E) Robitussin-DM   (Ref. 2)

48. Thrombocytopenia often results from the administration of

   (A) vitamin B_{12}
   (B) thiamine
   (C) folic acid
   (D) vitamin E
   (E) alcohol   (Ref. 73)

49. Minocycline can be used for chemoprophylaxis of

   (A) acne vulgaris
   (B) tuberculosis
   (C) typhoid fever

(D) meningococcal meningitis

(E) gonorrhea   *(Ref. 74)*

50. Which of the following is a measure for primary prevention?

    (A) serologic test for syphilis
    (B) blood pressure measurements
    (C) yellow fever immunization
    (D) isoniazid (INAH) chemoprophylaxis
    (E) tight control of diabetes   *(Ref. 3)*

51. Sickle cell anemia in an adult is usually associated with

    (A) splenomegaly
    (B) normal reticulocyte count
    (C) hemoglobin A
    (D) normal shape of erythrocyte except in crisis
    (E) gallstones   *(Ref. 73)*

52. One would expect to find which of the following in thalassemia minor?

    (A) an increased amount of fetal and A2 hemoglobin
    (B) increased osmotic fragility of the red cells
    (C) absent bone-marrow iron
    (D) increased macroglobulins in the serum
    (E) small amounts of S hemoglobin   *(Ref. 73)*

53. A 46-year-old woman complains of pain in her left leg of 2 days' duration. There is no peripheral edema. Examination shows redness, increased warmth, and tenderness, which is confined to a narrow area (3 to 5 cm in width) on the medial side of the leg from the ankle almost to the knee. Pressure on the posterior aspect of the calf and dorsiflexion of the foot produce no pain. A blood count shows a slight increase in the number of leukocytes. The most likely diagnosis is

    (A) deep venous thrombophlebitis
    (B) phlegmasia cerulea dolens
    (C) lymphangitis

(D) superficial venous thrombophlebitis

(E) acute obstruction of the superficial femoral artery   *(Ref. 2)*

54. An 18-year-old man of Italian descent is found to have a hypochromic microcytic anemia with a hemoglobin of 10 g%. In addition, there is a fair degree of anisocytosis, poikilotosis, and targeting on the smear. The white blood count is 9500; the platelet count is 240,000; and the reticulocyte count is 7%. The spleen is palpated 5 cm below the left costal margin. Which of the following is the most likely diagnosis?

    (A) sickle cell trait
    (B) thalassemia minor
    (C) hemoglobin S-C disease
    (D) iron deficiency anemia
    (E) hereditary spherocytosis   *(Ref. 73)*

55. The most common cause of lung cancer is

    (A) asbestosis
    (B) radon
    (C) uranium
    (D) chromium
    (E) cigarette smoking   *(Ref. 2)*

56. Which of the following medications may increase the risk of falls in the elderly?

    (A) anticoagulants
    (B) antibiotics
    (C) antacids
    (D) benzodiazepines
    (E) vitamins   *(Ref. 7)*

57. Where on the adult chest would you place the heel of your hand in order to perform cardiopulmonary resuscitation (CPR) chest compression?

    (A) two or three fingers above the lower end of the sternum
    (B) on the upper third of the sternum
    (C) where the sternum and collarbone meet
    (D) on the middle of the sternum
    (E) on the xiphoid process   *(Ref. 22)*

58. What too frequently happens to an unconscious person when he is lying on his back with a pillow under his head?

    (A) He aspirates vomitus into his airway.
    (B) His tongue falls back in his throat and blocks his airway.
    (C) It is the position easiest to start effective mouth-to-mouth breathing.
    (D) He clears his airway better.
    (E) His whole body is easily exposed for close observation.   *(Ref. 22)*

59. A 26-year-old nurse who previously had a negative purified protein derivative (PPD) (intermediate strength) skin test is found to have a positive PPD skin test 3 months after in-hospital exposure to a patient with active tuberculosis. The nurse is asymptomatic and a chest x-ray discloses no abnormalities. Sputum concentrates for *Mycobacterium tuberculosis* are negative. The most appropriate management would consist of

    (A) repeat chest x-rays at annual intervals
    (B) administration of INH for 12 months
    (C) administration of rifampin for 3 months
    (D) administration of isoniazid and ethambutol for 12 months
    (E) repeating chest x-rays every 3 months and institution of treatment if roentgenographic evidence of tuberculosis appears   *(Ref. 2)*

60. A 32-year-old pregnant woman is admitted to the hospital because of severe dyspnea and cyanosis. The patient has had a skin rash for the past 5 days. Her two children had a febrile exanthem for 14 days and 9 days, respectively, prior to the patient's illness. Which of the following is the most likely diagnosis?

    (A) lupus erythematosus
    (B) varicella pneumonia
    (C) amniotic fluid emboli
    (D) staphylococcal pneumonia
    (E) mycoplasmal pneumonia   *(Ref. 2)*

61. A patient is suspected of having allergic alveolitis secondary to inhalation of thermophilic *Actinomyces* (farmer's lung). Useful diagnostic findings would include

    (A) demonstration of serum-precipitating antibody to an extract of *Blastomyces*
    (B) a specific histologic reaction evident on a biopsy of the lung
    (C) production of dyspnea, fever, and pulmonary infiltrates 5 to 6 hours after an inhalation challenge with thermophilic *Actinomyces*
    (D) reduction in diffusing capacity with a normal vital capacity
    (E) an increase in diffusing capacity with a normal vital capacity   *(Ref. 22)*

62. Glyburide is effective in treating patients with

    (A) ketosis-prone, insulin-dependent diabetes
    (B) morbid obesity
    (C) non–insulin-dependent (type II) diabetes
    (D) pregnant diabetes
    (E) insulinoma   *(Ref. 43)*

63. Which of the following sulfonylureas has the longest duration of action?

    (A) tolbutamide
    (B) chlorpropamide
    (C) glipizide
    (D) glyburide
    (E) tolazamide   *(Ref. 43)*

64. The deficiency of α_1-antitrypsin (AAT) is associated with

    (A) hypertension
    (B) diabetes mellitus
    (C) hepatoma
    (D) pulmonary fibrosis
    (E) cholelithiasis   *(Ref. 75)*

65. An 18-year-old girl has developed nausea and vomiting followed by cramping abdominal pain, flatulation, and diarrhea with mucus and blood in the stool. She has also experi-

enced fever. There is no evidence of dehydration; however, the stool culture has identified *Salmonella enteritidis*. The choice treatment is

(A) chloramphenicol

(B) ampicillin

(C) trimethoprim-sulfamethoxazole (Septra or Bactrim)

(D) a liquid diet with adequate hydration

(E) diphenoxylate with atropine sulfate (Lomotil)   *(Ref. 75)*

66. The most likely clinical presentation of early left colonic cancer is

(A) anemia

(B) euphoria

(C) cough

(D) bowel change

(E) weight gain   *(Ref. 22)*

67. Twenty-four hours after admission, intubation, and the institution of mechanical ventilation in a 70-year-old man with chronic obstructive pulmonary disease (COPD), hypotension occurs, "coffee-ground" material comes from the nasogastric tube, and his hematocrit (HCT) falls to 28%. The most likely cause is

(A) cirrhosis of the liver

(B) chronic peptic ulcer

(C) stress ulcer

(D) pulmonary tuberculosis

(E) peptic esophagitis   *(Ref. 72)*

68. Twelve days after the successful treatment of an episode of acute respiratory failure in a 60-year-old man with COPD, he begins to cough up a purulent sputum and develops a temperature of 104°F. A chest x-ray reveals an area of consolidation in the right lower lobe. The most likely complication encountered at present is

(A) pulmonary infarction

(B) congestive heart failure

(C) staphylococcal empyema

(D) *Pseudomonas* pneumonia

(E) *Escherichia coli* septicemia   *(Ref. 74)*

69. The most common side reaction of zidovudine (AZT) is

(A) headache

(B) gingival hypertrophy

(C) constipation

(D) erythema nodosum

(E) muscular weakness   *(Ref. 43)*

70. Side reactions of thiazide diuretics include all of the following EXCEPT

(A) hyperkalemia

(B) hyperglycemia

(C) hyperuricemia

(D) hypercholesterolemia

(E) hypertriglyceridemia   *(Ref. 43)*

71. A 45-year-old male complains of back pain. His serum calcium is found to be 15 mg/100 mL, serum phosphorus 1.3 mg/100 mL, and alkaline phosphatase 14 Bodansky units. X-ray of the spine shows demineralization. The most likely diagnosis is

(A) osteitis deformans

(B) osteoporosis

(C) hyperparathyroidism

(D) hyperthyroidism

(E) hypothyroidism   *(Ref. 2)*

72. In elderly patients, postural hypotension may be caused by

(A) methyldopa

(B) digoxin

(C) ampicillin

(D) ibuprofen

(E) chlorpropamide   *(Ref. 2)*

73. A 20-year-old Japanese-American college student recently converted his PPD to a positive result. In prescribing INH, you would advise him to avoid

(A) rice

(B) oranges

(C) tuna sashimi

(D) spinach

(E) bread   *(Ref. 22)*

74. A patient presents with lethargy. His serum chemistries reveal Na^+ 150, Cl^- 100, K^+ 3.0, CO_2 40, albumin 3.5 g/100 mL, and pH 7.55. He displays 3^+ pitting edema of the extremities. This situation is caused by

    (A) secondary aldosteronism due to diuretics
    (B) vomiting
    (C) primary aldosteronism
    (D) ingestion of alkali
    (E) licorice ingestion   *(Ref. 22)*

75. A 60-year-old man presents with weakness of several days' duration. Serum chemistries reveal Na^+ 135, K^+ 2.5, Cl^- 115, CO_2 10, and pH 7.30. The first step in correction of the electrolytes in this patient is administration of

    (A) $NaHCO_3$ (sodium bicarbonate)
    (B) NaCl (sodium chloride)
    (C) KCl (potassium chloride)
    (D) sodium lactate
    (E) D_5W (5% dextrose in water)   *(Ref. 22)*

76. Methyldopa may produce

    (A) cold syndrome
    (B) anxiety syndrome
    (C) pulmonary fibrosis
    (D) lupus syndrome
    (E) peptic esophagitis   *(Ref. 43)*

77. A patient is suspected of having Rocky Mountain spotted fever. You would now

    (A) perform a blood culture
    (B) order a Weil–Felix test
    (C) perform bone marrow aspirations
    (D) order a CT scan of the skull
    (E) order a human lymphocyte antigen (HLA) test   *(Ref. 22)*

78. A 22-year-old college girl developed tingling and burning in the back of the neck, radiating to the upper back, arms, and front of the chest 20 minutes after eating at a Chinese restaurant. She also complains of throbbing pain in the temples and infraorbital region. The most likely cause of her symptoms is

    (A) monosodium glutamate
    (B) monosodium urate

    (C) monosodium pyrophosphate
    (D) monosodium oxalate
    (E) monosodium citrate   *(Ref. 2)*

79. A 40-year-old man, diabetic since age 25, has previously been stable on insulin. His blood chemistries have been normal. Six days before admission, he developed fever and nausea with continuous vomiting. Three days before admission, he stopped taking insulin. He continued to urinate six to eight times a day. On the day of admission, he became lethargic. Physical examination reveals: blood pressure 95/70, pulse 115, respiration 28, mental dullness, and decreased skin turgor. Lab values are as follows: HCT 52, blood urea nitrogen (BUN) 60, blood sugar 560, Na^+ 152, K^+ 5.2, Cl^- 108, HCO_3^- 16. Urine studies revealed: 50 mL/hour, specific gravity 1.020, glucose 4+, ketones 2+, protein 2+. His acid–base status is best described as

    (A) metabolic acidosis
    (B) normal
    (C) metabolic alkalosis
    (D) respiratory alkalosis
    (E) respiratory acidosis   *(Ref. 2)*

80. A 30-year-old female complains of a sore throat lasting 2 days. Physical examinations reveal an infected pharynx without any other findings. You would now

    (A) prescribe oral penicillin
    (B) order SMA-14
    (C) order a chest x-ray
    (D) give a penicillin shot
    (E) perform a throat culture   *(Ref. 74)*

81. Amantadine is effective for the treatment of

    (A) influenza A infections
    (B) respiratory syncytial virus infections
    (C) influenza B infections
    (D) parainfluenza infections
    (E) adenovirus infections   *(Ref. 43)*

82. The side reactions of amantadine include

    (A) diplopia
    (B) depression

(C) bloody stools

(D) dyspnea

(E) joint pain   *(Ref. 43)*

83. The most powerful method of reducing mortality in the United States is

   (A) building more hospitals

   (B) iodizing salts

   (C) smoking cessation

   (D) developing an AIDS vaccine

   (E) popularizing a prudent diet   *(Ref. 2)*

84. An elderly patient on thiazide therapy for hypertension was found to have a low serum sodium level of 120 mEq/L. The preferred treatment is

   (A) potassium-restriction diet

   (B) high-purine diet

   (C) zinc-restriction diet

   (D) fluid-restriction diet

   (E) high-carbohydrate diet   *(Ref. 22)*

85. A 33-year-old family practice resident complained of widespread aching pain, fatigue, depression, anxiousness, and difficulty in falling asleep. Pain on palpation of all 18 tender points (occiput, low cervical, trapezius, supraspinatus, second rib, lateral epicondyle, gluteal, greater tronchanter, and knee) can be elicited. You made a diagnosis of fibromyalgia. The most useful drug is

   (A) codeine

   (B) amitryptyline (Elavil)

   (C) ascorbic acid

   (D) propranolol (Inderal)

   (E) amphetamine   *(Ref. 2)*

86. A recent immigrant from Southeast Asia is suspected of malaria. Prior to antimalarial therapy, you will order

   (A) stool culture

   (B) Guthrie bacterial inhibition test

(C) sweat test

(D) microassay of enzyme glucose-6-phosphate dehydrogenase (G6PD)

(E) hepatitis B profile   *(Ref. 74)*

87. One of your middle-aged Indochinese patients believes in the yin-yang theory. For 3 days he took lemon and ginger slices for his sore throat, without improvement, and now appears at your urban family practice office. The streptococcal screening is negative, and the physical examination is essentially negative, except for the infected pharynx. You will now

   (A) perform acupuncture to treat his yin-yang imbalance

   (B) order expiratory ceremonies to expel evil spirits

   (C) prescribe oral penicillin 250 mg qid for 20 days

   (D) instruct him that next time he should visit you as soon as the symptoms develop

   (E) accuse him of using home remedies
                                           (Ref. 5)

88. Recurrent genital herpes may be treated with

   (A) bretylium

   (B) acyclovir

   (C) propranolol

   (D) metronidazole

   (E) erythromycin   *(Ref. 43)*

89. When a patient expresses his desire to seek a second opinion, you

   (A) accept his demand

   (B) terminate the professional relationship with him

   (C) accuse him of being a clinician shopper

   (D) diagnose him as a schizophrenic

   (E) express your anger and frustration to him   *(Ref. 2)*

90. A postmenopausal woman has had a long history of varicose veins in both lower extremities. She has developed an erythematous, scaling plaque with superficial ulcer at the medial aspect of the right ankle. It is painful and mildly itching. The most likely diagnosis is

    (A) consequence of hormone replacement
    (B) stasis dermatitis
    (C) filariasis
    (D) rodent ulcer
    (E) Buerger's disease   (Ref. 55)

91. A 24-year-old female received a normal pre-employment physical; however, the screening laboratory test revealed a total serum bilirubin level of 1.7 mg/dL with an indirect level of 1.0 mg/dL. You ordered liver enzymes (glutamic oxaloacetic transaminase [GOT], glutamic pyruvic transaminase [GPT]), and serum alkaline phosphatase, all of which were within normal limits. Hepatitis B surface antigen (HBsAg) was also negative. The most likely condition is

    (A) liver cirrhosis
    (B) acute cholecystitis
    (C) hepatocellular adenoma
    (D) Gilbert's syndrome
    (E) cytomegalovirus disease   (Ref. 72)

92. A patient with a history of asthma has developed hypertension. The drug to be avoided is

    (A) alpha blockers
    (B) alpha agonists
    (C) beta blockers
    (D) beta agonists
    (E) angiotensin-converting enzyme (ACE) inhibitors   (Ref. 3)

93. Which of the following is NOT a routine health maintenance procedure?

    (A) chest x-ray
    (B) tetanus toxoid
    (C) influenza immunization
    (D) mammogram
    (E) Pap smear   (Ref. 3)

94. Which of the following diets is recommended for a patient with hypertension?

    (A) low potassium (<100 mg/d)
    (B) low calcium (<200 mg/d)
    (C) low protein (<20 mg/d)
    (D) low sodium (<2 mg/d)
    (E) low fiber (<12 mg/d)   (Ref. 3)

95. In ambulatory care, at each visit the medical record should document all problems addressed. This will

    (A) increase the cost
    (B) decrease the quality
    (C) annoy the patient
    (D) burden the staff
    (E) improve the quality   (Ref. 2)

96. Asymptomatic hyperuricemia may be caused by

    (A) hypoparathyroidism
    (B) megaloblastic anemia
    (C) high-dose salicylate intake
    (D) diuretic therapy
    (E) INH therapy   (Ref. 48)

97. In an average female adult aged 23 to 50 years, the daily caloric requirement in the nonpregnant state is

    (A) 1200 kcal
    (B) 2000 kcal
    (C) 2700 kcal
    (D) 3000 kcal
    (E) 3500 kcal   (Ref. 2)

98. In an average male adult aged 23 to 50 years, the daily caloric requirement is

    (A) 1800 kcal
    (B) 2000 kcal
    (C) 2700 kcal
    (D) 3400 kcal
    (E) 4000 kcal   (Ref. 2)

99. Which of the following patient characteristics is most likely to be encountered in the urban family practice?

    (A) The presenting problems are usually at the early stage.
    (B) The patients' cultural beliefs are usually homogeneous.
    (C) Psychosocial problems are less likely to be encountered.
    (D) The lifelong environmental stresses are often interwoven into illness.
    (E) Most families fit into the mold of two parents and two children, as shown on the family practice logo   *(Ref. 5)*

100. Digitalis toxicity may produce ECG changes of

    (A) bigeminy
    (B) tall P
    (C) deep Q
    (D) ST elevation
    (E) elevation of U   *(Ref. 43)*

101. An 84-year-old male has had a pressure ulcer on the sacral area, involving full-thickness skin loss over the base of visible fatty tissue. The sore is classified as a

    (A) stage 0 ulcer
    (B) stage 1 ulcer
    (C) stage 2 ulcer
    (D) stage 3 ulcer
    (E) stage 4 ulcer   *(Ref. 2)*

102. The most important element in the successful management of an urban patient's illness is

    (A) a computerized information system
    (B) a therapeutic alliance
    (C) a problem-oriented medical record (POMR)
    (D) high-tech equipment
    (E) a modern office facility   *(Ref. 5)*

103. Which of the following strategies is most useful in improving the therapeutic alliance in urban patients?

    (A) a physician-controlled physician–patient interaction
    (B) patient education activity
    (C) the use of safety locks on pill containers
    (D) color-coded drugs without revealing the nature of the drugs prescribed
    (E) varied drug-dosage schedule streamlined by a computer program   *(Ref. 5)*

104. The most likely reason for noncompliance in the urban setting is

    (A) convenient and supportive care
    (B) mutual participation type of doctor–patient interaction
    (C) short waiting-room times
    (D) an open, nonjudgmental interview style
    (E) dropping out of regular office appointments   *(Ref. 5)*

105. A 40-year-old male fisherman developed an itching, burning, and throbbing pain in his right index and middle fingers. There are multiple painful, purplish-red, swollen plaques on the fingers. The most likely causative organism is

    (A) *Staphylococcus aureus*
    (B) *Erysipelothrix rhusiopathiae*
    (C) *Streptococcus hemolyticus*
    (D) *Streptococcus pneumoniae*
    (E) *Candida albicans*   *(Ref. 55)*

106. Hypocalcemia may show ECG changes of

    (A) prolongation of PR interval
    (B) prolongation of QT interval
    (C) shortening of PR interval
    (D) prolongation of QRS complex
    (E) shortening of QT interval   *(Ref. 2)*

107. You are the urgent-care doctor at the family health center. A 64-year-old female comes to see you, complaining of lower leg cramping pain and general weakness of 1 week's duration. She is a poor historian, but she remembers that she has had "high blood pressure" and has been on medication for almost 2 months. She cannot remember the name of the medication, but it is most likely

   (A) atenolol (Tenormin) 50 mg qd
   (B) benazepril (Lotensin) 10 mg qd
   (C) hydrochlorothiazide 25 mg qd
   (D) felodipine (Plendil) 5 mg qd
   (E) doxazosin (Cardura) 4 mg qd   (Ref. 3)

108. First-generation immigrants often concentrate in urban centers. Immigrants from the Mediterranean are at higher risk to have which of the following diseases?

   (A) thalassemias
   (B) sickle cell anemias
   (C) Tay–Sachs disease
   (D) hepatitis B
   (E) tuberculosis   (Ref. 5)

109. In hypokalemia, the ECG may show

   (A) U waves
   (B) broad P
   (C) tall P
   (D) tall R
   (E) deep Q   (Ref. 2)

110. Widening of QRS complex in the ECG may be caused by

   (A) penicillin
   (B) quinidine
   (C) INH
   (D) thiamine
   (E) theophylline   (Ref. 2)

111. Hyperchromic macrocytic anemia is most likely produced by

   (A) azotemia
   (B) sickle cell disease
   (C) diabetes mellitus
   (D) theophylline administration
   (E) malabsorption syndrome   (Ref. 73)

112. Acute pericarditis may show ECG changes of

   (A) notched P
   (B) tall P
   (C) lengthening of PR interval
   (D) ST elevation
   (E) ST depression   (Ref. 2)

113. A family physician practicing in the urban setting usually provides

   (A) sickness-oriented care
   (B) single-person-oriented care
   (C) injury-oriented care
   (D) family-oriented care
   (E) crisis-oriented care   (Ref. 5)

114. In North American family practice, about 50% of the problems belong to

   (A) 10 diagnoses
   (B) 25 diagnoses
   (C) 50 diagnoses
   (D) 100 diagnoses
   (E) 170 diagnoses   (Ref. 5)

115. The most common endocrine problem seen in the urban family practice setting is

   (A) thyroid storm
   (B) Hashimoto's thyroiditis
   (C) primary hyperparathyroidism
   (D) diabetes mellitus
   (E) Addison's disease   (Ref. 5)

116. Among the following conditions, the most common problem for home visits in urban family practice is

   (A) cardiovascular accident (CVA)
   (B) eczema
   (C) vaginitis
   (D) warts
   (E) obesity   (Ref. 5)

117. In the POMR used by the urban family practice office, the prognosis is derived by

    (A) profile of symptoms
    (B) natural history
    (C) physical signs
    (D) available medications
    (E) diagnostic process   (Ref. 5)

118. Which of the following problems is the so-called "hidden illness" in the elderly?

    (A) stroke
    (B) pressure sores
    (C) flu syndrome
    (D) dental caries
    (E) Parkinson's disease   (Ref. 2)

119. In the urban family practice setting, which of the following diagnoses is most commonly seen?

    (A) URI
    (B) acute myeloblastic leukemia
    (C) AIDS
    (D) colon cancer
    (E) dermatomyositis   (Ref. 5)

120. Compared to white men, black men have a lower mortality in

    (A) bladder cancer
    (B) esophageal cancer
    (C) prostatic cancer
    (D) gastric cancer
    (E) oral cancer   (Ref. 5)

121. Which of the following diseases is more prevalent in Hispanic populations?

    (A) lung cancer
    (B) diabetes mellitus
    (C) heart diseases
    (D) breast cancer
    (E) prostatic cancer   (Ref. 5)

122. Which of the following statements is true concerning the tuberculin skin test for Indochinese refugees in the inner city?

    (A) Everyone should be tested.
    (B) If a child is inoculated with bacillus Calmette–Guérin (BCG), the test is not needed.
    (C) If a child was inoculated with BCG 10 years ago, a positive test can be ignored.
    (D) When the tine test (the multiple puncture test) produces 5 to 9 mm induration, it indicates that the individual has never had tuberculous infection.
    (E) All children living in a community with tuberculin sensitivity exceeding 1% should be tested.   (Ref. 5)

123. Which of the following statements is true regarding sickle cell traits?

    (A) Only persons voluntarily seeking sickle cell screening should be tested.
    (B) Order sickle cell screening for all black patients in the urban family practice.
    (C) Individuals with the positive sickle cell trait are advised to change their jobs.
    (D) Individuals with the positive hemoglobin D trait have a life expectancy half that of an unaffected individual.
    (E) Individuals of German or Irish descent have a prevalence of 10%.   (Ref. 5)

124. The health risks of inner-city populations are increased by

    (A) crowding
    (B) poor nutrition
    (C) inadequate heat during winter
    (D) poverty
    (E) all of the above   (Ref. 5)

125. Acute disseminated gonococcal infection is characterized by

    (A) penile ulcers
    (B) palmar erythema
    (C) symmetrical joint involvement
    (D) hemorrhagic pustular eruption of distal extremities
    (E) strawberry cervix   (Ref. 55)

126. One of your elderly, black, hypertensive patients is well controlled with a diuretic regimen; the patient has attributed this normal pressure to his concomitant use of garlic water. You will now

    (A) allow the patient to continue the dual practice
    (B) order the patient to discontinue garlic water
    (C) instruct the patient to discontinue the diuretics and to continue the garlic water
    (D) tell the patient that he is ignorant and unscientific to believe in voodoo practice
    (E) refer the patient to a psychiatrist to evaluate his mental status   *(Ref. 5)*

127. A patient with a history of gouty arthritis developed hypertension. You will avoid

    (A) beta blockers
    (B) ACE inhibitors
    (C) diuretics
    (D) calcium-channel blockers
    (E) alpha blockers   *(Ref. 3)*

128. Lactose intolerance is commonly seen in

    (A) Arabs
    (B) Italians
    (C) Russians
    (D) Asians
    (E) those of Mediterranean ancestry   *(Ref. 5)*

129. Among the following conditions, which is the most common problem seen in the Indochinese?

    (A) diabetes mellitus
    (B) ascariasis
    (C) essential hypertension
    (D) ischemic heart disease
    (E) multiple sclerosis   *(Ref. 5)*

130. ECG changes in cor pulmonale reveal

    (A) peaked P
    (B) shortened PR
    (C) prolonged PR
    (D) wide notched P
    (E) peaked T   *(Ref. 2)*

131. The prevalence of tuberculosis among Indochinese refugees is estimated to be

    (A) 0%
    (B) 1%
    (C) 10%
    (D) 25%
    (E) 45%   *(Ref. 5)*

132. In Wolff–Parkinson–White syndrome, the most typical ECG change is

    (A) tall T
    (B) tall U
    (C) delta wave
    (D) prolonged PR
    (E) prolonged QT   *(Ref. 2)*

133. Left ventricular hypertrophy LVH may show ECG changes of

    (A) $S_1 + R_5 > 3.5$ mv
    (B) $Q_2 + T_6 > 3.5$ mv
    (C) $S_3 + T_6 > 3.5$ mv
    (D) $S_1 + U_5 > 3.5$ mv
    (E) $S_1 + T_5 > 3.5$ mv   *(Ref. 2)*

134. Right bundle branch block (RBBB) shows ECG changes of

    (A) SS′ in V_1–V_2
    (B) RR′ in V_1–V_2
    (C) TT′ in V_5–V_6
    (D) QQ′ in V_5–V_6
    (E) PP′ in I–II   *(Ref. 2)*

135. Most anterior or anteroseptal infarctions are seen in ECG as

    (A) ST elevation and QS in V_1–V_2
    (B) ST elevation and QS in V_5–V_6
    (C) ST depression and QS in V_1–V_2
    (D) ST depression and QS in V_5–V_6
    (E) ST depression and QS in I–II   *(Ref. 2)*

136. The murmur for aortic stenosis is

   (A) systolic murmur variable with respiration at the left second interspace
   (B) crescendo–decrescendo systolic murmur at the right second interspace transmitted to the neck and apex
   (C) decrescendo diastolic murmur at the right second interspace
   (D) mid-diastolic rumbling at the apex
   (E) holosystolic murmur at the apex radiated to the left axilla   (Ref. 2)

137. In posterior infarction, the ECG may show

   (A) ST depression and prominent R in V_1–V_2
   (B) ST elevation and prominent R in V_5–V_6
   (C) ST elevation and small R in V_5–V_6
   (D) ST elevation and prominent R in V_1–V_2
   (E) ST depression and prominent P in V_5–V_6 (Ref. 2)

138. Wenckebach phenomenon is the progressive lengthening of

   (A) PR
   (B) PP
   (C) QRS
   (D) QT
   (E) ST   (Ref. 2)

139. Mitral regurgitation may produce

   (A) continuous murmur
   (B) midsystolic murmur
   (C) holosystolic murmur
   (D) late systolic murmur
   (E) middiastolic murmur   (Ref. 2)

140. The murmur of mitral stenosis is a

   (A) holosystolic murmur
   (B) continuous murmur
   (C) late systolic murmur
   (D) diastolic rumbling murmur
   (E) midsystolic murmur   (Ref. 2)

141. A patient with the following lab results

pH	Pco_2	HCO_3^-
7.10	80	24

   probably is suffering from

   (A) metabolic acidosis
   (B) normal status
   (C) respiratory alkalosis
   (D) respiratory acidosis
   (E) metabolic alkalosis   (Ref. 2)

142. The atrial rate in paroxysmal atrial tachycardia is

   (A) 45
   (B) 70
   (C) 100
   (D) 180
   (E) 300   (Ref. 2)

143. In sinus bradycardia, the heart rate is most likely

   (A) 45
   (B) 75
   (C) 105
   (D) 135
   (E) 165   (Ref. 2)

144. A 42-year-old male patient complains of racing of the heart. The pulse rate is regular and is 140 beats/min. He is most likely suffering from

   (A) paroxysmal atrial tachycardia
   (B) sinus bradycardia
   (C) sinus tachycardia
   (D) atrial flutter
   (E) ventricular fibrillation   (Ref. 2)

145. The atrial rate in atrial flutter is

   (A) 45
   (B) 72
   (C) 40
   (D) 80
   (E) 280   (Ref. 2)

146. The topical solution of minoxidil, an antihypertensive, is used for

    (A) severe hypertension
    (B) angina pectoris
    (C) alopecia androgenetica
    (D) contact dermatitis
    (E) carbuncle   (Ref. 43)

147. A 36-year-old family physician consults you about his general health status. Physical examinations are essentially normal, and he does not have any special complaints. However, he told you that he was originally from the Philippines, received a BCG vaccination in his childhood, and he has always had a positive PPD skin test. His chest x-ray shows a calcified granuloma in the right upper lobe. He is currently working at a county medical center serving multicultural underserved populations. In the hospital where he works, there were six active tuberculous patients admitted last year. You would tell him that

    (A) he is in perfect health without any health risk
    (B) because of his age, no INH is needed
    (C) he needs INH for a year
    (D) he has had immunity to tuberculosis and does not need further surveillance for tuberculosis
    (E) he needs repeated PPD every 2 months to determine the need for INH   (Ref. 74)

148. The most common helminth infestation in the United States is

    (A) schistosomiasis
    (B) strongyloidiasis
    (C) clonorchiasis
    (D) enterobiasis
    (E) ascariasis   (Ref. 74)

149. The treatment of gastroesophageal reflux disease (GERD) includes

    (A) alcoholic beverages
    (B) frequent coffee drinks
    (C) vagotomy
    (D) sucralfate 1 g bid
    (E) ranitidine 150 mg bid   (Ref. 72)

150. Clubbing of the finger is most likely an early sign of

    (A) thrombocytopenia
    (B) lung cancer
    (C) colon cancer
    (D) osteoarthritis
    (E) depression   (Ref. 33)

151. A 56-year-old female has suffered from frostbite in her feet while ice fishing. You will

    (A) start rapid rewarming in a water bath at 104°F to 108°F
    (B) slowly rewarm in a water bath at 115°F to 120°F
    (C) order dry heat thermotherapy
    (D) perform sympathectomy
    (E) prescribe thyroxine 100 µg qd for 4 weeks   (Ref. 2)

152. Interstitial cystitis is characterized by

    (A) recurrent *E. coli* infections
    (B) association with trichomonal vaginitis
    (C) suprapubic pain relieved by voiding
    (D) positive exfoliative cytology
    (E) absence of dysuria   (Ref. 15)

153. A 25-year-old male presents for an employment physical. He has no complaints, and the history and physical (H&P) are unremarkable. You would order

    (A) nonfasting cholesterol and high-density lipoprotein (HDL)
    (B) fasting cholesterol
    (C) chest x-rays
    (D) ECG
    (E) fasting blood sugar   (Ref. 3)

154. To perform an annual health screening for an asymptomatic 52-year-old male whose H&P are essentially negative, you will order

(A) ECG

(B) chest x-rays

(C) serum cholesterol

(D) urinalysis

(E) complete blood count (CBC)   *(Ref. 3)*

155. A healthy 70-year-old male is recommended for

(A) BCG

(B) influenza vaccine

(C) smallpox vaccine

(D) typhoid vaccine

(E) cholera vaccine   *(Ref. 3)*

156. The use of topical chemical sunscreens most likely

(A) promotes erythema

(B) allows deeper tanning

(C) decreases wrinkles

(D) protects photosensitivity

(E) decreases sunburn   *(Ref. 27)*

157. A patient you have seen twice before for non-specific complaints calls for an appointment. At the outset of the interview, which of the following responses on your part is likely to bring the most thorough and personal information?

(A) a focused question such as "Can you describe your pain?"

(B) a closed question or series of questions such as "Where is it?," "How long does it last?," and "Does it affect your sleep?"

(C) a leading question such as "You are having some pain, aren't you?"

(D) an open-ended question such as "What brought you in today?" or "Tell me about your problem."

(E) a compound question(s) such as "Do you have some pain or are you feeling better, or has it been the same since your last visit?"   *(Ref. 4)*

158. Meningococcal meningitis may show

(A) cerebrospinal fluid (CSF) cell 120; lymphocytes: neutrophils (L:N) = 95:5; sugar 70

(B) CSF cell 1200; L:N = 5:95; sugar 20

(C) CSF cell 120; L:N = 60:40; sugar 20; chloride 400 mg/100 mL

(D) CSF protein 150; albuminocytologic dissociation

(E) CSF cell 30, mostly lymphocytes; protein 30; sugar 60; pressure 250 mm H_2O *(Ref. 74)*

159. The CSF findings in aseptic meningitis include

(A) pleocytosis

(B) cell count of 10,000

(C) polys dominate

(D) decreased proteins

(E) elevated glucose   *(Ref. 74)*

160. Which of the following statements is true regarding influenza?

(A) It is caused by a deoxyribonucleic acid (DNA) virus.

(B) Its symptoms are mostly in gastrointestinal (GI) areas.

(C) It lasts for 2 to 3 days.

(D) Its incubation period is 10 to 14 days.

(E) It is treated by metronidazole.   *(Ref. 74)*

161. Influenza vaccine is indicated for

(A) infants

(B) healthy athletes

(C) adolescents

(D) the elderly

(E) schoolchildren   *(Ref. 74)*

162. Influenza vaccine is given

(A) annually

(B) once in a lifetime

(C) in a series of three shots

(D) in combination with *Haemophilus influenzae*

(E) to prevent pulmonary tuberculosis

(Ref. 7)

163. A 60-year-old hypertensive male developed congestive heart failure (CHF). The drug of choice is

    (A) propranolol
    (B) labetalol
    (C) captopril
    (D) metoprolol
    (E) atenolol   (Ref. 4)

164. Metoclopramide (Reglan) may

    (A) decrease the serum prolactin level
    (B) decrease GI motility
    (C) lower the lower esophageal sphincter pressure
    (D) produce infertility
    (E) develop akathisia   (Ref. 43)

165. Treatments of lead poisoning include

    (A) D-penicillamine
    (B) dimercaprol (BAL)
    (C) calcium disodium edetate (EDTA)
    (D) avoidance of further industrial exposure of lead
    (E) all of the above   (Ref. 43)

166. A normal CSF glucose can be compatible with all of the following EXCEPT

    (A) viral meningitis
    (B) partially treated bacterial meningitis
    (C) fungal meningitis
    (D) brain abscess
    (E) meningoencephalitis   (Ref. 74)

167. Which of the following clinical manifestations will arouse suspicion of lead poisoning?

    (A) increased libido
    (B) convulsion
    (C) improved memory
    (D) gum hypertrophy
    (E) iritis   (Ref. 1)

168. According to the family system theory

    (A) psychotherapeutic intervention must include the entire family
    (B) the individual's psychic life and his behavior can only be understood in the family context
    (C) the family physician's behavior may contribute to the development of a new family system that governs the behavior of its members
    (D) the family physician's behavior may change the family system
    (E) all of the above   (Ref. 3)

169. A 60-year-old construction worker complains of progressive dyspnea on exertion, a dry cough, and a "tight" feeling in the chest for 10 months. Physical examination reveals fine inspiratory rales in the posterior and posterolateral lung bases. A chest x-ray shows interstitial fibrosis in the lower lung fields and pleural thickening with calcification. The most likely diagnosis is

    (A) COPD
    (B) sarcoidosis
    (C) AIDS
    (D) asbestosis
    (E) chronic bronchitis   (Ref. 22)

170. Which of the following individuals might encounter significant exposure to asbestos?

    (A) auto mechanics
    (B) Korean war veterans
    (C) schoolteachers
    (D) librarians
    (E) bus drivers   (Ref. 22)

171. Interstitial fibrosis in the lung is associated with

    (A) aspirin
    (B) captopril
    (C) nitrofurantoin
    (D) INH
    (E) codeine   (Ref. 43)

172. Characteristic pulmonary function test findings in asbestosis may show

    (A) increased total lung capacity
    (B) increased residual volume
    (C) decreased vital capacity
    (D) increased forced vital capacity
    (E) increased forced expiratory flow rate
    (Ref. 22)

173. A patient with asbestosis is at higher risk to develop

    (A) hepatoma
    (B) leukemia
    (C) breast cancer
    (D) cervical cancer
    (E) lung cancer   *(Ref. 22)*

174. Mesothelioma is associated with

    (A) radon exposure
    (B) asbestosis
    (C) hepatitis B
    (D) schistosomiasis
    (E) psoriasis   *(Ref. 22)*

175. The complications of asbestosis include

    (A) hypertension
    (B) diabetes insipidus
    (C) dementia
    (D) cataracts
    (E) cardiac failure   *(Ref. 22)*

176. The patient with asbestosis should

    (A) stop automobile driving
    (B) smoke two packs of cigarettes per day
    (C) receive BCG vaccinations
    (D) take aspirin 325 mg one tablet per day
    (E) avoid pulmonary irritants   *(Ref. 22)*

177. A patient with PUD is well controlled by an H2 blocker. The prolonged use of the H2 blocker may be associated with

    (A) decreased creatine phosphokinase (CPK)
    (B) gynecomastia

    (C) polycythemia
    (D) decreased aspartate transaminase (AST)
    (E) depressed alanine transaminase (ALT)
    (Ref. 2)

178. Which of the following therapeutic approaches is NOT recommended for patients with PUD

    (A) histamine H2-receptor antagonists
    (B) cigarette smoking
    (C) mucosal coating agent (coating ulcer craters)
    (D) proton pump inhibitors
    (E) *Helicobacter pylori* eradication   *(Ref. 2)*

179. The major source of radon exposure is from

    (A) vegetables imported from abroad
    (B) animal meats ingested
    (C) water supplies
    (D) soil beneath the dwelling
    (E) drinking river water   *(Ref. 22)*

180. Radon exposure is a risk factor for

    (A) pancreatic cancer
    (B) malignant melanoma
    (C) lung cancer
    (D) thyroid cancer
    (E) retinoblastoma   *(Ref. 22)*

181. Concerning radon exposure in homes, which of the following statements is true?

    (A) Radon concentrations are at the same level in homes within a radius of 20 miles.
    (B) All inhabitants are required to receive yearly chest x-rays and sputum cytology for radon exposure.
    (C) Third floors will have higher radon concentrations than the ground floor.
    (D) Indoor radon concentration is one half that of the outdoor concentration.
    (E) The highest radon concentration is in the basement.   *(Ref. 22)*

182. Which of the following statements is true of radon effect?

    (A) The physiologic effect of radon is derived from its tissue stimulation characteristic.
    (B) Radon daughters account for most tracheobronchial damages.
    (C) Cigarette smoking antagonizes radon's physiologic action.
    (D) Radon induces hepatocellular enzyme systems.
    (E) Radon mothers cause neurophysiologic serotonin reduction.   (Ref. 22)

183. Indoor concentrations of radon can be measured by

    (A) charcoal canisters
    (B) humidifiers
    (C) thermometers
    (D) mathematic models
    (E) chromatographers   (Ref. 22)

184. The indoor radon concentration can be reduced by

    (A) opening windows
    (B) spending more time in the basement
    (C) cigarette smoking
    (D) establishment of fireplaces
    (E) increasing room temperature   (Ref. 22)

185. Corrective actions are recommended for indoor radon concentrations of

    (A) 0.2 pci/L (pico curies per liter)
    (B) 1 pci/L
    (C) 1 working level (WL)
    (D) 0.005 (WL)
    (E) 0.01 (WL)   (Ref. 22)

186. The area with a high background level of natural radiation is

    (A) the Hawaiian islands
    (B) the Reading Prong physiographic province
    (C) Southern California

    (D) the Great Plains
    (E) the Nevada desert   (Ref. 22)

187. Which of the following facts about radon is true?

    (A) New homes are immune to radon exposure.
    (B) Radon exposure is nonexistent in the United States.
    (C) There are no remedies available for indoor radon accumulations.
    (D) Radon may enter the building through cracks in the floor.
    (E) The elderly are at higher risk of radon exposure than children.   (Ref. 22)

188. A 40-year-old male welding-factory worker complains of sudden onset of malaise, fever, dyspnea, nonproductive cough, and nausea at noon and lasting the entire afternoon, for a period of 3 to 6 months. However, during the weekends he is often symptom-free and is able to pursue his golf activities. The most useful information for assessing his problem is

    (A) occupational history
    (B) family history
    (C) family genogram
    (D) dietary history
    (E) golfing history   (Ref. 22)

189. Farmer's lung is caused by

    (A) zinc oxide
    (B) *Bacillus subtilis* enzyme
    (C) *Trichosporon cutaneum*
    (D) *Aspergillus fumigatus*
    (E) *Micropolyspora faeni*   (Ref. 22)

190. Malt worker's disease is caused by

    (A) *Mycoplasma pneumoniae*
    (B) copper fumes
    (C) *A. fumigatus*
    (D) *Legionella pneumophila*
    (E) *Candida albicans*   (Ref. 22)

191. Bagassosis is caused by

    (A) fumes of lead
    (B) radon radiation
    (C) thermodegradation of polytetrafluo-
        roethylene (Teflon)
    (D) *Cryptococcus neoformans*
    (E) *Thermoactinomyces sacchari*   (Ref. 22)

192. Metal fume fever is characterized by

    (A) a coin lesion on the chest roentgenogram
    (B) a metallic taste in the mouth
    (C) leukopenia
    (D) positive cold agglutinins
    (E) urethritis   (Ref. 22)

193. The appropriate work-up for a patient sus-
    pected of polymer fume fever is

    (A) BCG
    (B) antinuclear antibody (ANA)
    (C) BUN
    (D) white blood count (WBC)
    (E) thyroid-stimulating hormone (TSH)
            (Ref. 22)

194. The causal agent of hypersensitivity pneu-
    monitis can be identified by

    (A) urine analysis
    (B) joint fluid analysis
    (C) fungal cultures of the particulate parti-
        cles for inhalation
    (D) blood bacterial cultures for staphylococ-
        cus
    (E) stool ova examinations   (Ref. 22)

195. The diagnosis of hypersensitivity pneumoni-
    tis is aided by the positive test of

    (A) cold agglutinins
    (B) serologic test for syphilis (STS)
    (C) immunoglobulin G (IgG) precipitating
        antibodies
    (D) human immunodeficiency virus (HIV)
    (E) alpha-fetoprotein (AFP)   (Ref. 22)

196. The finding of bronchoalveolar lavage for hy-
    persensitivity pneumonitis is most likely
    showing

    (A) malignant cells
    (B) atypical epithelial cells
    (C) neutrophils
    (D) Langhans' giant cells
    (E) mononuclear cells   (Ref. 22)

197. The best treatment of hypersensitivity pneu-
    monitis is

    (A) Septra DS (trimethoprim-sulfamethoxa-
        zole) 1# bid for 10 days
    (B) Vibramycin 100 (doxycycline hyclate) 1#
        bid for 10 days
    (C) Flagyl 250 (metronidazole) 1# bid for 5
        days
    (D) antigen avoidance
    (E) Ventolin (albuterol) inhaler 17 g 2 puffs
        q4h   (Ref. 22)

198. The most common complication of silo-
    filler's disease is

    (A) nasopharyngeal carcinoma
    (B) bronchiolitis obliterans
    (C) mesothelioma
    (D) arrhythmia
    (E) amenorrhea   (Ref. 22)

199. A characteristic chest x-ray finding in silico-
    sis is

    (A) enlarged right ventricle
    (B) Kerley B lines
    (C) hilar eggshell calcification
    (D) pleural effusion
    (E) peripheral coin lesion   (Ref. 22)

200. Patients with silicosis are at higher risk to
    contract

    (A) tuberculosis
    (B) asbestosis
    (C) syphilis
    (D) erythema nodosum
    (E) rheumatoid arthritis   (Ref. 22)

201. Most patients with chronic silicosis exhibit

(A) cyanosis
(B) hepatomegaly
(C) no symptoms
(D) cachexia
(E) frequent syncopal episodes   *(Ref. 22)*

202. The most common clinical presentation in acute beryllium disease is

(A) clubbing of fingers
(B) hepatomegaly
(C) splenomegaly
(D) renal calculi
(E) bronchiolitis   *(Ref. 22)*

203. The clinical manifestation of chronic beryllium disease is characterized by

(A) posterior uveitis
(B) systemic granulomatosis
(C) cerebral calcification
(D) dermatitis arthritis syndrome
(E) presbycusis   *(Ref. 22)*

204. The treatment choice for berylliosis is

(A) corticosteroids
(B) sulfa drugs
(C) cephalosporins
(D) antidepressants
(E) minor tranquilizers   *(Ref. 22)*

205. A 42-year-old nonpregnant, obese female complains of dyspepsia for 4 months. Cimetidine (Tagamet) is helpful but does not completely relieve the symptom. There is a tenderness at the right upper quadrant without other remarkable findings. The most productive procedure is

(A) pelvic ultrasound
(B) upper GI series
(C) liver function tests
(D) serum amylase levels
(E) right upper quadrant abdominal ultrasounds   *(Ref. 2)*

DIRECTIONS (Questions 206 through 279): Each question consists of an introduction followed by some statements. Mark T (true) or F (false) after each statement.

206. Side reactions of misoprostol (Cytotec) include

(A) diarrhea
(B) vaginal spotting
(C) flatulence
(D) constipation
(E) headache   *(Ref. 43)*

207. Pancreatitis is associated with the use of

(A) estrogen
(B) furosemide
(C) thiazide
(D) ethanol
(E) sulfonamides   *(Ref. 43)*

208. Polycythemia may be associated with

(A) hypernephroma
(B) hepatoma
(C) uterine myoma
(D) pheochromocytoma
(E) high altitude   *(Ref. 22)*

209. A diabetic patient was found to have hypercholesterolemia. Following administration of new medications for a month, the patient returns complaining of severe muscle soreness. The patient is taking

(A) niacin (nicotinic acid)
(B) fish oil
(C) pravastatin (Provacol)
(D) probucol (Lorelco)
(E) neutral protamine Hagedorn (NPH) insulin   *(Ref. 3)*

210. Which of the following should be used to eradicate *H. pylori*?

(A) Septra DS 1# bid for 2 weeks
(B) Pepto-Bismol 2# qid for 2 weeks
(C) tetracycline 500 mg 1# qid for 2 weeks

(D) metronidazole 250 mg 1# tid for 2 weeks

(E) INH 300 mg 1# hs for 3 weeks

(Ref. 43)

211. Drugs that may induce orthostatic hypotension include

(A) corticosteroids

(B) hydrochlorothiazide

(C) clonidine (Catapres)

(D) amitriptyline (Elavil)

(E) erythromycin   *(Ref. 43)*

212. Complications of prosthetic heart valves include

(A) infection

(B) hemolytic anemia

(C) thromboembolism

(D) heart failure

(E) angina pectoris   *(Ref. 2)*

213. Which of the following statements is true concerning immunoglobulins?

(A) IgG comprises approximately 80% of normal serum gamma globulin; this group includes most of the acquired antibodies.

(B) IgA makes up approximately 15%, exhibited with a variety of antimicrobial activities, and is the principal type of antibody present in external secretions.

(C) IgM, comprising perhaps 5%, includes such antibodies as heterophil.

(D) IgE antibodies appear responsible for immediate hypersensitivity reactions such as atopic dermatitis and allergic asthma.

(E) IgD is a specific antibody to AIDS and is very useful for treatment of AIDS.

(Ref. 22)

214. Chronic constrictive pericarditis may be caused by which of the following?

(A) coxsackie B viral infections

(B) mediastinal irradiation

(C) pneumococcal infections

(D) uremia

(E) diabetes mellitus   *(Ref. 74)*

215. Clinical manifestations of acute pancreatitis include

(A) decrease of serum calcium

(B) rectal tenderness

(C) pneumoperitoneum

(D) leukopenia

(E) cholelithiasis   *(Ref. 62)*

216. Laboratory findings in multiple myeloma show

(A) elevated erythrocyte sedimentation rate (ESR)

(B) a monoclonal spike at gamma globulin

(C) plasma cell infiltration in bone marrow

(D) lytic lesions in the spine x-rays

(E) normocytic normochromic anemia

(Ref. 73)

217. The etiology of aortic regurgitation includes

(A) hypertension

(B) Marfan syndrome

(C) rheumatoid spondylitis

(D) blunt trauma to the chest

(E) syphilis   *(Ref. 2)*

218. Which of the following features are frequently associated with Hodgkin's disease?

(A) lymph node biopsy showing characteristic Reed–Sternberg giant cells

(B) herpes zoster

(C) pruritus

(D) pain in the region of enlarged lymph nodes after drinking alcohol

(E) fever   *(Ref. 73)*

219. The high-risk groups for syphilis include

(A) sexually active teens

(B) drug users

(C) persons with multiple sexual partners

(D) women of childbearing age

(E) individuals who have sex with prostitutes   *(Ref. 74)*

220. The urban homeless are at higher risk of developing

    (A) tuberculosis
    (B) lice infestations
    (C) malnutrition
    (D) personality disorders
    (E) seizure disorders   (Ref. 5)

221. The barriers for the inner-city elderly in seeing a physician include

    (A) lack of financial resources
    (B) long waiting time
    (C) no one to take the patient to visit the physician
    (D) fear of being victimized once out of the house
    (E) lack of transportation   (Ref. 5)

222. Family physicians are particularly suited to detect and manage high-risk urban patients because the excess urban risk is most likely due to

    (A) biologic insults
    (B) environmental impacts
    (C) psychosocial issues
    (D) political influences
    (E) economic hardships   (Ref. 5)

223. High-risk groups for tuberculosis include

    (A) minority populations
    (B) AIDS patients
    (C) patients with Hodgkin's disease
    (D) the homeless
    (E) long-term steroid users   (Ref. 74)

224. An 82-year-old Mexican-American male complains of low-grade afternoon fever, productive cough, night sweats, anorexia, and weight loss for 2 months. You suspect tuberculosis and perform the tuberculin test, which is negative. You will now

    (A) order sputum cytology studies for lung cancer
    (B) order sputum smears and cultures for acid-fast bacilli
    (C) order sputum smears and cultures for common bacterial pathogens
    (D) order fungal sputum smears and cultures
    (E) order blood cultures for brucellosis   (Ref. 2)

225. Coccidioidomycosis

    (A) is associated with erythema nodosum
    (B) may produce arthralgia
    (C) may show a coin lesion on the chest x-ray
    (D) may cause cough, chest pain, and fever
    (E) may cause meningitis   (Ref. 74)

226. The priority groups for HBsAg screening among Indochinese patients include

    (A) pregnant women
    (B) women of reproductive age
    (C) orphans
    (D) preschool children
    (E) drug abusers   (Ref. 5)

227. Which of the following statements concerning bronchopulmonary aspergillosis is/are true?

    (A) Significant eosinophilia is usually present.
    (B) Serum precipitins are frequently found against *A. fumigatus.*
    (C) Patchy infiltrates may be seen on the chest x-ray.
    (D) Patients often expectorate small brown plugs in the sputum.
    (E) *A. fumigatus* is always isolated from sputum.   (Ref. 74)

228. Which of the following statements is/are true concerning antihypertensive agents?

    (A) Beta blockers are best suited for asthmatic patients.
    (B) Verapamil is the drug of choice in third-degree heart block.
    (C) Thiazide is the drug of choice in hypertensive patients who develop acute gouty arthritis.

(D) Alpha-receptor blockers are to be used for the hypertensive elderly complaining of lightheadedness.

(E) Dysgeusia may be produced by ACE inhibitors.   *(Ref. 43)*

229. For travelers, the precautions against HIV infection include

(A) engagement in frequent casual sexual activities

(B) receiving immunoaugmentative therapies

(C) receiving acupuncture therapies

(D) tatooing the body with colorful paints

(E) receiving penicillin injections for URIs   *(Ref. 74)*

230. Symptoms of food reactions include

(A) urinary frequency

(B) constipation

(C) pruritus

(D) dyspnea

(E) headache   *(Ref. 72)*

231. Foods causing IgE-mediated allergic reactions include

(A) shellfish

(B) chicken

(C) melons

(D) eggs

(E) corn   *(Ref. 72)*

232. In Lyme disease

(A) most cases have been reported from the Pacific coast area

(B) the treatment of choice for children under 8 years of age is tetracycline

(C) the most common vector is the dog tick *Dermacentor variabilis*

(D) the cutaneous manifestation is characterized by erythema chronicum migrans

(E) arthralgia and arthritis may occur in stage 3   *(Ref. 74)*

233. Malignant hyperthermia is associated with

(A) dantrolene (Dantrium)

(B) succinylcholine (Anectine)

(C) trauma

(D) viral infections

(E) heat stress   *(Ref. 2)*

234. Factors that may delay recovery from occupational injuries include

(A) refusal to refill narcotic prescriptions

(B) secondary gain

(C) depression

(D) physician's supporting attitudes

(E) life crises   *(Ref. 3)*

235. The management of scombroid poisoning involves

(A) corticosteroids

(B) phenobarbital

(C) diphenhydramine (Benadryl)

(D) cimetidine (Tagamet)

(E) Mylanta (an antacid)   *(Ref. 43)*

236. Travelers who are visiting malarious areas where *Plasmodium falciparum* is not known to be resistant to chloroquine should

(A) start chloroquine 2 weeks before travel

(B) start chloroquine 4 weeks before travel

(C) take chloroquine 500 mg once weekly during their stay in the area

(D) continue chloroquine for 2 weeks after departure from the malarious area

(E) continue chloroquine for 4 weeks after departure from the malarious area   *(Ref. 43)*

237. Which of the following statements is/are correct in regard to polychlorinated biphenyls (PCBs)?

    (A) A major source of low-level exposure is from eating fish.
    (B) In animal studies, PCBs are associated with malignant melanomas.
    (C) Some newborns of pregnant women who ingested PCB-contaminated rice oils are called "seven-up babies."
    (D) Exposure to sewage sludge contaminated with PCBs is correlated with severe hyperglycemia.
    (E) It has been suggested that the fetal PCB syndrome seen in Japan was actually due to exposure to PCDFs (polychlorinated dibenzofurans).   *(Ref. 76)*

238. Which of the following occupations are at higher risk to develop brucellosis?

    (A) meat-packing plant employees
    (B) fishermen
    (C) pet shop owners
    (D) veterinarians
    (E) slaughterhouse employees   *(Ref. 43)*

239. Brucellosis is commonly transmitted from infected

    (A) cattle
    (B) patients
    (C) hogs
    (D) fish
    (E) soil   *(Ref. 43)*

240. The correct agent/host teams are

    (A) *Brucella abortus*–monkey
    (B) *Brucella suis*–swine
    (C) *Brucella melitensis*–cattle
    (D) *Brucella canis*–dogs
    (E) *Brucella hominis*–humans   *(Ref. 43)*

241. A 30-year-old recent immigrant from Central America has worked at a slaughterhouse for 9 months. He complains of an insidious onset of general malaise, fatigue, myalgia, weakness, depression, sweats, headache, and loss of appetite during the last 2 to 3 weeks. He also experienced a fever pattern of rising in the afternoon and falling at night. The most likely diagnosis is

    (A) adjustment disorder
    (B) depression
    (C) brucellosis
    (D) tuberculosis
    (E) syphilis   *(Ref. 43)*

242. Diagnosis of brucellosis is aided by

    (A) a positive serology
    (B) a positive blood culture
    (C) a characteristic pulmonary infiltrate pattern
    (D) a positive abnormal ultrasound
    (E) a characteristic synovial fluid finding   *(Ref. 43)*

243. Toxoplasmosis

    (A) is transmitted by hogs
    (B) resembles the clinical symptoms of infectious mononucleosis
    (C) is caused by HIV
    (D) may cause congenital dislocation of the hip in a fetus
    (E) may increase the risk of infertility   *(Ref. 74)*

244. Anthrax is

    (A) transmitted by shellfish
    (B) a rickettsial disease
    (C) an occupational disease for weavers
    (D) characterized by necrotic skin ulcer
    (E) associated with wool-sorter's disease   *(Ref. 74)*

245. Common complications of brucellosis include

    (A) endocarditis
    (B) hypersplenism
    (C) spondylitis
    (D) osteosarcoma
    (E) labrynthitis   *(Ref. 43)*

246. Treatment of brucellosis is by

(A) Flagyl (metronidazole) 2 g PO stat
(B) Flagyl 250 mg tid PO for 10 days
(C) Vibramycin (doxycycline) 100 mg PO bid for 6 weeks
(D) streptomycin 1.0 g IM qd for 2 weeks
(E) aspirin 325 mg PO qd for 3 weeks

(Ref. 43)

247. Effective preventive measures for brucellosis include

(A) appropriate personal hygiene
(B) immunizations of susceptible animals
(C) isolation of brucellosis patients
(D) chemoprophylaxis with rifampin for 3 months
(E) use of *Brucella* immune serum every 6 months for high-risk individuals

(Ref. 43)

248. In the diagnosis of syphilis

(A) the VDRL (Venereal Disease Research Laboratory) test is 100% positive for primary syphilis
(B) the CSF VDRL test is nearly 100% specific for neurosyphilis
(C) the FTA-ABS (fluorescent treponemal antibody-absorption) test will remain positive after treatment of syphilis
(D) the most specific diagnosis of syphilis is by the culture of *T. pallidum*
(E) the Wassermann test is the most commonly used serologic test for syphilis nowadays

(Ref. 74)

249. Cysticercosis

(A) is most commonly encountered in the Midwest in the United States
(B) affects only Americans who travel to Mexico City
(C) is caused by eating beef containing cysts of *Taenia saginata*
(D) is always manifested by central nervous system (CNS) abnormalities
(E) can be treated by pyrantel pamoate (Antiminth)

(Ref. 74)

250. Normocytic anemia may be caused by

(A) acute blood loss
(B) renal disease
(C) pregnancy
(D) hypothyroidism
(E) macroglobulinemia

(Ref. 73)

251. Alteplase (Activase) is contraindicated in

(A) recent intracranial surgery (within 2 months)
(B) age beyond 70 years
(C) abdominal aneurysm
(D) diabetes mellitus
(E) coronary thrombosis

(Ref. 43)

252. Antihistamines may cause

(A) blurred vision
(B) impotence
(C) difficulty sleeping
(D) hypertension
(E) dry mouth

(Ref. 43)

253. Side reactions of cyclosporine (Sandimmune) include

(A) acute tubular necrosis
(B) hypertension
(C) hypertrichosis
(D) gingival hyperplasia
(E) hair loss

(Ref. 43)

254. Common side reactions of lovastatin (Mevacor) include

(A) increased serum transaminases
(B) myalgia
(C) skin rashes
(D) rhabdomyolysis
(E) gastrointestinal upset

(Ref. 43)

255. Common side effects of theophylline include

(A) drowsiness
(B) vomiting
(C) diarrhea
(D) palpitation
(E) agitation

(Ref. 43)

256. Clinical presentation of Crohn's disease includes

   (A) sclerosing cholangitis
   (B) uveitis
   (C) ankylosing spondylitis
   (D) erythema nodosum
   (E) aphthous stomatitis   (Ref. 22)

257. Digitalis toxicity is frequently manifested by

   (A) constipation
   (B) nausea and vomiting
   (C) blurring of vision
   (D) ventricular ectopy with frequent couples on ECG
   (E) hypermagnesemia   (Ref. 43)

258. Which of the following statements is/are true for smoking cessation?

   (A) Eighty to 90% of smokers consider quitting.
   (B) Physician's advice yields a 1-year quit rate of 5% in asymptomatic smokers.
   (C) Most smoking cessation programs yield 1-year abstinence rates of approximately 25%.
   (D) Withdrawal symptoms can be prevented by gradual reduction of smoking.
   (E) Nicorette (2 mg nicotine gum) is the drug of choice for pregnant smokers who decide to quit.   (Ref. 4)

259. Managements of infectious mononucleosis include

   (A) analgesics for pain relief
   (B) ampicillin for exudative pharyngitis
   (C) corticosteroids for pharyngeal obstruction
   (D) avoidance of heavy lifting and strenuous exercise
   (E) resting for malaise   (Ref. 74)

260. Which of the following individuals are at high risk to develop iron deficiency anemia?

   (A) infants on iron supplementation diets
   (B) 12-month-old infants on a diet consisting predominantly of cow's milk
   (C) pregnant women
   (D) infants with pica
   (E) premenarcheal girls   (Ref. 73)

261. Cardiac myxomas

   (A) may lead to embolism
   (B) may present with syncope
   (C) are metastatic tumors of the breast
   (D) show a marked decrease of gamma globulin level which is pathognomonic
   (E) arise from right ventricle in 95% of cases   (Ref. 33)

262. Which of the following agents may cause QT widening in ECG?

   (A) quinidine
   (B) procainamide
   (C) tocainide
   (D) disopyramide
   (E) calcium   (Ref. 43)

263. In providing the influenza immunization to your elderly patient, you will explain that influenza vaccines

   (A) are useful in protecting the infection caused by *Haemophilus influenzae*
   (B) should be received from May through July
   (C) can be given to patients who are allergic to eggs
   (D) do not cause any side reactions
   (E) should be received annually   (Ref. 2)

264. The management of patients with *Campylobacter fetus* gastroenteritis includes

   (A) symptomatic treatment
   (B) replacement of water loss
   (C) correction of any electrolyte imbalance
   (D) administration of nitrofurantoin
   (E) administration of vancomycin   (Ref. 74)

265. Clinical presentations of infectious mononucleosis include

   (A) exudative pharyngitis
   (B) megaloblastic anemia

(C) atypical large monocytes

(D) puffy eyelids

(E) elevated cold agglutinin titer *(Ref. 74)*

266. NSAIDs

(A) enhance prostaglandin synthesis

(B) may cause upper GI bleeding

(C) may be useful in the treatment of osteoarthritis

(D) may cause headaches

(E) are muscle relaxants *(Ref. 43)*

267. Traveler's diarrhea

(A) is caused by high zinc content of the water

(B) is caused by the enterotoxin producing *E. coli*

(C) is treated by amphotericin B

(D) is treated by penicillin K

(E) is prevented by immunizations prior to travel *(Ref. 72)*

268. To assess the risk of protein–calorie malnutrition in a nursing home patient, you will order which of the following tests?

(A) serum potassium

(B) serum cholesterol

(C) serum calcium

(D) serum albumin

(E) serum triglyceride *(Ref. 33)*

269. Complications of PUD include

(A) bleeding

(B) perforation

(C) obstruction

(D) metabolic alkalosis

(E) dumping syndrome *(Ref. 72)*

270. Which of the following adults are recommended for pneumococcal vaccines?

(A) patients with cirrhosis of the liver

(B) individuals who received pneumococcal vaccines 5 years ago

(C) elderly, healthy individuals who are eligible for Medicare

(D) patients with diabetes mellitus

(E) healthy pregnant women *(Ref. 74)*

271. Which of the following statements concerning the use of drugs in the elderly is/are true?

(A) The dosage of tetracyclines should be increased 1.5 times the usual dose.

(B) Diazepam may prolong the elimination half-life in the elderly.

(C) Increased digoxin dosage may take 2 weeks to show the effect.

(D) The lidocaine dosage needs to increase two-fold because of the increase in liver clearance.

(E) The sensitivity to CNS depressants is increased. *(Ref. 43)*

272. Which of the following side reactions is/are commonly seen in the lipid-lowering drugs?

(A) Clofibrate (Atromid-S) may cause flu-like syndrome.

(B) Gemfibrozil (Lopid) may cause anemia.

(C) Nicotinic acid (Nicolar) results in hypertension.

(D) Resins (Colestid) may cause bleeding.

(E) Probucol (Lorelco) may prolong QT interval in the ECG. *(Ref. 43)*

273. Increased adverse drug reactions in the elderly are associated with

(A) decreased creatinine clearance

(B) normal serum creatinine

(C) increased hepatic metabolic capacity

(D) increased production of gastric acid

(E) increased lean body mass *(Ref. 3)*

274. Complications of infectious mononucleosis include

(A) cervical polyp

(B) renal rupture

(C) meningoencephalitis

(D) peritonsillar abscess

(E) hepatitis *(Ref. 74)*

275. Which of the following statements is/are true for pneumonias?

    (A) The most common pneumonia acquired in the community is caused by *Klebsiella pneumoniae*.
    (B) In the elderly, the most likely etiologic organism for community-acquired pneumonia is *E. coli*.
    (C) Most pediatric pneumonias acquired in the community are viral pneumonias.
    (D) Pneumocystis pneumonia is associated with AIDS.
    (E) Penicillin is empirically the drug of choice for pneumonias caused by the beta-lactamase–producing *H. influenzae*.
    (Ref. 74)

276. Side reactions of calcium-channel blockers include

    (A) atrioventricular heart block
    (B) bradycardia
    (C) hypotension
    (D) constipation
    (E) peripheral edema   *(Ref. 43)*

277. To lower the cholesterol, the following diets are recommended:

    (A) coconut oil
    (B) palm kernel oil
    (C) chicken liver
    (D) lean beef
    (E) peach   *(Ref. 2)*

278. The side reactions of sumatriptan (Imitrex) include

    (A) lightheadedness
    (B) chest tightness
    (C) warmth throughout the body
    (D) vertigo
    (E) tingling sensations   *(Ref. 43)*

279. In the treatment of asthma

    (A) beta blockers should be used vigorously
    (B) cromolyn is to be used only during the acute attacks
    (C) oral theophylline is the cornerstone of the therapy
    (D) inhaled beta agonists are used for mild asthma
    (E) oral corticosteroids are the first-line medications for all patients with mild asthma
    (Ref. 43)

DIRECTIONS (Questions 280 through 288): The following clinical set problem consists of clinical information presented in the format of questions or incomplete statements followed by a group of numbered options.

Indicate T if the option is true;
Indicate F if the option is false.

A 27-year-old male complained of sore throat, nonproductive cough, nausea, anorexia, occasional epigastric discomfort, and general malaise for a week. He worked as an engineer in a government agency for 2 years; 3 months ago a new administrator arrived with multiple new directives, which gave him a lot of stress. He has been married for a year, and his wife is in the second trimester of pregnancy. Physical examinations were unremarkable, and he was supported with compassion and encouragement. One week later, the patient returned with dark urine and yellow skin. His liver was enlarged and tender. GOT and GPT were in the range of 1000 IU, with positive HBsAg. The appropriate treatments include

280. administration of corticosteroids

281. megadose acetaminophen

282. methotrexate 15 mg IM bid for 10 days

283. high-protein, high-fat, low-carbohydrate diet during the acute phase

The patient's colleagues at work

284.   are at higher risk to develop hepatitis D

285.   all need to receive hepatitis B immune globulin (HBIG)

286.   all need to receive hepatitis B vaccine

The patient's wife was found to be HBsAg positive and hepatitis B antigen (HBeAg) negative. You should recommend

287.   the wife to receive 3 doses of hepatitis B vaccine

288.   the newborn baby to receive HBIG and hepatitis B vaccine   *(Ref. 72)*

Answers and Explanations

1. **(B)** Condyloma latum is secondary syphilis caused by *T. pallidum,* a spirochetal organism. Granuloma inguinale is caused by protozoan Donovan bodies. Condyloma acuminatum is multiple papillary proliferation on the vulva, vagina, or cervix and is associated with papillomavirus. Herpes progenitalis is caused by the type II herpesvirus hominis.

2. **(B)** Ciguatera poisoning is caused by the toxin derived from migratory reef fish, especially grouper, jack, snapper, and barracuda. The toxin is called ichthyosarcotoxic because it is in the body parts (musculature, viscera, skin, and mucus) of fish. Cooking cannot prevent the poisoning, and the cignatoxic fish cannot be identified by odor or color. It usually causes nausea, vomiting, diarrhea, and abdominal pain within 36 hours after ingestion, and the patient may develop numbness and tingling of the lips, hands, and feet; reversal of cold to hot sensations in touch and taste; and arthralgia and myalgia of the legs and thighs. Emesis, gastric lavage, and cathartic administration are used to remove unabsorbed toxin; atropine and intravenous fluids are administered for symptomatic relief. There are no antidotes available yet.

3. **(D)** In the elderly, an infectious process may not present with fever, pain, tachycardia, or even leukocytosis. Confusion or disorientation is often the first clue of serious infections. A high index of suspicion of infection is the usual hypothesis when an elderly deteriorates clinically without adequate explanation.

4. **(C)** Hypertension, hyperlipidemia, and hypothyroidism are associated with tinnitus; however, tinnitus is most commonly associated with high-frequency sensorineural hearing loss (such as presbycusis). Tinnitus is also associated with Ménière's disease, acoustic neuroma, and pontine tumor.

5. **(E)** A complete and accurate medical record is the basis of good documentation. The records should be legible, consistent, and timely completed. A change of record is to be dated, with an explanation.

6. **(C)** Approximately one third of community-residing elderly report at least one fall a year; 45% of nursing home residents and 20% of hospitalized elderly experience a fall. Decline in visual function places the elderly at risk of falling. Patients with diuretics, cardiotonics, hypnotics, antihypertensives, sedatives, and psychotropics are at a higher risk of falling.

7. **(C)** Neurosyphilis is the third stage of syphilis, characterized by general paresis and tabes dorsalis; chancre is the first stage of syphilis. In general paresis, the patient depicts symptoms of diffuse dementia involving memory, judgment, emotional life, and conation. Argyll–Robertson pupils are miotic pupils that accommodate to near vision without light reaction. In tabes dorsalis, the patient may show ataxic gait, absent knee jerks, and loss of position sensation in the lower extremities. VDRL is positive in serum and in CSF.

8. **(D)** Erythromycin is the drug of choice in penicillin-allergic patients with probable streptococcal sore throat. Oral clindamycin, though effective, has a serious side effect of pseudomembranous enterocolitis. Tetracycline-resistant strains of streptococci are now being reported. Oral cephalexin offers an expensive way of treating strep throat.

9. **(D)** Bacterial pneumonia complicating influenza most often occurs on day 5; early treatment of influenza with antibiotics usually does not prevent bacterial pneumonia. Pneumonia is commonly due to bacterial infection with pneumococci or staphylococci. As a nurse, the patient most likely has a penicillin-resistant *S. aureus* pneumonia.

10. **(D)** HDL is increased in exercise and estrogen, and alcohol intake. HDL is cardioprotective, and hypercholesterolemia needs to fractionate low-density lipoprotein (LDL) and HDL for risk analysis. HDL is also increased in niacin, hepatic hydroxymethylglutaryl coenzyme A (HMG-CoA) reductase inhibitors, bile acid-binding resin, and fibric acid derivatives.

11. **(A)** Many hypertensive elderly patients are characterized by a low cardiac output and a very high total peripheral resistance. Renal blood flow is usually low, intravascular volume becomes contracted, and plasma renin level is usually low.

12. **(A)** The first step in utilizing antibiotics is to determine whether the patient has a microbial infection that can be influenced by antimicrobial drugs.

13. **(A)** The most common side reaction of thiazide diuretics is hypokalemia. It can also produce hyperglycemia, hypertrigleridemia, hyperuricemia, hyponatremia, hypomagnesemia, and hypercalcemia.

14. **(E)** Beta blockers are recommended for a hypertensive patient with concomitant conditions of angina, tachyarrhythmias, migraine headache, mitral prolapse, asymmetric septal hypertrophy, and postmyocardial infarction.

They should be used with caution in bronchial asthma, congestive heart failure, depression, diabetes mellitus, impotence, and Raynaud's phenomenon.

15. **(D)** Due to the popularity of air travel and scuba diving, barotrauma is a common condition in modern society. Barotrauma most commonly occurs in the middle ear, followed by the paranasal sinus, particularly the frontal sinus. It is more likely to occur in small, private aircraft without pressurized cabins. Even in the commercial aircraft with pressurized cabins, if the patient has a congested upper respiratory tract that prevents pressure equalization in the sinuses, barosinusitis may result.

16. **(A)** Cigarette smoking causes many cancers including cancers of the lung, larynx, bladder, uterine cervix, and pancreas. Coronary artery disease, acute bronchitis, COPD, osteoporosis, and PUD are also associated with cigarette smoking.

17. **(D)** This man most likely has mycoplasmal pneumonia. Erythromycin is now considered the drug of choice in this infection and is best used for three weeks. Tetracycline is also effective. *Mycoplasma pneumoniae* infection is often associated with bullous myringitis.

18. **(B)** Women approximately 27 years of age with community-acquired pneumonias are usually sensitive to erythromycin; infants to 5-year-olds are usually sensitive to ampicillin; for anyone over 5 years of age, the drug of choice is erythromycin.

19. **(E)** Since this patient is asymptomatic, chemotherapy administered either systemically or by hepatic artery catheter is not indicated. Treatment with serotonin antagonists and antihistamines is not appropriate, since these are palliative antihormonal therapies. Hepatic irradiation is valueless in a patient with no symptoms of malignant hepatomegaly. The most reasonable approach is careful follow-up with consideration of cytoreductive surgery, including partial hepatectomy if the patient becomes symptomatic.

It would also be possible to use chemotherapy or antihormonal therapy if symptoms develop. It should be emphasized that patients with carcinoid tumors metastatic to the liver can have a long indolent course and survive for years with no significant symptoms.

20. **(C)** AIDS is characterized by a profound reduction in cellular immunity that predisposes to both recurrent opportunistic infections and Kaposi's sarcoma. While the latter neoplasm may be fulminant in the setting of AIDS with widespread visceral metastases, affected patients typically are beset by many concurrent infectious diseases. These typically include those caused by *Pneumocystis carinii*, cytomegalovirus, *M. avium intracellulare*, and hepatitis virus, which ultimately prove to be the major cause of death. The use of cytotoxic chemotherapy to treat Kaposi's sarcoma carries the theoretic risk of further reducing immune defenses and worsening the almost universal underlying infectious complications. Progressive cutaneous ulceration by Kaposi's sarcoma, in itself, is rarely of sufficient severity to be judged the principal cause of death.

21. **(D)** Common symptoms in heart failure include the following: (1) Dyspnea: usually the earliest symptom of left-ventricular failure, seen especially on exertion; caused by elevated left-ventricular filling pressure with comparable rises in pulmonary venous and pulmonary capillary bed (wedge) pressure. Engorgement of the pulmonary capillary bed occurs. (2) Orthopnea: the sensation of dyspnea while the patient lies flat in bed; patient may need several pillows under the head to elevate the upper body to avoid orthopnea, caused by increased venous return from dependent parts of the body during recumbency. (3) Paroxysmal nocturnal dyspnea (PND): a sensation of smothering or gasping for breath that awakens the patient three to four hours after he or she falls asleep, relieved by assumption of the upright position. (4) Nocturnal cough: another symptom of pulmonary congestion. (5) Hemoptysis: sputum is pink streaked or frothy in pulmonary edema, may contain bright red blood in tight mitral stenosis, may be rusty or dark red in pulmonary embolism, and may contain dark red blood streaks in chronic bronchitis. (6) Weight gain: caused by retention of salt and water. (7) Edema: occurs in the dependent portions of the body, unlikely to be due to heart failure if central venous pressure is not elevated. (8) Abdominal swelling: due to leakage of edema fluid or transudate from the hepatic capsule into the abdominal cavity. (9) Fatigue: easy fatigability and chronic tiredness caused by low cardiac output. (10) Nocturia: caused by an easing of renal vascular constriction during sleep.

22. **(E)** A serum iron determination would be most helpful. Iron stores in thalassemia are greatly increased, as in most chronic hemolytic anemias.

23. **(A)** Nitrofurantoin should be taken with food to improve absorption and tolerance. Because of the risk of hemolytic anemia, it is contraindicated for pregnant women at term and for newborns less than 1 month of age. Renal insufficiency increases its toxicity, and it is not recommended. Nitrofurantoin may cause interstitial pneumonitis and agranulocytosis.

24. **(D)** Patients with vestibular causes of dizziness often present with tinnitus and hearing inpairment; nystagmus is usually elicited. Dysphagia with dizziness is usually seen in patients with central causes.

25. **(B)** NSAIDs are frequently used by the elderly for pain control (including osteoarthritis). Side reactions include interstitial nephritis and PUD. In the elderly, melena is often the presenting symptom of PUD. Misoprostol (cytotec) may be used with the NSAIDs to reduce the risk of PUD.

26. **(A)** Common causes of chronic cough include postnasal drip syndrome, asthma, gastroesophageal reflux, chronic bronchitis, bronchiectasis, and the use of ACE inhibitors.

27. **(B)** Silo-filler's disease is characterized by pulmonary edema, hypotension, and bronchiolitis fibrosa obliterans. The symptoms of URIs and bronchitis (cough, wheezing, and dyspnea) are the results of inhalation of toxic nitrogen dioxide.

28. **(A)** Accumulation of lactic acid is a relatively common cause of metabolic acidosis. Lactic acidosis is frequently encountered in patients with circulatory failure caused by dehydration, hemorrhage, or endotoxic or cardiogenic shock. Hypoxemia shifts the aerobic metabolism of the tissue to anaerobic glycolysis, which produces lactic acid. Spontaneous lactic acidosis is usually associated with diabetes, hepatic failure, subacute bacterial endocarditis (SBE), and leukemia. Phenformin therapy and accidental ingestion of 15 to 20 g of INH may also cause lactic acidosis. Plasma expanders and sodium bicarbonate are used for treatment.

29. **(B)** Marker infections of AIDS are commonly caused by the following microorganisms: cytomegalovirus, herpes simplex virus, Epstein–Barr virus, *M. avium intracellulare*, *Mycobacterium tuberculosis*, *Candida albicans*, *Cryptococcus neoformans*, *Pneumocystis carinii*, *Toxoplasma gondii*, *Entamoeba histolytica*, and cryptosporidium.

30. **(D)** High-risk groups include homosexual men (promiscuity; anal intercourse; enteric parasitic infestations; non-A, non-B hepatitis; syphilis; use of illicit drugs), intravenous drug abusers, hemophiliacs (receiving blood products before 1985), intimate contacts (sexual partners) of AIDS patients, infants born to mothers infected with HIV, and parents of AIDS children.

31. **(A)** In chronic renal failure, sodium needs to be equal to daily urinary output, fluids equal to daily urinary output plus insensible loss. The patient needs a caloric intake of 30 calories/kg; adequate vitamins, and restriction of potassium (1500 to 2000 mg/d), protein (0.50 to 0.75 g/kg/d), and phosphorus (restriction of dairy products). Calcium supplementation may often be necessary.

32. **(B)** Acute viral pericarditis is characterized by substernal or precordial pain radiating to the left neck, which is worsened by supine position and accentuated by swallowing. Pericardial friction rub and ST elevation with upward concavity in ECG may develop.

33. **(B)** Vitamin D deficiency causes rickets. Children with malabsorption syndromes, pancreatitis, cystic fibrosis, hepatic diseases, kidney diseases, and corticosteroid administration are at higher risk of developing vitamin D deficiency. Black children and children who are rarely exposed to ultraviolet irradiation are also at high risk of developing vitamin D deficiency.

34. **(E)** The poor nutrition of alcoholics often results in vitamin deficiencies. Niacin deficiency (pellagra) may cause diarrhea, dermatitis, and dementia; riboflavin (B_2) deficiency may cause dermatitis, cheilosis, and stomatitis; pyridoxine (B_6) deficiency may cause sideroblastic anemia; folic acid deficiency may cause macrocytic anemia; and vitamin C deficiency (scurvy) may cause perifollicular hemorrhages and gingival hemorrhages. However, the most common vitamin deficiency of alcoholics is thiamine (B_1) deficiency, which may result in Wernicke's encephalopathy (nystagmus, diplopia, abducens palsy) and beriberi (circulatory collapse, high-output heart failure).

35. **(C)** The most common side reaction is peripheral neuropathy. A pyridoxine supplement may be helpful. Convulsions, memory impairment, and psychosis may occur. Optic neuritis, agranulocytosis, hemolytic anemia, gynecomastia, rheumatic syndrome, and lupus syndrome are rare occurrences. GOT and GPT may be elevated, and jaundice and hepatitis may develop.

36. **(D)** Clindamycin therapy is associated with severe life-threatening diarrhea (pseudomembranous enterocolitis), which may be caused by the toxins produced by clostridia. Vancomycin may be helpful.

37. **(A)** Neurologic symptoms without infarction, often manifested as TIAs, most often arise from embolization of small fragments from areas of proximal arterial disease (microemboli) to the cerebral cortex. Momentary weakness or numbness of the contralateral arm or leg and temporary partial or complete loss of vision of the ipsilateral eye or both eyes (amaurosis fugax) are common manifestations.

38. **(A)** The lesion is often located in the extracranial arteries in segmental distribution. The areas most often involved are the common carotid bifurcation, the origin of the vertebral artery, and the intrathoracic segments of the aortic arch branches.

39. **(D)** Malignancies that cause thrombocytosis include Hodgkin's disease, lymphoreticular disorders, and various carcinomas. Other causes include osteoporosis, nephrotic syndrome, renal cysts, and Cushing syndrome.

40. **(D)** The recovery of elderly patients with stroke sequelae depends on their willingness to participate in comprehensive rehabilitation programs to restore personal and professional functional status. Family members need to recognize the slow process of recovery and to provide unconditional, continuing support.

41. **(C)** The clinical presentation is CHF with pansystolic murmur of ventricular septal defect. The signs of CHF in acute myocardial infarction (MI) include S3 gallop, rales, congestion on chest x-ray, peripheral edema, and neck vein distention.

42. **(D)** Patients with ASD are usually asymptomatic until the fourth decade. The symptoms developed include pulmonary hypertension, atrial arrhythmias, bidirectional and then right-to-left shunting of blood, and cardiac failure.

43. **(D)** Normal pressure hydrocephalus is characterized by dementia, urinary incontinence, and ataxic gait disturbance without signs of increased intracranial pressure. Magnetic resonance imaging (MRI) may show diffuse white matter lesions.

44. **(B)** Howell–Jolly bodies, a feature of the post-splenectomy state, or hyposplenism, are also characteristically seen in the erythrocytes of patients with megaloblastic anemia due either to folate deficiency or to vitamin B_{12} deficiency. They may provide a clue to the presence of those disorders. A quantity of blood sufficient to raise the HCT to normal will not correct megaloblastic abnormalities of the erythroid precursors in the bone marrow of patients with vitamin B_{12} deficiency. The effect of such transfusions is a suppression of erythropoiesis; megaloblastic abnormalities of the erythroid precursors in the marrow persist, as do the morphological abnormalities of the myeloid series.

In patients with vitamin B_{12} deficiency, the serum folic acid levels are usually normal or elevated, whereas erythrocyte folate levels are often reduced. If the serum folic acid level is low, a low serum B_{12} level alone cannot be used to establish vitamin B_{12} deficiency as the cause of a megaloblastic anemia.

Vitamin B_{12} is extracted from food during digestion in the stomach, and in that acid environment it binds not to intrinsic factor but to other B_{12} binders (R proteins). The R protein–B_{12} complex is broken up in the alkaline environment of the small intestine by pancreatic proteases; this action allows the B_{12} to be bound by intrinsic factor in patients with chronic exocrine pancreatic protein–B_{12} complex. Consequently, the vitamin is not available for binding to intrinsic factor subsequent to absorption in the terminal ileum. In some patients with chronic pancreatic insufficiency, the defect in protease activity is sufficient to cause B_{12} malabsorption and megaloblastic anemia.

One of the great values of the Schilling test is that it can be used to confirm the presence of vitamin B_{12} malabsorption in patients with vitamin B_{12} deficiency who have been treated with the vitamin. Parenteral treatment with vitamin B_{12} will not correct any of the malabsorption defects responsible for vitamin B_{12} deficiency.

45. **(D)** Hemoglobin C characteristically produces targeting in the peripheral blood. Targeting is also seen in liver disease and may represent redundant membrane.

46. **(E)** Long-term exposure to the PCBs may result in chloracne appearing behind the ears and on the trunk, thighs, and genitalia. PCBs remain toxic for many years, especially in waste dumps. PCBs also can cause hyperpigmentation of the skin, conjunctiva, gingiva, and nails. Occupational exposure includes workers at the railroad repair factories, electric cable repair shops, metal finishing shops, and transformer/capacitor repair agencies.

47. **(A)** The drug use of patients with dyspepsia must be ascertained. Many patients fail to report OTC medications, and the use of NSAIDs has to be requested specifically. OTC iron tablets also cause dyspepsia.

48. **(E)** Thrombocytopenia can be caused by folic acid and vitamin B_{12} deficiency, and by the administration of alcohol, quinidine, quinine, gold, and heroin. In addition, thrombocytopenia is associated with aplastic anemia, leukemia, and disseminated tuberculosis.

49. **(D)** Minocycline 100 mg 1# bid PO for 5 days can be used for chemoprophylaxis of the meningococcal carrier state. Minocycline is also frequently used for acne vulgaris. The side reactions include dizziness, nausea, vomiting, unsteady gait, and agranulocytosis.

50. **(C)** Primary prevention is the prevention of disease occurrence, such as immunizations, cessation of smoking habits, prudent diets, contraception, and exercises. Secondary prevention is the early detection of diseases including STS, blood pressure measurement, and health screening procedures (mammograms, Pap smears). Tertiary prevention is the stopping or slowing of disease progression, including INAH chemoprophylaxis, rehabilitation, and the treatment of diseases.

51. **(E)** In adult patients with sickle cell anemia, the spleen is autosplenectomized with frequent infections. Since sickle cell anemia is a chronic hemolytic anemia, the reticulocyte is chronically elevated except in aplastic crises. The HCT is usually around the mid-twenties. The hemoglobin is S with some F without A. The red blood cells (RBCs) are characteristically sickle cells. Pigment gallstones are common, and thrombotic pain crisis is frequent.

52. **(A)** An increased amount of fetal and A2 hemoglobin would be expected. Since beta chains are decreased, the alpha chains combine with gamma and delta chains to make F and A2.

53. **(D)** The features of superficial thrombophlebitis include mass or cord purpura, rubor, edema, dolor, history of trauma, and preexisting varicose veins. The treatment consists of application of an elastic bandage or stocking from the toes to the knee and continued ambulatory activity.

54. **(B)** Thalassemia minor usually represents a heterozygous state and is often asymptomatic.

55. **(E)** Cigarette smoking is estimated to be related to 80 to 90% of lung cancers. Other causes are mainly industrial exposures (asbestos, chromium, uranium, nickel, zinc, arsenic, chloroethyl ether, iron oxide, and beryllium) and radon. The risk of smokers to develop lung cancer is 20 times higher than nonsmokers, and even for "passive" smokers the risk is twice higher than for nonsmokers. Lung cancer is a "family" disease.

56. **(D)** Sedatives, benzodiazepines, phenothiazines, antidepressants, antihypertensives, antiarrhythmics, anticonvulsants, vasodilators, diuretics, and alcohol all increase the risk of falls. Falls often cause fractures of the wrist, hip, and vertebrae, resulting in disability.

57. **(A)** The rescuer feels the tip of the xiphoid and places the heel of his hand on the lower half of the sternum about 1 to $1^1/2$ inches

away from the tip of the xiphoid and toward the victim's head for chest compression. The depth should be $1^1/_2$ to 2 inches, and the ratio to be used for adult CPR is 15 compressions with two ventilations. The contraindication of CPR is numerous rib fractures and a "flail" chest. To start cardiac compression, the patient should be put on a firm surface, such as a floor.

58. **(B)** The most common cause of airway obstruction is from the tongue. Thus, tilting the head back to hyperextend the patient's head adequately is important in order to lift the tongue away from the back of the throat.

59. **(B)** Chemotherapy with INH for a year has been shown to reduce the risk of the development of dormant infection into active tuberculosis by 75%. Close contacts of an infectious tuberculous patient and persons whose tuberculin conversion has occurred within the previous year or two should be put on chemoprophylaxis.

60. **(B)** Varicella pneumonia may cause hemoptysis. Extensive bilateral nodular opacities of the lung are usually seen on chest x-rays of severely ill patients. Respiratory failure should be avoided, for the mortality is 10 to 25% if untreated.

61. **(C)** There is a fall in lung compliance, vital capacity, and Po_2.

62. **(C)** Glyburide is not effective in ketosis-prone insulin-dependent diabetes or in obesity. It is not recommended for pregnant diabetics or diabetic women who are likely to become pregnant.

63. **(B)** The duration of the sulfanylureas is as follows: chlorpropamide (Diabinese), 48 hours; glyburide (Micronase), 24 hours; glipizide (Glucotrol), 18 hours; tolazamide (Tolinase), 18 hours; acetohexamide (Dynelor), 10 hours; tolbutamide (Orinase), 9 hours. Because of their long duration of action, chlorpropamide and glyburide are given once a day.

64. **(C)** The deficiency of AAT leads to pulmonary emphysema, neonatal hepatitis, chronic active hepatitis, cholestasis, cirrhosis, and hepatoma.

65. **(D)** *Salmonella* gastroenteritis is commonly caused by eating uncooked food (such as homemade ice cream, eggs, or meats) contaminated with *Salmonella*. The symptom usually develops in 8 to 48 hours. The treatment is symptomatic. Antidiarrheal agents (paregoric or Lomotil) are used only for severe cases to relieve diarrhea and abdominal pain. Intravenous fluid replacement is indicated when dehydration is significant (10% of body loss in children). Antibiotics are not indicated because they do not shorten the course of illness and they may actually prolong the bacterial colonization; they are reserved only for bacteremia.

66. **(D)** Colonic cancer is usually adenocarcinoma. Carcinoma of the left colon is usually annular, characterized by the symptoms of obstruction due to the smaller size of the lumen and the solidity of the contents. A change in bowel habits may be the first symptom noted, with a progressive decrease in the caliber of the stools. Blood and mucus is seen in or on the stool.

67. **(C)** Stress ulcer, with hemorrhage, develops frequently in patients with severe acute respiratory failure. Bleeding may be massive, frequently leading to shock. H2 blockers and sucralfate may be used for prophylaxis.

68. **(D)** Hospital-acquired pulmonary infections caused by gram-negative organisms (especially *Pseudomonas*) are very common and probably result in part from contaminated respiratory therapy equipment. The danger of gram-negative *Pseudomonas* pneumonia stems from the frequent complication of septicemia, with endotoxin shock, disseminated intravascular coagulation, and, later, renal failure. Since hospital-acquired gram-negative infections are major complications of treatment for acute respiratory failure, and since gram-negative septicemia has a 50%

mortality, it is essential that everything possible be done to prevent these infections.

69. (A) AZT is a thymidine analog that is an inhibitor of the in vitro replication of HIV retrovirus. It is useful in reducing mortality and prolonging the survival of adult AIDS patients. Common side reactions include severe headache and significant anemia. Its long-term effect is still unknown, and it does not reduce the risk of transmission of HIV to others.

70. (A) Thiazide diuretics often cause hypokalemia, which may precipitate arrhythmia and sudden death. Thiazide diuretics cause an increase in serum total cholesterol and triglycerides and a decrease in HDL. There is a decrease of the ratio of HDL to total cholesterol. Thiazide diuretics also impair glucose tolerance.

71. (C) Hyperparathyroidism is usually associated with back pain, renal stone, hypercalcemia, hypophosphatemia, and hypercalciuria.

72. (A) In the elderly, postural hypotension may lead to falls. Drugs that may induce postural hypotension include nitroglycerin, barbiturates, phenothiazines, levodopa (Dopar, Larodopa), carbidopa–levodopa (Sinemet), tricyclic antidepressants, diuretics, vasodilators and other antihypertensives, benzodiazepines, monoamine oxidase inhibitors, procainamide (Pronestyl), and anticholinergics (including OTC preparations).

73. (C) INH may inhibit diamine oxidase and may cause exaggerated responses (headache, palpitations, sweating, hypotension, flushing, diarrhea, itching) to foods containing histamine (tuna, sauerkraut juice, yeast extract).

74. (D) This is a condition of metabolic alkalosis. Diuretics should be used with water replacements of urine losses (D_5W).

75. (C) Serum K^+ is elevated by acidosis and depressed by alkalosis due to anion shift.

Thus, a pH of 7.30 with K^+ of 2.5 means the patient's K^+ is depleted. Serum K^+ should be replaced while correcting acidosis to prevent its sudden fall.

76. (D) Many elderly hypertensives on methyldopa receive good blood pressure control, but a few may develop orthostatic hypotension and may increase the risk of falls, often serious in the osteoporotic elderly female. Long-term use may cause impotence, depression, hemolytic anemia, and lupus-like syndrome.

77. (B)

Disease	Pathogen	Vector	Positive Weil–Felix Test
Rocky Mountain spotted fever	*Rickettsia rickettsii*	Ticks	OX19, OX2
Epidemic typhus	*R. prowazekii*	Body lice	OX19
Scrub typhus	*R. tsutsugamushi*	Mites	OXK
Endemic typhus	*R. mooseri*	Fleas	OX19

78. (A) Chinese restaurant syndrome is probably caused by monosodium glutamate used as seasoning in Chinese food, although evidence is not conclusive. The symptoms are usually self-limited and last for 45 minutes to 2 hours. Reassurance can be provided for the patient.

79. (A) His arterial pH is close to 7.30, with high serum osmolarity. During the period of acute illness, he has sustained losses of Na^+, K^+, and HCO_5^-. Hypopotassemia is common.

80. (E) Acute pharyngitis is an extremely common complaint in family practice. The cause is usually viral in origin, and the treatment is symptomatic—rest, warm gargles, and adequate fluid intake. Analgesics are used when indicated. Antibiotics are prescribed when there is evidence of bacterial infections, which can be confirmed by throat culture.

81. **(A)**   Amantadine (Symmetrel) is a synthetic cyclic primary amine effective for the prevention and treatment of influenza A infections.

82. **(B)**   Most of the side effects of amantadine are related to CNS disturbances, such as nervousness, irritability, fatigue, depression, insomnia, and inability to concentrate. Side effects may appear after the first few doses or after the patient has been receiving the drug for a prolonged period. From 5 to 33% of patients develop side reactions. Once the drug is stopped or, in some patients, the dosage reduced, the side reactions will resolve.

83. **(C)**   Cigarette smoking is the chief avoidable cause of death. Each year, smoking is responsible for 19% of the total deaths in the United States. Approximately 40% of cancer deaths and 21% of cardiovascular deaths are related to smoking. Smoking contributes to about 400,000 deaths annually in the United States.

84. **(D)**   Syndrome of inappropriate secretion of antidiuretic hormone (SIADH) is a real possibility; work-ups include urine osmolarity, sodium excretion, and serum osmolarity. SIADH is characterized by hyponatremia with hyposmolarity of the serum, high urine osmolarity, and high urine sodium content. SIADH is associated with oat cell lung carcinoma, GI cancers, pancreatic carcinoma, thymoma, lymphoma, head injury, tuberculosis, pneumonia, meningitis, subarachnoid hemorrhage, psychosis, myxedema, Addison's disease, hypopituitarism, acute intermittent porphyria, vasopressin, oxytocin, vincristine, chlorpropamide (Diabinese), clofibrate, cyclophosphamide (Cytoxan), carbamazepine, and thiazide. Treatments include fluid restriction, management of the underlying causes, and administration of demeclocycline (Declomycin).

85. **(B)**   In fibromyalgia, psychotropic drugs such as amitriptyline and other tricyclic antidepressants are used at bedtime. Small doses of amitriptyline (10 to 50 mg hs) may be used. Depression often accompanies fibromyalgia, and such patients may benefit from antidepressant doses of amitriptyline.

86. **(D)**   G6PD deficiency in southeast Asians is 10 to 12%, justifying screening prior to antimalarial therapy.

87. **(D)**   The treatment of the common cold (acute pharyngitis) is bedrest and abundant fluid intake. However, the patient needs to be educated to come to your office as soon as the symptoms develop for appropriate needed care. The patient and his or her family needs to come for health maintenance services during the asymptomatic period.

88. **(B)**   Acyclovir (Zovirax) is useful in genital herpes. Five percent ointment can be applied to decrease viral shedding and pruritus. Recurrent infections can be treated by 200 mg oral acyclovir capsules five times a day. Side reactions include headache, nausea, vomiting, vertigo, arthralgia, and inguinal adenopathy.

89. **(A)**   The reasons for referral include diagnosis and/or management, reinforcement or confirmation of diagnosis and/or management, and patient/family request. It is better to ask for a consultation whenever the patient or family expresses doubt or shows lack of confidence in diagnosis and/or management. It is often wise to obtain a second opinion for a life-threatening condition or a disease with a poor prognosis.

90. **(B)**   Varicose veins cause venous hypertension that leads to edema, skin pigmentation, and stasis dermatitis. Stasis dermatitis may develop acute inflammation and cellutitis. Ulceration occurs with the slightest trauma.

91. **(D)**   Gilbert syndrome is a benign syndrome caused by hereditary glucuronyl transferase deficiency. The patient may show slight scleral icterus but is usually asymptomatic with mild, persistent unconjugated hyperbilirubinemia. The syndrome is present in 7% of the population and is relatively common in family practice.

92. **(C)** Beta blockers may produce mood changes, depression, heart block, nightmares, sleep disturbances, and decreased cardiac output. It increases bronchospasm and is best to be avoided for a patient with a history of bronchial asthma.

93. **(A)** At present, there are no effective ways of screening for lung cancers and routine chest x-rays are not recommended.

94. **(D)** Obese patients need to reduce weight, and a low-sodium diet is helpful (less than 500 mg/d is ideal but less than 2 g/d is acceptable). A diet rich in potassium, calcium, and fiber will be helpful. Protein restriction is not recommended. Coffee restriction is not necessary, and moderate alcohol use is permitted. Tobacco use should be eliminated.

95. **(E)** The problem list is the basis of providing a comprehensive and continuous total health care for the patient and the family. Each problem is numbered and constantly updated at each visit to reflect the current status for appropriate diagnostic and therapeutic actions.

96. **(D)** Asymptomatic hyperuricemia may be caused by hematologic malignancy, hemolytic anemia, hyperparathyroidism, polycythemia vera, psoriasis, small dosage of salicylate, diuretic therapy, nicotinic acid, ethambutol, and cytolytic chemotherapeutic agents.

97. **(B)** In an average female aged 23 to 50 years with a body weight of 58 kg, the daily caloric requirement in the nonpregnant state is 2000 kcal (1600 to 2400 kcal).

98. **(C)** In an average adult male aged 23 to 50 years with a body weight of 70 kg, the daily caloric requirement is 2700 kcal, within a variation of ± 400 kcal (ie, 2300 to 3100 kcal).

99. **(D)** Common patient characteristics in urban family practice include (1) psychosocial problems that are obvious and critical for management; (2) clinical presentation that is likely to be at an advanced state; (3) illnesses that often reflect lifelong environmental stresses; and (4) a large variety of cultural, racial, ethnic, and family configurations.

100. **(A)** Digitalis causes gradual downward sloping of the ST segment. Excess digitalis causes atrioventricular (AV) block (Wenckebach); digitalis toxicity may cause bigeminy, premature ventricular contractions (PVCs), and ventricular tachycardia.

101. **(D)**

Stage	Involvement
1	Erythema
2	Epidermis
3	Subcutaneous
4	Muscle/bone

102. **(B)** Therapeutic alliance (ie, the primary-care team) conveys a sense of partnership between a family physician and a patient and his or her family.

103. **(B)** Patient education produces patient adherence through patient understanding. Every contact with patients is an educational process for appropriate health-care behavior.

104. **(E)** Approximately 50% of patients with chronic diseases are noncompliant. Complex dose regimen, poor doctor–patient relationship, inadequate confidence in therapeutic efficacy, and intolerable side reactions of the therapy are correlated with noncompliance. The largest portion of noncompliant patients is those who drop out of regular medical care.

105. **(B)** Erysipeloid is an acute skin infection caused by the gram-positive bacillus. It is common in fishermen, meat handlers, butchers, farmers, and veterinarians. It responds to penicillin.

106. **(B)** With hypocalcemia, the QT interval becomes prolonged.

107. **(C)** Common side effects of hydrochlorothiazide are hypokalemia (which may cause cramping leg pain and general weakness),

hyperuricemia, hyperglycemia, and elevation of LDL.

108. **(A)** Tay–Sachs disease is most common among Jews; sickle cell diseases and hypertension are common in blacks; tuberculosis and hepatitis B are common in Southeast Asians; thalassemias are common in Mediterranean people. Parasites are common among recent immigrants from tropical or subtropical regions.

109. **(A)** Hypokalemia causes sagging ST, T depression, and U elevation. U-wave amplitude is larger than T-wave amplitude.

110. **(B)** Quinidine causes notching of a wide P wave and widening of the QRS complex. There is often an ST depression, prolonged QT interval, prolonged PR interval, and U waves. Procainamide can also induce widening of QRS complexes.

111. **(E)** Hyperchromic macrocytic anemia is frequently seen in pernicious anemia, liver disease, and malabsorption syndrome (sprue-like), and folic acid deficiency.

112. **(D)** In pericarditis, ST elevation in all leads preserves normal upward concavity; in acute myocardial infarction, ST elevation is concave downward or depressed. In acute pericarditis, ST segment elevation is most pronounced in lead II or III; it subsequently may return to normal. The T may become flattened and then inverted in all leads except AVR. With effusion, QRS voltage is decreased.

113. **(D)** A family physician in an urban setting provides family-oriented care and community-oriented primary care. Sickness-oriented single-person care is a component of family-oriented care or community-oriented primary care.

114. **(B)** Approximately 160 to 170 diagnoses account for 90% of all problems, and 25 diagnoses account for 50% of all problems. These 25 diagnoses are medical examination, URI, forms (letters, certificates), hypertension, gynecologic examination (Pap smear), obesity, strep throat, acute otitis media, medical–surgical procedure, prenatal care, low back pain, nonspecific abdominal pain, warts, depressive neurosis, allergic rhinitis, acne, diabetes, eczema, osteoarthritis, anxiety neurosis, marital problems, family relationship problems, serous otitis, UTI, and vaginitis. These top 25 diagnoses are essentially the same in urban as well as in rural settings.

115. **(D)** Diabetes mellitus accounts for 0.9 to 2.4% of total problems in family practice. The prevalence of undiagnosed non–insulin-dependent diabetes mellitus is 2.5% in the general population (range 1 to 6%).

116. **(A)** Common problems for home visits include CVA, CHF, arteriosclerotic heart disease (ASHD), hypertension, degenerative joint disease (DJD), rheumatoid arthritis (RA), diabetes mellitus, COPD, and cancer.

117. **(B)** The POMR usually includes the following components: (1) subjective data: qualitative data (history), profile of symptoms, explanation of problems, perception of resources; (2) objective data: direct observations (signs), indirect observations (quantitative data); (3) assessment: the diagnostic process; (4) prognosis: knowledge of the natural history of the problem; and (5) plan: education, intervention, and further data collection.

118. **(D)** Many elderly individuals tolerate treatable illnesses even when they have access to health care. These untreated "hidden illnesses" include depression, incontinence, musculoskeletal stiffness, falling, alcoholism, hearing loss, dementia, dental problems, poor nutrition, and sexual dysfunction. Dental caries are common dental problems, followed by periodontal disease, missing teeth, and the use of dentures. The prevalence of dental caries may be related to dietary changes, decreased salivary flow, drug effects, vitamin deficiencies, and poor oral hygiene.

119. **(A)** URI syndromes account for almost 25% of ambulatory family practice diagnoses, and

among the listed five disease entities, it is the most commonly seen in the urban family practice setting.

120. **(A)** The overall cancer mortality was higher in black men than in white men. The rate was higher in black men for esophageal cancer, stomach cancer, larynx cancer, and oral cancer, in that order. Black men were lower in mortality rate in bladder cancer and kidney cancer.

121. **(B)** The incidence of diabetes in the Hispanic population is $2\frac{1}{2}$ times higher than that in whites. This may be related to dietary and genetic factors.

122. **(E)** All children who have had contact with tuberculous patients and who live in the community where tuberculous sensitivity exceeds 1% should be tested (if exceeding 2%, test is performed annually). The BCG immunization produces a positive test for 5 to 8 years. When the induration is beyond 10 mm, it is indicative of a tuberculous infection. Positive and doubtful tine test (induration 5 to 9 mm) should be retested with Mantoux.

123. **(A)** Approximately 8 to 10% of blacks and a much smaller portion of Greeks, Italians, and Latin Americans from coastal areas of the Caribbean and South America carry the sickle cell trait. The frequency of hemoglobin C is 3%; hemoglobin D is less than 0.3%.

124. **(E)** Poverty limits the access of many inner-city people to health care. Many persons may not be eligible for Medicaid or other public assistance programs and yet cannot afford even ambulatory visits to family physicians' offices. Poverty is often associated with crowded housing without adequate heat in winter, poor nutrition, crime, and drugs. Moreover, poverty usually increases the health risks of those inner-city populations.

125. **(D)** Acute disseminated gonorrheal infection is characterized by migratory polyarthralgias, tenosynovitis, and hemorrhagic pustular eruptions on distal extremities.

Oligoarticular or monoarticular arthritis of the knees or elbows will develop.

126. **(A)** If the treatment regimen is successful, concomitant use of traditional medicine can be allowed.

127. **(C)** Diuretics may cause hypokalemia, hyperglycemia, and elevated LDL. It also causes hyperuricemia, and it is best to be avoided in a patient with a history of gouty arthritis.

128. **(D)** About 90% of Asians have lactose intolerance.

129. **(B)** Intestinal parasites are common in Indochinese, ranging from 15 to 78%. The most common parasites include *Trichuris*, *Giardia lamblia*, *Ascaris*, hookworm, *Entamoeba histolytica*, and *Strongyloides*.

130. **(A)** In cor pulmonale, there is peaked P, right axis deviation, and deep S in V_6. Q may be present in II, III, and F, but it is not deep or wide.

131. **(B)** The prevalence of tuberculosis among Indochinese refugees is estimated to be 0.7 to 1.5%.

132. **(C)** Wolff–Parkinson–White syndrome is characteristic for delta wave (slurred QRS complex) and shortened PR.

133. **(A)** LVH is characterized by $S_1 + R_5 > 3.5$ mv. In LVH, QRS is more than 0.08 seconds and less than 0.12 seconds.

134. **(B)** In RBBB, there are RR´ in lead V_1 or V_2 and wide S in leads V_5 to V_6. In left bundle branch block (LBBB), there are RR´ in leads V_5 or V_6 and wide S in leads V_1 to V_2.

135. **(A)** ST elevation in V_1–V_2, or even V_3–V_4 are characteristic for acute anterior or anteroseptal infarctions. With time, T will be inverted and Q will develop in V_1–V_2. R will show poor progression.

136. **(B)** The classic triad of aortic stenosis is syncope, angina, and dyspnea on exertion.

137. **(A)** Acute posterior infarction is characterized by ST depression in V_1–V_2; in time, positive T and prominent R will develop in V_1, and possibly V_2 also.

138. **(A)** In Wenckebach phenomenon, the PR interval progressively prolongs in the successive beats until there is a dropped QRS complex. The PP interval is equal. RR is progressively shortened, but when the complete block occurs, there is a long RR interval.

139. **(C)** Mitral regurgitation produces holosystolic murmur heard best at the apex with radiation to the left axilla. Mitral regurgitation is often associated with mitral valve prolapse, rheumatic valve disease, calcification of mitral valve anulus, papillary muscle dysfunction, and dilatation of mitral ring. In mitral prolapse, a midsystolic click followed by a late systolic murmur may be noted.

140. **(D)** In mitral stenosis, an accentuated S_1, opening snap, and diastolic rumbling may develop, which is best heard when the patient is in the left lateral position.

141. **(D)**

	pH	Pco$_2$	HCO$_3^-$
Normal	7.4	40	24
Respiratory acidosis	Decreased	Increased	—
Respiratory alkalosis	Increased	Decreased	—
Metabolic acidosis	Decreased	—	Decreased
Metabolic alkalosis	Increased	—	Increased

142. **(D)** In paroxysmal atrial tachycardia, the patient may complain of palpitation, shortness of breath, fluttering, and thumping. The rate is 160 to 220 beats/min. Carotid sinus massage may bring the rate abruptly to 75. Verapamil may be useful.

143. **(A)** In sinus bradycardia, the heart rate is slower than 60 beats/min. Dizziness and syncope may occur.

144. **(C)** The heart rate for sinus tachycardia is 100 to 160 beats/min. PP and RR intervals are equal. The PR interval may be shortened but is appropriate for the rapid rate. Carotid sinus massage can slowly decrease the rate.

145. **(E)** The atrial rate is 250 to 350 beats/min. The P wave is clearly visible, almost identical, and in a saw-tooth pattern of F waves. Digitalis, verapamil, or procainamide may be useful.

146. **(C)** Minoxidil (Loniten) may cause weight gain, edema, tachycardia, and hypertrichosis. The topical agent (Rogaine) may be useful for treatment of male pattern baldness.

147. **(C)** He has been infected with the tubercle bacilli, and even though there is no sign of active tuberculous disease at present, he is at increased risk for reactivation; thus, he needs INH for a year, when the liver function test is normal.

148. **(D)** Enterobiasis, also called oxyuriasis, is the most common helminth infestation in the United States. It is estimated that 200 million people are suffering from this infestation worldwide, with around 18 million patients in North America. Thirty to 80% of all American children are infected at some time during their school years.

149. **(E)** GERD is treated by: (1) life-style modifications—avoid coffee, alcohol, citrus juices, cola drinks, and chocolate; (2) antacids as needed; (3) H2-receptor antagonists, regular or double doses: ranitidine 150 mg bid or qid; (3) proton pump inhibitors (omeprazole) 20 mg qd for 6 weeks; (4) prokinetic agents (metoclopramide).

150. **(B)** Clubbing of the finger is often due to hypoxia, cirrhosis of the liver, chronic diarrhea, chronic obstructive lung diseases, cyanotic cardiac diseases, and carcinoma of the lung. It can also be an hereditary condition seen in the other members of the same family.

151. **(A)** Frostbite should be prevented by avoidance of cold exposure and wearing of adequate insulated, dry, loose-fitting clothes. It occurs most frequently on the distal extremities, the nose, and the ears. Rapid rewarming in a water bath at 100°F to 110°F is the treatment of choice. The water temperature should not exceed 112°F. Alcoholism may increase the risk of frostbite.

152. **(C)** Interstitial cystitis is characterized by persistent dysuria, continuous frequency urgency, and suprapubic pain relieved by voiding. Pyuria and hematuria are usually present, but culture and cytology are normal. Cystoscopy reveals reduced bladder capacity and presence of multiple petechiae-like hemorrhages or ulcers.

153. **(A)** For an asymptomatic, low-risk individual, the screening for hypercholesterolemia and hyperlipidemia should start at age 20 to 24 years. If the test value is normal, the patient can be rescreened every 4 to 5 years.

154. **(C)** An adult male in the United States has a 1 in 5 chance of having a myocardial infarction by 60 years of age, which is twice the incidence in females. All male patients at age 50 should initiate dietary therapy if serum cholesterol and lipid levels exceed the normal value.

155. **(B)** Approximately 10,000 deaths per year result from influenza infections, with 80 to 90% percent of the excess mortality in individuals older than 65 years. All elderly beyond 65 years of age are recommended for influenza immunization annually.

156. **(E)** Topical chemical sunscreens decrease erythema and tanning by absorption of ultraviolet light in decreasing sun-burning radiation. However, they may cause contact dermatitis, photosensitivity, and allergic reactions to thiazides, benzocaine, and sulfonamides. The commonly used para-aminobenzoic acid (PABA) chemical sunscreens absorb ultraviolet radiation in the range of 290 to 320 nm.

157. **(D)** The open-ended question is a question asking for information from the patient and specifying the content in general terms. During the opening of the interview, it will facilitate the establishment of rapport with the patient, let the patient initiate a wide variety of topics, and provide or discuss various kinds of problems. Support is provided to assist the patient to narrate and to focus on specific issues for obtaining needed information to formulate diagnostic possibilities and therapeutic approaches.

158. **(B)** In (A), aseptic meningitis should be considered; in (C) tuberculous meningitis needs to be considered; (D) is typical for Guillain-Barré syndrome; brain tumor may show a CSF picture of (E).

159. **(A)** Bacterial meningitis is most frequently confused with aseptic meningitis due to a variety of viruses. Differentiation by spinal fluid findings is at times difficult, but usually possible. When patients present with ambiguous CSF findings, they usually should be treated as if they have bacterial meningitis with suboptimal antibiotic therapy. The CSF of aseptic meningitis is pleocytosis with a cell count of 200 or less (can reach 1200). Mononuclear cells predominate and if polys dominate, bacterial meningitis needs to be considered. Protein is elevated and sugar is normal. Smears and cultures are important in differentiating from the bacterial insults.

160. **(C)** Influenza virus is a ribonucleic acid (RNA) virus; the incubation period is 18 to 36 hours, and the illness lasts for 2 to 3 days. The symptoms are mostly myalgia, fever, headache, sore throat, sneezing, and cough. When symptoms last for more than 1 week, the possibility of complications such as pneumonia should be considered.

161. **(D)** Influenza vaccine is indicated for individuals older than 65; for individuals with diabetes, cancers, HIV, asplenia, renal diseases, cardiopulmonary diseases; nursing home residents; and health-care workers.

162. **(A)** Influenza vaccine is given annually, usually in early October or November. The protection of the influenza immunization lasts for about 6 months. Its effectiveness is 60 to 70%.

163. **(C)** Initial therapy for antihypertensives during congestive heart failure is ACE inhibitors and diuretics. Beta blockers, calcium antagonists, and labetalol (an alpha and beta blocker) are to be avoided.

164. **(E)** Metoclopramide stimulates GI motility, increases the lower esophageal sphincter pressure, and is used for symptomatic GERD. It increases the prolactin level and may produce galactorrhea, reversible amenorrhea, nipple tenderness, and gynecomastia (male). It does not have evidence for impaired fertility. It can cause drowsiness, fatigue, extrapyramidal reactions, akathisia, anxiety, and depression.

165. **(E)** D-penicillamine may cause taste impairment, nephrotic syndrome, and optic neuritis; BAL (dimercaprol) can produce lacrimation, blepharospasm, hypertension, and paresthesia; EDTA (calcium disodium edetate) may produce hypercalcemia and renal tubular necrosis.

166. **(B)**

| Disease | CSF | | |
	Cell Count	Glucose	Protein
Bacterial meningitis	Increased (polys)	Low	High
Partially treated meningitis	Increased (polys)	Low	High
Tuberculous meningitis	Increased (lymphs)	Low	High
Viral meningitis	Increased (lymphs)	Normal	High
Fungal meningitis	Increased (lymphs)	Normal or low	Normal or high
Brain abscess	Normal or increased (variable)	Normal	High
Lead encephalopathy	Normal or increased (lymphs)	Normal	High
Meningismus	Normal	Normal	Normal

167. **(B)** Lead poisoning usually causes fatigue, anorexia, musculoskeletal pains, difficulty concentrating, weakening memory, abdominal pain, headache, seizure, and delirium. Anemia, Burtonian bluish lead line on the gums, and weakness of wrist extensors may also develop.

168. **(E)** All family members occupy appropriate positions in the family system. Their interactions produce satisfactory family functions to support growth of all family members: adaptation, partnership, growth, affection, and resolve. When the family is in trouble, the family physician, as a most powerful therapeutic agent, will be able to change the family behaviors into adequate coping behaviors through family counseling/therapy to facilitate the family's continuous growth through satisfactory family life-cycle stages.

169. **(D)** Asbestosis is pulmonary interstitial fibrosis of the pleural or parenchymal tissue. A radiographic finding of pleural plaques is characteristic, but open lung biopsy is the only definitive diagnostic test.

170. **(A)** Individuals at risk for asbestos exposure include: asbestos miners, manufacturers of asbestos products, construction workers, auto repair mechanics exposed to brake and clutch linings, carpenters, utility workers, electricians, pipefitters, steel mill workers, sheet metal workers, boilermakers, and laborers. During World War II, 4 to 5 million shipyard workers were exposed when a relatively small number of insulation workers applied asbestos to ships' pipes and hulls. Asbestos-related diseases have occurred in family members whose only contact was dust from an exposed worker's clothes. Similar diseases were also found in persons who grew up within one-half mile of an asbestos factory.

171. **(C)** Pulmonary fibrosis may be caused by drugs such as nitrofurantoin, bleomycin, busulfan, cyclophosphamide, and methysergide.

172. **(C)** Characteristic pulmonary function tests in asbestosis reveal restrictive defects including decreased (25 to 75% reduction) forced expiratory flow rates, reduced vital capacity,

decreased total lung capacity with normal residual volume, decreased forced vital capacity, reduced P_{O_2}, and normal to high air flows.

173. **(E)** Asbestosis is associated with lung cancers, with a latency period of 10 to 30 years. Asbestosis may also increase a slight risk of developing gastrointestinal (esophageal, gastric, colonic, and rectal) cancers.

174. **(B)** Both pleural and peritoneal mesotheliomas are seen in patients with asbestosis. The latency period for mesothelioma is 20 years or more. Mesotheliomas are rapidly invasive; the one-year survival rate is less than 30%.

175. **(E)** Asbestosis often complicates pulmonary hypertension, cor pulmonale, and cardiac failure. Asbestosis depresses cell-mediated immunity, and autoantibodies (rheumatoid factor, antinuclear antibodies) are present. Caplan syndrome may develop.

176. **(E)** Respiratory infections should be prevented through influenza and pneumococcal vaccinations and avoidance of pulmonary irritants, including cigarette smoking; respiratory infections should be treated vigorously.

177. **(B)** H2 blockers may cause gynecomastia, mental confusion, hepatitis, and agranulocytosis. PUD is a chronic disease, and many patients may take H2 blockers for a prolonged period; consequently, drug side reaction often becomes the reason for the patient's visit.

178. **(B)** The treatment of PUD includes reduction of acidity; reduction of psychologic stresses; avoidance of cigarettes, salicylates, and NSAIDs; and the use of mucosal defense medications (sucralfate). To reduce acid production, histamine H2-receptor antagonists are recommended. When H2 blockers fail, proton pump inhibitors (omeprazole) can be utilized. When *H. pylori* is identified, eradication is instituted (eg, Pepto-Bismol, metronidazole, tetracyclines, or omeprazole and biaxin).

179. **(D)** Radon is a radioactive decay product of uranium 238 with immediate precursor of radium 226. Radon itself is not particularly harmful, but its alpha-emitting polonium radioactive decay products account for most radiation exposure. Radiation from food consumption or well drinking water is low. Outdoors, the radon concentrations are likewise trivial. The major source of radon is the soil beneath the dwelling.

180. **(C)** At present, the only recognized late effect from excessive radon exposure is lung cancer. It is estimated that 6,000 to 25,000 bronchogenic carcinomas developed (7% of total cases of bronchogenic carcinoma) each year are due to radon. In uranium miners and radon chemists, the risk of developing sinus cancers are also increased.

181. **(E)** Radon and its daughter products can accumulate in substantial concentrations in homes. Homes in the same community can vary markedly in radon indoor concentrations. Outdoor concentrations are usually insignificant compared to indoor concentrations. Radon concentrations are highest in the basement and lowest at the top floor. At present, asymptomatic inhabitants require no special screening procedures.

182. **(B)** Inhalation of radon daughters (mostly polonium-218 and polonium-214) results in radiation exposure to the tracheobronchial epithelium. The energy deposited directly or indirectly in DNA may cause breaks in strands or chromosomes. Some alterations may be premalignant, and the alterations may be passed to succeeding generations of cells.

183. **(A)** The radon level in the home can be measured through commercially available charcoal canisters and alpha track detectors. Local government agencies may provide a radon indoor detector at no cost.

184. **(A)** Control methods of radon concentrations in the house include: smoking cessation, opening windows, improving ventilation (particularly crawlspaces), sealing the

foundations, spending less time in the basement, and using fans and air cleaners.

185. **(C)** The average indoor radon concentration is around 1.5 pci/L. It is recommended that correction measures be taken when a level beyond 4 pci/L is detected. An indoor radon concentration of pci/L is equivalent to about 0.005 WL. Ten pci/L concentrations should be corrected within a few years, 20 to 100 pci/L concentrations need to be corrected in a few months, and concentrations beyond 200 pci/L need to be corrected in a few weeks.

186. **(B)** Many homes in the physiographic province of the Reading Prong, where the background level of natural radiation is high, have had radon concentrations beyond 4 pci/L (0.02 WL).

187. **(D)** It is estimated that around 8 million homes in the United States have radon levels above 4 pci/L (requiring remedial actions). Hazardous radon levels may be present even in new, well-constructed homes. Radon can enter into homes through foundations. Children increase the risk of radon exposures due to longer potential period of exposure.

188. **(A)** The clinical presentation is typical for hypersensitivity pneumonitis ("extrinsic allergic alveolitis"), which is often manifested mainly as an occupational disease. The symptoms appear on Monday morning when the patient reports to work (ie, exposure to the offensive agent) and the symptoms recur.

189. **(E)** Farmer's lung is the prototype of hypersensitivity pneumonitis. It is caused by *M. faeni*, a thermophilic actinomyces, existing in moldy hay. *M. faeni* can also cause mushroom worker's disease (or mushroom picker's disease) through moldy mushroom compost.

190. **(C)** *A. fumigatus* usually results in acute bronchopulmonary aspergillosis; it also exists in moldy barley to cause malt worker's disease, a type of hypersensitivity pneumonitis.

191. **(E)** Bagassosis is caused by the *Thermoactinomyces sacchari* existing in moldy bagasse (sugarcane fiber residue).

192. **(B)** Metal fume fever is caused by the inhalation of fumes of zinc oxide, copper, or magnesium. It presents symptoms similar to those of hypersensitivity pneumonitis. It causes leukocytosis and begins with thirst and a metallic taste in the mouth. Chest x-rays may be normal in the initial stage. Welding, melting of copper and zinc in electric furnaces and zinc smelting, and galvanizing frequently cause metal fume fever. The analysis of metallic ion concentrations during metal processing procedures will aid in the identification of metal fume fever.

193. **(D)** Polymer fume fever occurs with exposure to fumes produced from thermodegradation of polytetrafluoroethylene (Teflon). The patient may exhibit sweating, chills, fever, chest tightness, malaise, headache, dyspnea, and nonproductive cough 4 to 6 hours after exposure. The appropriate work-ups include WBC determination for leukocytosis and work environment evaluation to measure the metallic ion concentrations.

194. **(C)** In susceptible individuals of any age, repetitive inhalation of antigenic material may precipitate hypersensitivity pneumonitis, characterized by a granulomatous inflammatory reaction in the pulmonary alveolar and interstitial spaces. Although it can be induced by animal antigens (furrier's lung, caused by animal fur; bird breeder's lung, caused by avian protein), bacterial antigens (detergent worker's lung, caused by *Bacillus subtilis*), inorganic haptens (isocyanate lung, caused by toluene disocyanate; vineyard sprayer's lung, caused by copper sulfate) and fungal antigens, but the term is customarily reserved for fungal origins (most commonly micropolyspora and thermoactinomyces). Bacterial and fungal cultures of inhaled particles, as well as metallic ion analysis, are useful in identification.

195. **(C)** In hypersensitivity pneumonitis, leukocytosis with excess neutrophils may be seen

in the acute phase but is less prominent in chronic cases. Eosinophilia is not common. Serum immunoglobulin levels (except IgE levels) are elevated. Examination for serum precipitins against suspected antigens is useful in diagnosis.

196. (E) The fluid from the bronchoalveolar lavage for hypersensitivity pneumonitis shows an increased concentration of IgG, increased number of mononuclear cells (mostly T lymphocytes), and precipitating antibodies. Lymphocytes will proliferate when exposed to the appropriate antigen in vitro, but the results are only suggestive; pulmonary function test shows a restrictive pattern with decreased diffusion. Chest x-rays show interstitial fibrosis, and when in doubt, open lung biopsy will establish the diagnosis.

197. (D) Antigen avoidance is the mainstay in the therapy. This can be accomplished by the removal of the agent from the source in the environment. The patient is recommended to wear protective devices, and the workplace should be ventilated adequately.

198. (B) Silo-filler's disease may cause cough, dyspnea, fever, myalgia, and pulmonary edema in 4 to 12 hours following exposure to nitrogen dioxide, and in 2 to 6 weeks, bronchiolitis obliterans with pulmonary insufficiency may develop. Bronchiolitis obliterans may be prevented by early treatment of acute reaction with corticosteroids. Extensive exposure to silage gas may cause sudden death.

199. (C) In silicosis, the presence of multiple, small, rounded opacities (silicotic nodules) throughout the lung is characteristic. Moreover, calcification of the periphery of hilar lymph nodes ("eggshell" calcification) is typical.

200. (A) Patients with chronic silicosis are at an increased risk for infections with tuberculosis and nontuberculous mycobacteriosis. When PPD is positive, silicosis patients should be treated with (INAH) chemoprophylaxis. Tuberculosis should be suspected in silicosis patients with markedly asymmetric infiltrates,

progressive unilateral infiltrates, or cavitation. Patients with silicosis are also associated with respiratory failure and cor pulmonale in severe cases. The association of silica exposure with lung cancer is controversial.

201. (C) Most patients with chronic silicosis have no symptoms. In patients with progressive massive pulmonary fibrosis, dyspnea may be present. Cough is common but may be due to chronic bronchitis or superimposed infection. Chest pain and clubbing are not common; their presence calls for consideration of alternative disease conditions, including coronary artery diseases and chronic obstructive lung diseases.

202. (E) Intense exposure to beryllium may produce acute disease that results in lung injury characterized by bronchiolitis, pneumonia, and pulmonary edema, with symptoms of dyspnea, cough, weight loss, and diffuse alveolar consolidation on chest x-rays. The mortality rate is claimed to be as high as 10%.

203. (B) Chronic beryllium disease may have a latent period of 5 to 15 years. Beryllium salts are absorbed through the respiratory tract and are distributed throughout the body to produce systemic noncaseating granulomatosis in the lung, lymph nodes, liver, spleen, adrenal glands, and kidney. Skin granulomas are usually due to direct exposure. Berylliosis is also associated with hyperostosis and hypercalcemia.

204. (A) Avoidance of beryllium salts is the best treatment and prevention. The acute and chronic disease of berylliosis should be recognized promptly to remove patients from further beryllium exposure. The treatment of acute berylliosis is usually symptomatic, and prolonged therapy with corticosteroids is often recommended for chronic exposure.

205. (E) Dyspepsia and epigastralgia can often be the chief complaint of patients with cholelithiasis. The most useful procedure is the ultrasound of the right upper abdomen.

206. **(A)-T, (B)-T, (C)-T, (D)-T, (E)-T.** Misoprostol is indicated to prevent NSAID-induced gastric ulcer, particularly for patients who have had debilitating diseases. It should be used during the entire period of NSAID therapy. Side reactions include GI symptoms and menstrual problems.

207. **(A)-T, (B)-T, (C)-T, (D)-T, (E)-T.** Acute pancreatitis is associated with hyperlipoproteinemia (types I and V), pancreatic carcinoma, duodenal ulcer, hypercalcemia, gallstones, hyperparathyroidism, abdominal surgery, abdominal trauma, group B coxsackievirus infection, pregnancy, alcoholism, and the administration of drugs, including corticosteroids, estrogen, furosemide, thiazide, azathioprine, and acetaminophen.

208. **(A)-T, (B)-T, (C)-T, (D)-T, (E)-T.** Secondary polycythemia can be caused by congenital cardiovascular disease, pulmonary arteriovenous fistulas, high-altitude residence, Pickwickian syndrome (obesity, hypoventilation), erythropoietin-producingmalignancies (ovarian carcinoma, CNS malignancies, hypernephroma), renal cysts, adrenal hypercorticism, virilizing tumors, and the use of androgens, sulfonamides, nitrites, and alcohol. In 1% of cases, it can progress to acute myelogenous leukemia.

209. **(A)-F, (B)-F, (C)-T, (D)-F, (E)-F.** Pravastatin is an inhibitor of 3-hydroxy-3-methyglutaryl-coenzyme A (HMG-CoA) reductase. This enzyme catalyzes the conversion of HMG CoA to mevalonate, which is an early and rate-limiting step in cholesterol biosynthesis. Headache and GI disturbance are common, and myositis may occur (0.1% in pravastatin and 0.5% in lovastatin). Liver enzyme elevation may develop and cataract is a remote possibility. Gemfibrozil (Lopid) may also develop myositis, but cholestyramine (Questran) rarely causes myositis.

210. **(A)-F, (B)-T, (C)-T, (D)-T, (E)-F.** Anti-*H. pylori* therapy improves ulcer healing and markedly reduces recurrences. Triple therapy with Pepto-Bismol, tetracyclines, and metronidazole for 2 weeks is successful for 85% to 90% of patients.

211. **(A)-F, (B)-T, (C)-T, (D)-T, (E)-F.** Drugs that may induce orthostatic hypotension include: (1) antihypertensives: diuretics, vasodilators, alpha-adrenergic blockers, and beta-adrenergic blockers; (2) antidepressants: tricyclics and monoamine oxidase inhibitors (MAOIs); (3) major tranquilizers: phenothiazines and butyrophenones; (4) alcohol; (5) narcotics; (6) antiparkinsonism agents: levodopa; and (7) OTC decongestants: phenylephrine and oxymetazoline.

212. **(A)-T, (B)-T, (C)-T, (D)-T, (E)-T.** Patients with prosthetic heart valves are at high risk of developing infective endocarditis, and prophylactic antibiotics should be instituted during dental or minor surgical procedures. Homograft and heterograft valves have lowered the incidence of thromboembolism. Paravalvular leak may occur, and regurgitation murmur may develop. Heart failure, syncope, angina, and embolization may occur in prosthesis malfunction. Chronic hemolysis may cause hemolytic anemia with iron deficiency.

213. **(A)-T, (B)-T, (C)-T, (D)-T, (E)-F.** Immunoglobulins are gamma globulins synthesized by different classes of plasma cells. They are classified into four groups: IgG, IgA, IgM, and IgE.

214. **(A)-T, (B)-T, (C)-T, (D)-T, (E)-F.** Coxsackie B viral infections of the heart may cause chest pain and fever. Myocarditis is fairly common in patients who develop pericarditis. Cardiac tamponade is an uncommon complication. Pleurodynia is characteristic. Classic cases are usually due to tuberculosis. Rheumatoid arthritis often is associated with chronic constrictive pericarditis.

215. **(A)-T, (B)-F, (C)-F, (D)-F, (E)-T.** Acute pancreatitis is associated with cholelithiasis, alcoholism, mumps, hyperparathyroidism, and intra-abdominal operations. Moderate leukocytosis (10,000 to 30,000/mL), elevated serum

lipase (normal 0 to 1.5 Cherry–Crandall units), hyperamylasemia (300 Somogyi units), and lowered serum calcium level (7.5 mg/100 mL) are frequently helpful in the diagnosis of acute pancreatitis. Pneumoperitoneum is characteristic of perforated peptic ulcer and is rarely seen in pancreatitis.

216. (A)-T, (B)-T, (C)-T, (D)-T, (E)-T. Multiple myeloma is characterized by low back pain, anemia, and infection (eg, pneumonia). The laboratory tests will show elevated ESR, proteinuria, hypercalcemia, paraprotein in serum protein electrophoresis, and bone marrow infiltration by plasma cells.

217. (A)-T, (B)-T, (C)-T, (D)-T, (E)-T. Aortic regurgitation is most commonly of rheumatic origin. Less commonly, bacterial endocarditis may result in aortic regurgitation. There is a wide pulse pressure, and the difference of blood pressure at the brachial and femoral arteries is exaggerated.

218. (A)-T, (B)-T, (C)-T, (D)-T, (E)-T. The complications of Hodgkin's disease include hemolytic anemia, intractable itching, superior vena cava obstruction, and pleural effusion.

219. (A)-T, (B)-T, (C)-T, (D)-T, (E)-T. There were 50,000 cases of primary and secondary syphilis cases reported in 1990. Most patients were from the inner city and from rural areas. Cases of congenital syphilis were increased.

220. (A)-T, (B)-T, (C)-T, (D)-T, (E)-T. In 1992, it was estimated that there were 250,000 to 3,000,000 homeless persons in the United States, many of them located in the urban cities. They are at higher risk to develop schizophrenia, severe personality disorders, mild retardation, gender-identity disorders, alcoholism, drug abuse, social breakdown syndrome (withdrawal, aggressive behavior, apathy, negativism), tuberculosis, skin problems (scabies, lice, leg ulcers), and malnutrition.

221. (A)-T, (B)-T, (C)-T, (D)-T, (E)-T. Lack of money, lack of faith in doctors, perceived inadequacy in care (waiting too long, inconvenient hours, insensitivity of health-care personnel), and difficulties in getting to a doctor (too far, no one to take them) are some of the barriers that prevent the inner-city elderly from seeing a physician.

222. (A)-T, (B)-T, (C)-T, (D)-T, (E)-T. The urban family physician has first contact with and has the primary opportunity to recognize the high-risk urban patient. As a provider of long-term continuous care, the family physician is responsible for ensuring that the management of the patient is rational, coordinated, and compassionate. The multidisciplinary training of urban family physicians enables them to understand multifaceted excess urban risk and to begin intervention.

223. (A)-T, (B)-T, (C)-T, (D)-T, (E)-T. Tuberculosis is traditionally more susceptible for postpubertal adolescents who contacted infectious cases; the high-risk groups include minority individuals, the homeless, the institutionalized, and individuals in corrective institutions. Patients with HIV, lymphomas, diabetes, chronic renal failure, and malnutrition, and patients on immunosuppressors are at higher risk.

224. (A)-F, (B)-T, (C)-F, (D)-F, (E)-F. In elderly tuberculosis often presents with negative tuberculin test. The tuberculin test should be repeated in 1 to 2 weeks for increased positive rate (booster or recall phenomenon). Sometimes a third test may be needed to elicit a positive test. A positive acid-fast bacilli (atypical microbacteria should be excluded) on sputum smears and cultures is diagnostic of tuberculosis.

225. (A)-T, (B)-T, (C)-T, (D)-T, (E)-T. In a suspected patient, positive sputum examination with potassium hydroxide (KOH) and culture, a positive coccidioidin skin test result, and a rising complement fixation titer of 1:16 are helpful in establishing diagnosis. Amphotericin B is effective.

226. (A)-T, (B)-T, (C)-T, (D)-T, (E)-T. HBsAg carriers are highly prevalent among Indochinese, and a screening test is needed for the patient over 15 years of age.

227. (A)-T, (B)-T, (C)-T, (D)-T, (E)-F. Allergic bronchopulmonary aspergillosis may develop in patients with a history of asthma. It is characterized by a cough that is often productive of brownish, rubbery sputum, fever, wheezing, pulmonary infiltrates, elevation of serum IgE levels, serum precipitins against *A. fumigatus*, and occasionally, but not always, *A. fumigatus* in the sputum. Positive wheal and erythema skin test results with late reactions at 6 to 8 hours are found. Response to corticosteroid therapy is usually excellent.

228. (A)-F, (B)-F, (C)-F, (D)-F, (E)-T.

Drugs	Side Reactions
Thiazides	Hypokalemia, hyperglycemia, hypercholesterolemia, hyperuricemia
Beta blockers	Bronchospasm, CHF exacerbation, masking hypoglycemia
Alpha-receptor blockers	Orthostatic hypotension
ACE inhibitors	Cough, angioneurotic edema, dysgeusia
Calcium antagonists Dihydropyridines: Nifedipine	Peripheral edema, tachycardia, gingival hyperplasia
Verapamil	Constipation, AV block, bradycardia
Centrally acting alpha-2 agonists	Sedation, dry mouth, fatigue, orthostatic dizziness

229. (A)-F, (B)-F, (C)-F, (D)-F, (E)-F. To prevent HIV infection when traveling, do not (1) engage in casual sexual encounters; (2) have sexual relations with prostitutes, members of other high-risk groups for AIDS, or individuals who have multiple sexual partners; (3) get a tattoo or have ears pierced when out of the United States; (4) resort to experimental or acupuncture treatments when traveling abroad; (5) obtain injectable treatments, medications, vaccines, or gamma globulins in less developed regions of the world; (6) receive transfusion of blood or blood products when overseas, unless it is a true medical emer-

gency; or (7) use illicit injectable drugs or needles and syringes that might have been used previously.

When traveling, do (1) associate socially with the indigenous population, since AIDS is not transmitted by casual contact; (2) visit local hotels, swimming pools, and restaurants; (3) use a condom during a spontaneous sexual liaison, and employ such protection during vaginal, anal, and oral sex (both men and women should have ready access to reliable brands of condoms); (4) use a spermicidal jelly in addition to a condom during vaginal intercourse; (5) obtain appropriate vaccines and other inoculations before leaving the United States; and (6) in seeking potentially life-saving treatment in the face of serious illness or injury, the closest U.S. embassy or consulate should be consulted.

230. (A)-F, (B)-F, (C)-T, (D)-T, (E)-T. Symptoms of food reactions can be categorized as follows: (1) Systemic: anaphylaxis; pallor, fatigue, and irritability; headaches; cardiac arrhythmias; and hypertension. (2) Gastrointestinal: angioneurotic edema of lips, mouth, and throat; nausea and vomiting; abdominal pain and cramping; malabsorption; abdominal distention; diarrhea; flatulence; occult fecal blood loss; and protein-losing enteropathy. (3) Respiratory: dyspnea, rhinitis, and asthma. (4) Dermatologic: pruritus, urticaria, eczema, and erythema.

231. (A)-T, (B)-T, (C)-T, (D)-T, (E)-T. Foods causing IgE-mediated allergic reactions include cow's milk, eggs, nuts, whitefish, shellfish, soy products, wheat, corn, bananas, chicken, and melons.

232. (A)-F, (B)-F, (C)-T, (D)-T, (E)-T. Lyme disease is the most common tick-borne disease in the United States, being most prevalent in New England, Minnesota, and Wisconsin. It is caused by the spirochete *Borrelia burgdorferi*, which is transmitted by the *Ixodes* tick. In stage 1, erythema chronicum migrans is present; in stage 2, neurologic (meningitis, radiculoneuritis, and myelitis) and cardiac (myocarditis and conduction abnormalities) symptoms develop; in stage 3, arthralgia and arthritis develop. Treatment is by tetracycline or by amoxicillin in children.

233. **(A)-F, (B)-T, (C)-T, (D)-T, (E)-T.** Malignant hyperthermia is an autosomal dominant metabolic disease that can result in sudden death. Exaggerated anxiety and muscle fasciculations are frequently present. It is associated with succinylcholine and halothane anesthetics. Trauma, exercise, heat, and viral infections may precipitate the condition, which elevates creatine kinase. Dantrolene is used for the treatment.

234. **(A)-F, (B)-T, (C)-T, (D)-F, (E)-T.** Factors that may delay recovery from occupational injuries include depression, secondary gain, pending litigation, alcoholism, substance abuse, divorce or other life crisis, family history of disability, "doctor shopping," and impending plant closure or layoff.

235. **(A)-F, (B)-F, (C)-T, (D)-T, (E)-F.** Scombroid poisoning is a food-borne illness that can occur with consumption of dark-meat fish, including tuna, albacore, mackerel, bonito, mahi-mahi, and bluefish. Patients taking INH are at a higher risk. Antihistamines and H2-blockers are used for therapy.

236. **(A)-T, (B)-F, (C)-T, (D)-F, (E)-T.** Travelers visiting any malarious areas should take chloroquine 500 mg once weekly beginning 2 weeks before travel and continuing until 4 weeks after departure from the malarious area. Those who travel to areas with the chloroquine-resistant *P. falciparum* strains should take the above chloroquine chemoprophylaxis for nonfalciparum strains. In addition, a one-time dose of three Fansidar tablets (25 mg pyrimethamine and 500 mg sulfadoxine) should be taken if fever occurs. For prolonged exposure of more than 3 weeks, once-weekly Fansidar prophylaxis should be considered, along with side reactions.

237. **(A)-T, (B)-F, (C)-F, (D)-F, (E)-T.** Toxic effects of PCBs to animals are variable with age, sex, and species. Liver cancers developed in mice and rats fed with high doses of PCBs. Some pregnant women who ingested PCB-contaminated foods in Japan delivered "Coca-Cola" babies with transient dark skin pigmentation. This fetal PCB syndrome may be caused by PCDFs. People exposed to PCB-contaminated sewage sludge showed positive correlation of hypertension and elevated triglyceride with PCB body levels. No adverse effects have been identified for those who regularly eat fresh-water fish, which is the main source of PCB exposure.

238. **(A)-T, (B)-F, (C)-F, (D)-T, (E)-T.** Brucellosis is often called "hog fever" and is common in areas with meat-packing industries or slaughterhouses. Employees working for livestock producers are at higher risk to contract the illness; veterinarians, hunters, and laboratory workers are also at increased risk. Brucellosis is the most commonly reported laboratory-associated bacterial infection. Individuals who drink raw milk or eat unpasteurized imported goat cheese are at increased risk.

239. **(A)-T, (B)-F, (C)-T, (D)-F, (E)-F.** Brucellosis is commonly transmitted by blood, urine, vaginal discharges, milk, secretions, and tissues (particularly aborted tissues) of infected cattle, swine, hogs, sheep, goats, dogs, and caribou. Brucellosis is common in animals from rural areas of Third World countries.

240. **(A)-F, (B)-T, (C)-F, (D)-T, (E)-F.** Brucellosis is caused by gram-negative bacteria with animal-specific species: *B. abortus*—cattle, *B. suis*—swine, *B. melitensis*—goats and sheep, and *B. canis*—dogs.

241. **(A)-F, (B)-F, (C)-T, (D)-F, (E)-F.** Brucellosis is called "undulant fever" because of the characteristic fever pattern of rising in the afternoon and falling at night. The infection is systemic and may result in gastric, intestinal, neurologic, hepatic, or musculoskeletal involvement. There is usually an initial septicemic phase, followed by a more chronic stage that is characterized by low-grade fever, malaise, and psychoneurotic symptoms, including depression.

242. **(A)-T, (B)-T, (C)-F, (D)-F, (E)-F.** Diagnosis of brucellosis is by a positive brucella serology. Increased high titer is indicative of relapse, and a low serology titer may not indicate active disease. Definitive diagnosis is the recovery of *Brucella* organisms from blood culture. The brucella skin test is not useful in diagnosis.

243. **(A)-F, (B)-T, (C)-F, (D)-F, (E)-F.** Toxoplasmosis is caused by the protozoa *Toxoplasma gondii*. The disease is acquired primarily in tropical areas through contact with feces of infected cats; in the United States, the infection is acquired more commonly by ingestion of uncooked infected meat. It can accidentally inoculate into laboratory workers, during the transplantation of organs, or the transfusion of leukocytes from immunosuppressed donors. It is associated with mental retardation, microphthalmia, and micro- or macrocephaly of the fetus.

244. **(A)-F, (B)-F, (C)-T, (D)-T, (E)-T.** Anthrax is caused by *Bacillus anthracis,* which commonly infects cattle, goats, or sheep. It is transmitted to humans by the contaminated spores on wool, goat hair, and hides. Anthrax means "coal" in Greek, denoting the blackish, necrotic ulcer of the skin. Anthrax pneumonia is called "wool-sorter's disease." High-risk individuals include weavers; goat hair, wool, or hide handlers; butchers; veterinarians; and agricultural workers.

245. **(A)-T, (B)-T, (C)-T, (D)-F, (E)-F.** Brucellosis may be complicated by splenomegaly with persistent hypersplenism, which may produce recurrent fever and splenic calcifications. Brucella arthritis, spondylitis, prepatellar bursitis, and osteomyelitis may occur. Subacute endocarditis involving the aortic valve is a serious complication requiring immediate recognition for prompt antibiotics.

246. **(A)-F, (B)-F, (C)-T, (D)-T, (E)-F.** Treatment is according to the results of drug sensitivity tests. Initial treatment should start with tetracyclines or doxycycline. The recommended treatment regimen is doxycycline 100 mg PO bid for 6 weeks plus streptomycin (or gentamycin) 1.0 g IM qd for 2 weeks.

247. **(A)-T, (B)-T, (C)-F, (D)-F, (E)-F.** All livestock should be immunized; infected animals should be identified and treated or killed. Personal hygiene and protective precautions should be implemented to handle infected animal secretions and tissues (particularly those from abortions). Human brucella immunizations are still experimental. The serum of patients suspected of brucellosis should be handled with absolute caution by the laboratory personnel.

248. **(A)-F, (B)-T, (C)-T, (D)-F, (E)-F.** *T. pallidum* cannot be cultured, and serologic tests are used for diagnosis. The Kolmer and Wassermann tests are no longer used. In primary syphilis, VDRL is only 85% positive; however, if CSF VDRL test is positive, it is virtually diagnostic for neurosyphilis. Following treatments, VDRL can become negative, but FTA-ABS will remain positive for life.

249. **(A)-F, (B)-F, (C)-F, (D)-F, (E)-F.** Cysticercosis is caused by the ingestion of uncooked pork containing eggs of *Taenia solium*. The larval cysts remain silent in skeletal muscles with calcification. In the brain, they may cause headache and seizures, which can be identified by computed tomography (CT) scanning. Praziquantel (Biltricide) is effective in relieving cerebral hypertension and amelioration of seizures. In the United States, it is most commonly encountered in California and the Southwest. In Los Angeles, 4% of the cases occurred in Americans without a significant travel history.

250. **(A)-T, (B)-T, (C)-T, (D)-T, (E)-T.** In normocytic anemia, if the absolute reticulocyte count is elevated, it is probably due to acute blood loss, hemolysis (schistocytes), or hypersplenism. (It also shows pancytopenia with enlarged spleen.) If there are burr cells and the creatinine clearance is less than 30 mL/min, it is likely to be the anemia of renal disease. If the plasma volume is increased, it can be caused by pregnancy or

macroglobulinemia. Chronic diseases, iron deficiency, vitamin B_{12} deficiency, and hypothyroidism can be identified as the cause. Bone marrow infiltration with leukemia, fibrosis, and granuloma may also be the cause.

251. **(A)-T, (B)-F, (C)-T, (D)-F, (E)-F.** Alteplase is a tissue plasminogen activator used for coronary thrombosis. It is contraindicated in active internal bleeding, recent intraspinal or intracranial surgery (within 2 months), history of cerebrovascular accident, intracranial neoplasm, vascular aberrations (such as aneurysm), known bleeding diathesis, and severe uncontrolled hypertension.

252. **(A)-T, (B)-T, (C)-T, (D)-T, (E)-T.** The most common side reaction of antihistamines is drowsiness. However, dry mouth, blurred vision, difficulty voiding, and impotence (anticholinergic effects) are also common. Restlessness, nervousness, difficulty sleeping, hypertension, and decreased seizure threshold can also occur.

253. **(A)-T, (B)-T, (C)-T, (D)-T, (E)-T.** Cyclosporine is used for prophylaxis of organ rejection in kidney, liver, and heart allogeneic transplants. In addition, it may be promising in rheumatoid arthritis, systemic lupus erythematosus, insulin-dependent diabetes, Graves' ophthalmopathy, severe psoriasis, biliary cirrhosis, myasthenia gravis, multiple sclerosis, Crohn's disease, aplastic anemia, malaria, and schistosomiasis. Nephrotoxicity, hepatotoxicity, hypertension, hypertrichosis, hair loss, gingival hyperplasia, mild neurotoxic effects, gastrointestinal upset, infection, lymphoma, and epithelial malignancy may develop. Thus, the benfit–risk ratio must be carefully weighed.

254. **(A)-T, (B)-T, (C)-T, (D)-T, (E)-T.** Lovastatin is useful in patients with hypercholesterolemia. It is well tolerated; GI upset and CNS disturbances are mild and transient. However, skin rashes may occur, and increased serum transaminases and creatine kinase may develop.

255. **(A)-F, (B)-T, (C)-T, (D)-T, (E)-T.** At 15 to 25 mg/L (83 to 139 µmol/L), serum theophylline produces the following toxic effects: abdominal cramps, agitation, diarrhea, GI disturbances, headache, nausea, tremors, and vomiting; at 25 to 35 mg/L (139 to 194 µmol/L): occasional PVCs, sinus tachycardia (heart rate >120/min), and frequent PVCs; at >35 mg/L (>194 µmol/L): GI bleeding, grand mal seizures, and ventricular tachycardia.

256. **(A)-T, (B)-T, (C)-T, (D)-T, (E)-T.** Crohn's disease is characterized by intermittent abdominal pain and frequent diarrhea. Weight loss, anemia, and anal fissures develop; extraintestinal manifestations include pyoderma gangrenosum, iritis, arthritis, nephrolithiasis, and cholelithiasis.

257. **(A)-F, (B)-T, (C)-T, (D)-T, (E)-F.** Digitalis toxicity is often manifested by anorexia, nausea and vomiting, diarrhea, blurring of vision, ventricular ectopy with frequent couples, paroxysmal atrial tachycardia with block, and atrial fibrillation.

258. **(A)-T, (B)-T, (C)-T, (D)-F, (E)-F.** Approximately 80 to 90% of smokers are interested in quitting; with physician's suggestion, a 1 to 5% 1-year abstinence rate is accomplished. The formal smoking cessation programs yield a 1-year quit rate of 20 to 40%. Withdrawal symptoms (eg, cravings, difficulty in concentration, and tension) disappear more rapidly when quit abruptly. Nicorette is used as an adjunct to behavioral modification for smoking cessation. Its use during the last trimester has been associated with a decrease in fetal breathing movements.

259. **(A)-T, (B)-F, (C)-T, (D)-T, (E)-T.** Managements of infectious mononucleosis are symptomatic. Aspirin is associated with Reye syndrome, which is also a possible complication for infectious mononucleosis; acetaminophen is the preferred analgesic over aspirin. Ampicillin is associated with rashes in patients with infectious mononucleosis and is not recommended. When the spleen is enlarged, it

may rupture by heavy palpation or by bland impact, and patients should avoid contact sports and heavy lifting.

260. **(A)-F, (B)-T, (C)-T, (D)-T, (E)-F.** Iron deficiency anemias commonly occur in infants on an unsupplemented diet deficient in iron, in infants with pica, in 9- to 18-month-old children who grow rapidly, in teenage girls starting menstrual activity, in pregnant women, and in the elderly whose diets are deficient in iron intake. In adults with iron deficiency anemias, bleeding should be considered.

261. **(A)-T, (B)-T, (C)-F, (D)-F, (E)-F.** Cardiac tumors are mostly metastatic tumors from melanoma, leukemia, and lymphomas without significant problems. Primary tumors include myxomas, rhabdomyomas, fibromas, and methotheliomas. Myxomas may cause cachexia, fever, syncope, dyspnea, arrhythmia, and Raynaud's disease. The third heart sound varies in time after the second heart sound and can be diagnosed by ECGs, chest x-rays, and echocardiograms. Ninety-five percent arise from the atria, with 75% from the left atrium. It elevates ESR and serum gamma globulins.

262. **(A)-T, (B)-T, (C)-F, (D)-T, (E)-F.** Quinidine, procainamide, and disopyramide are used for atrial flutter/fibrillation and ventricular arrhythmia. Quinidine may cause cinchonism, hemolytic anemia, hepatitis, and thrombocytopenia. Procainamide (Pronestyl) may cause lupus syndrome and granulocytopenia; disopyramide (Norpace) may cause anticholinergic symptoms (urinary retention, dry mouth). Tocainide is used for ventricular arrhythmia; it may cause QT shortening in ECG, tremor, insomnia, and hallucination. Hypocalcemia may prolong the QT interval, and hypercalcemia may shorten the QT interval in ECG.

263. **(A)-F, (B)-F, (C)-F, (D)-F, (E)-T.** Immunizations recommended for the elderly include Td, pneumococcus (single dose), and influenza vaccines. Due to antigenic drift, influenza vaccines should be received yearly during September through November. Malaise, myalgia, and local swelling with redness may occur 6 to 12 hours after the vaccination, lasting 1 to 2 days. Guillain–Barré syndrome is a rare occurrence. It is not recommended for patients who are allergic to eggs. They can receive chemoprophylaxis with amantadine (Symmetrel) or rimantadine (Fumadine).

264. **(A)-T, (B)-T, (C)-T, (D)-F, (E)-F.** *Campylobacter* enteritis is usually self-limited and is treated symptomatically. In rare cases, correction of water and salt depletion is needed. In protracted or severe illness, a 7-day course of erythromycin 50 mg/kg/d in four divided doses) can be administered.

265. **(A)-T, (B)-F, (C)-F, (D)-T, (E)-F.** Characteristic presentations of infectious mononucleosis include fever, malaise, posterior cervical lymphadenopathies, exudative pharyngitis, puffy eyelids, splenomegaly, depression, atypical lymphocytes, and elevated heterophile antibody titer (>1:28); children under 4 years of age are less responsive to the heterophile test. In infectious mononucleosis, hemolytic anemias may develop.

266. **(A)-F, (B)-T, (C)-T, (D)-T, (E)-F.** NSAIDs are prostaglandin antagonists to synthetase. They may cause gastric irritation, acute gastritis, peptic ulcer, and upper GI bleeding. Headache, tinnitus, and dizziness may also occur. NSAIDs are used in patients with rheumatoid arthritis, osteoarthritis, bursitis, and tendinitis. Selected patients with gout or ankylosing spondylitis may also be responsive to NSAIDs.

267. **(A)-F, (B)-T, (C)-F, (D)-F, (E)-F.** Traveler's diarrhea is commonly caused by enterotoxigenic *E. coli*. Other pathogens include *Shigella, Salmonella,* and *Giardia lamblia.* The illness is usually self-limited and the treatment is symptomatic. Ingestion of bismuth subsalicylate (Pepto-Bismol) 60 mL qid may reduce the incidence of the illness. Trimethoprim-sulfamethoxazole (Septra) may be used for chemoprophylaxis in selected cases.

268. **(A)-F, (B)-F, (C)-F, (D)-T, (E)-F.** The risk of protein–calorie malnutrition is increased in those patients with dementia, the home-bound or bedridden, the poor, those discharged after long hospital stays, those with hip fractures, those in long-term institutional care (especially those with pressure sores), and persons with any long-term chronic illness. A serum albumin level less than 3.5 g/dL, anemia, lymphopenia (total lymphocyte count below 1220), and anergy may be frequent presentations.

269. **(A)-T, (B)-T, (C)-T, (D)-F, (E)-F.** Major complications include recurrences, hemorrhage, luminal pyloric and biliary obstructions, penetration, perforation, intractability, and pancreatitis. Metabolic alkalosis can develop following long-term therapy with antacids; and the dumping syndrome is a late complication of surgery.

270. **(A)-T, (B)-F, (C)-T, (D)-T, (E)-F.** Pneumococcal vaccines (pneumovax) are given to the following individuals to prevent pneumococcal pneumonias: (1) patients with chronic illnesses: diabetes mellitus, hepatic, cardiopulmonary and renal diseases; (2) patients with splenic dysfunctions: sickle cell diseases, asplenias, splenectomy; (3) individuals over 50 years of age; and (4) patients with Hodgkin's disease.

271. **(A)-F, (B)-T, (C)-T, (D)-F, (E)-T.** In the elderly, due to decreased muscle mass a normal serum creatinine level does not guarantee that the drug clearance is normal; it usually is reduced. Thus, the dosage of tetracyclines, sulfonamide, and cephalosporins should be reduced accordingly. The liver clearance is decreased in the elderly and the dosage of lidocaine should be reduced.

272. **(A)-T, (B)-T, (C)-F, (D)-T, (E)-T.** All lipid-lowering drugs cause gastrointestinal symptoms (abdominal pain, diarrhea, flatulence, nausea and vomiting). However, resins may also cause severe constipation requiring stool softener. Clofibrate and gemfibrozil may also be associated with cardiac arrhythmias. Nico-

tinic acid may cause hypotension and may activate peptic ulcer diseases.

273. **(A)-T, (B)-F, (C)-F, (D)-F, (E)-F.** Increased comorbidity in the elderly often results in polypharmacy in the elderly with three to seven times as many adverse drug reactions as in the 20- to 29-year-old group. Gastric acid production is decreased, but it does not affect drug absorption. The increased drug bioavailability (thus increased risk of adverse reactions) is related to decreased lean body mass, decreased hepatic clearance (decreased hepatic microsomal enzyme activity), and decreased renal clearance (decreased renal blood flow, diminished glomerular and tubular filtration). Due to reduced muscle mass, serum creatinine is not a good measure of renal function.

274. **(A)-F, (B)-F, (C)-T, (D)-T, (E)-T.** Complications of infectious mononucleosis include splenic rupture, meningitis, meningoencephalitis, necrotizing exudative pharyngitis, pharyngeal edema, airway obstruction, peritonsillar abscess, sinusitis, orbital cellulitis, hepatitis, rashes (particularly when the patient is treated with ampicillin), Bell's palsy, pancreatitis, depression, and Guillain–Barré syndrome.

275. **(A)-F, (B)-F, (C)-T, (D)-T, (E)-F.** The most common community-acquired pneumonia is caused by pneumococci; for the elderly, the most common is also pneumococci, followed by *Haemophilus. K. pneumoniae* is often associated with alcoholics and diabetics.

276. **(A)-T, (B)-T, (C)-T, (D)-T, (E)-T.** Common side reactions of calcium-channel blockers include hypotension, peripheral edema, AV block, bradycardia, fatigue, dizziness, constipation, elevated liver enzymes, abdominal discomfort, cough, and nervousness.

277. **(A)-F, (B)-F, (C)-F, (D)-T, (E)-T.** A low-cholesterol diet (300 mg or less daily) reduces blood cholesterol on average of 5 to 10%. Harmful oils (more than 30% saturated fats) include coconut oil and palm kernel oil. Better oils (less than 20% saturated fats) include peanut, olive, soybean, corn, sunflower, and canola oil. Cholesterol is present only in animal products, and thus vegetables, fruits, cereals, grains, and nuts are recommended. Red meats (lean beef, pork, lamb) and eggs (up to three per week) are permitted.

278. **(A)-T, (B)-T, (C)-T, (D)-T, (E)-T.** Sumatriptan is a serotonin agonist, which is effective in abolishing migraine headache in a rapid response. Side reactions include pressure in the head; feeling of heaviness, warmth, or tingling; vertigo; malaise; fatigue; and chest discomfort/tightness. A small rise in blood pressure may occur. Sumatriptan is also effective for cluster headaches; however, migraine headaches may recur.

279. **(A)-F, (B)-F, (C)-F, (D)-T, (E)-F.** All asthma patients should avoid drugs that worsen the symptoms (beta blockers may worsen bronchospasm; ACE inhibitors may aggravate cough). Mild asthma may be treated with inhaled beta agonists; if unable to use inhalers, oral beta agonists can be used. Moderate asthma patients can use inhaled corticosteroids and cromolyn. Beta-agonist inhalers are added for attacks. Theophylline is now a third-line drug, and cromolyn is not effective during attacks.

280. **(F)**

281. **(F)**

282. **(F)**

283. **(F)**

284. **(F)**

285. **(F)**

286. **(F)**

287. **(F)**

288. **(T)**

The treatment of acute hepatitis B is symptomatic, and the use of corticosteroids is unnecessary. Acetaminophen and methotrexate may damage liver cells and should be avoided. Diet is not critical for recovery, although a low-fat, high-carbohydrate diet may be used. Hepatitis B virus (HBV) is a DNA virus (Dane particle) but delta-virus is an RNA virus sharing the HBV outer coat. Unless the patient's colleagues maintain a close contact (such as sexual or blood contact) with the patient, they are not at a substantial higher risk to contract either hepatitis B or D. However, if there is sufficient interest among employees, an institution-wide screening for HBV can be instituted. Those individuals who are HBsAg-negative and HBsAb-negative (preferably also HBcAg- and HBeAg-negative) may receive hepatitis B vaccine.

Hepatitis B vaccine is not contraindicated during pregnancy; however, the pregnant wife has had a positive HBsAg, and hepatitis B vaccine is not indicated after delivery. The newborn baby needs HBIG and immunizations for hepatitis B vaccine immediately after birth, at 1 month, and at 6 months of age (three shots).

CHAPTER 8

Pediatrics
Questions

DIRECTIONS (Questions 1 through 75): Each of the numbered items or incomplete statements in this section is followed by answers or by completions of the statement. Select the ONE lettered answer or completion that is BEST in each case.

1. A newborn infant is found to have had no bowel movement for its first 36 hours and is vomiting green material. The x-ray shows a bubble-like appearance in the intestinal loops. The most likely diagnosis is

   (A) cystic fibrosis of the pancreas
   (B) Hirschsprung's disease
   (C) pyloric stenosis
   (D) intussusception
   (E) diaphragmatic hernia   *(Ref. 66)*

2. Two hours after birth, a 4-pound boy developed dyspnea and cyanosis. X-ray reveals a reticulogranular appearance in the lungs. The most likely diagnosis is

   (A) hyaline membrane disease
   (B) asthma
   (C) croup
   (D) pneumonia
   (E) pneumothorax   *(Ref. 66)*

3. In Turner syndrome, the number of Barr bodies is

   (A) 0
   (B) 1
   (C) 2
   (D) 3
   (E) 4   *(Ref. 66)*

4. In boys, the first sign of puberty is growth of the

   (A) testes
   (B) penis
   (C) nipples
   (D) pubic hair
   (E) Adam's apple   *(Ref. 3)*

5. Constitutional growth delay is characterized by

   (A) mental age far ahead of chronologic age
   (B) mental age equals the chronologic age
   (C) bone age equals the chronologic age
   (D) delayed puberty onset
   (E) borderline personality   *(Ref. 3)*

6. A young woman, the sister of one of your patients who has classic hemophilia, is considering marriage. Her boyfriend has been proved to have a deficiency of erythrocyte glucose-6-phosphate dehydrogenase (G6PD). If the young woman is not a carrier of G6PD deficiency, which of the following statements about their potential offspring is correct, if she decides to marry him?

   (A) Every daughter will be a carrier for hemophilia and G6PD deficiency.
   (B) Every son will have G6PD deficiency.
   (C) Some daughters and some sons will have G6PD deficiency.
   (D) None of the sons will have both hemophilia and G6PD deficiency.
   (E) All daughters are hemophiliacs.   *(Ref. 66)*

7. Burgundy-red urine is a sign of congenital

   (A) mumps
   (B) rubella
   (C) toxoplasmosis
   (D) porphyria
   (E) syphilis   *(Ref. 66)*

8. Evaporated milk: 6 oz
   Boiled water: 14 oz
   Carbohydrate: $^3/_4$ oz
   The caloric content per fluid ounce of the formula shown above is approximately

   (A) 4
   (B) 8
   (C) 10
   (D) 16
   (E) 25   *(Ref. 66)*

9. In a 2-year-old child with irritability, painful extremities, pallor, coarse hair, and x-rays revealing periosteal elevation, the most likely diagnosis is

   (A) vitamin A deficiency
   (B) hypervitaminosis D
   (C) hypervitaminosis A
   (D) vitamin D deficiency
   (E) vitamin E deficiency   *(Ref. 66)*

10. An infant usually triples its weight by

    (A) 3 months
    (B) 6 months
    (C) 12 months
    (D) 18 months
    (E) 24 months   *(Ref. 66)*

11. Most infants (75%) can sit alone by the age of

    (A) 1 month
    (B) 6 months
    (C) 12 months
    (D) 15 months
    (E) 24 months   *(Ref. 66)*

12. A dark-brown–stained diaper is a sign of

    (A) Hartnup's disease
    (B) alkaptonuria

   (C) phenylketonuria
   (D) cretinism
   (E) galactosemia   *(Ref. 68)*

13. A school-aged boy suffered from upper respiratory infection (URI) 3 weeks ago. Now he complains of fever, fatigue, and pain in both knee joints. The involved joints are tender, swollen, and hot. Tachycardia is also noted. The most likely diagnosis is

   (A) sickle cell anemia
   (B) acute glomerulonephritis
   (C) rheumatoid arthritis
   (D) rheumatic fever
   (E) acute pericarditis   *(Ref. 66)*

14. Blue-diaper syndrome is associated with

   (A) Hartnup's disease
   (B) congenital mumps
   (C) kernicterus
   (D) diabetes mellitus
   (E) congenital porphyria   *(Ref. 66)*

15. A 3-year-old girl was found to have feet that turn inwardly when she walks. The internal rotation of the hip is 75° and lateral rotation is 25°. You will

   (A) apply bilateral long leg casts for 4 weeks
   (B) instruct the use of medical shoe wedges
   (C) prescribe calcium carbonate 1 g/d for 6 months
   (D) schedule for surgical correction
   (E) provide continuous regular follow-up care   *(Ref. 25)*

16. An 8-month-old female infant has an umbilical hernia that measures approximately 1 cm in diameter. It protrudes with crying but is easily reducible. You will

   (A) schedule for surgical repair
   (B) apply silver nitrate sticks tid for 3 weeks
   (C) provide total health care for regular follow-ups
   (D) perform strapping as soon as possible
   (E) perform immediate laparotomy   *(Ref. 78)*

17. Retinitis pigmentosa is associated with

   (A) congenital porphyria
   (B) abetalipoproteinemia
   (C) Down syndrome
   (D) gargoylism
   (E) cerebral palsy   *(Ref. 66)*

18. The most common cause of amblyopia is

   (A) anisometropia
   (B) strabismus
   (C) pseudostrabismus
   (D) cataract
   (E) glaucoma   *(Ref. 2)*

19. A male infant who weighed 5 lb, 4 oz at term developed jitteriness, cyanosis, apathy, apnea, a weak and high-pitched cry, limpness, and eye rolling at 29 hours of age. The pregnancy had been complicated by albuminuria, excessive weight gain, and hypertension. However, the delivery was atraumatic and was not accompanied by any recognized trauma or anoxia. Despite his birthweight, the infant appeared quite mature. He was alert and was thought to have been normal at birth and for the first 24 hours of life. The most likely diagnosis is

   (A) hypoglycemia
   (B) congenital heart disease
   (C) intracranial bleeding
   (D) neonatal tetany
   (E) adrenal hemorrhage   *(Ref. 66)*

20. A 4-year-old boy suddenly developed a high fever, chills, and vomiting. On examination, he was found to have nuchal rigidity and positive Kernig's sign. Petechial lesions have been noted on both extremities and over the abdomen. The most likely diagnosis is

   (A) pneumococcal meningitis
   (B) encephalitis
   (C) brain tumor
   (D) meningococcal meningitis
   (E) aseptic meningitis   *(Ref. 66)*

21. An infant born with Apgar scores of 8 requires

   (A) immediate cardiopulmonary resuscitation (CPR)
   (B) endotracheal intubation
   (C) occasional suctioning of the oropharynx and nose
   (D) cardiac massage
   (E) administration of sodium bicarbonate
                                         (Ref. 66)

22. All of the following statements about febrile convulsions are true EXCEPT that

   (A) they occur in about 6 to 8% of all children
   (B) they frequently occur between 6 and 48 months
   (C) a family history of febrile convulsions is rarely obtained
   (D) seizures are symmetric and usually last less than 15 minutes
   (E) the child is neurologically normal before and after the convulsion   *(Ref. 66)*

23. Pseudohypertrophy of muscles is a sign of

   (A) myasthenia gravis
   (B) diabetes mellitus
   (C) Duchenne–Becker muscular dystrophy
   (D) hyperthyroidism
   (E) conversion reaction   *(Ref. 66)*

24. A 2-year-old girl is put to bed and she begins to cry. Her parents should

   (A) let her cry and ignore her
   (B) pick her up and kiss her
   (C) change her diaper
   (D) give her antihistamines
   (E) feed her baby food   *(Ref. 66)*

25. Evaluation of the emotional aspects of the child's life

    (A) is outside of the competence of the family physician
    (B) should be done only by pediatricians
    (C) should be done only by psychiatrists
    (D) is within the area of responsibility of the family physician
    (E) should be done only by child psychologists

    (Ref. 66)

26. The parental disciplinary behavior most conducive to delinquency is

    (A) excessive corporal punishment
    (B) avoidance of all corporal punishment
    (C) marked laxness
    (D) marked inconsistency
    (E) marked strictness   *(Ref. 66)*

27. If a child screams when he or she becomes angry, it is most likely due to

    (A) normal reaction
    (B) childhood schizophrenia
    (C) hyperkinesis
    (D) childhood neurosis
    (E) separation anxiety   *(Ref. 66)*

28. Kawasaki's disease is

    (A) geographically limited to Japan
    (B) a self-limited disease without complications
    (C) caused by fish tapeworms
    (D) associated with coronary aneurysms
    (E) predominantly a disease of the elderly
    (Ref. 66)

29. A 2-year-old boy was toilet trained at age 12 months but lost bladder and bowel control after his younger brother was born. His adjustment pattern is an example of

    (A) repression
    (B) suppression
    (C) projection
    (D) regression
    (E) rationalization   *(Ref. 7)*

30. Defiance, rebellion, antisocial feelings, and demands for independence in an adolescent boy

    (A) can usually be controlled by stricter rules and punishment
    (B) should be turned over to the courts for disposition
    (C) can be seen as the expected behavior during this stage of development
    (D) are usually accompanied by inner feelings of security, confidence, and masculinity
    (E) are psychotic behaviors   *(Ref. 66)*

31. A 10-year-old boy has been bitten by a skunk. To rule out rabies, which of the following is the rapid, reliable test?

    (A) antibody titer of the rabies
    (B) stain of the brain tissue of the skunk to find the Negri bodies
    (C) virus culture from the skunk's brain tissue
    (D) examination of the skunk's brain tissue by the fluorescent antibody test
    (E) immune fluorescent antibody titer of the boy

    (Ref. 66)

32. A 2-month-old baby is brought in for a well-baby visit. When the hips and knees are flexed 90° with the knees together in the midline, the left knee is lower than the right knee. This phenomenon is most likely due to

    (A) normal development
    (B) congenital dislocation of the left hip
    (C) congenital dislocation of the right hip
    (D) fracture of the right femur
    (E) congenital syphilis   *(Ref. 2)*

33. Which of the following groups of individuals are at higher risk to develop slipped capital femoral epiphysis?

    (A) tall, slim individuals
    (B) the elderly
    (C) infants who are not on vitamin D supplements

(D) females in the premenopausal stage

(E) males in puberty   *(Ref. 66)*

34. The treatment that has been most effective in the treatment of enuresis is

(A) hypnosis

(B) sleep interruption

(C) electric shocks

(D) imipramine

(E) psychotherapy   *(Ref. 66)*

35. Most full-term infants regain their birth weights by the age of

(A) 5 days

(B) 7 days

(C) 10 days

(D) 20 days

(E) 30 days   *(Ref. 66)*

36. An oblong right scrotal mass is seen in a 3-week-old male infant. It is nonreducible and transparent to light. The most likely diagnosis is

(A) testicular torsion

(B) orchitis

(C) hydrocele

(D) inguinal hernia

(E) epididymitis   *(Ref. 15)*

37. Recurrent abdominal pain in a child is most likely

(A) psychologic

(B) caused by worm infestation

(C) caused by peptic ulcer

(D) caused by abdominal epilepsy

(E) an indication for an intravenous pyelogram (IVP) study   *(Ref. 66)*

38. An 11-month-old girl has developed diarrhea that is watery in nature. No other symptoms are noted, and no abnormalities are found in the physical examination. You would now

(A) prescribe oral ampicillin

(B) advise that solid foods be discontinued

(C) start oral tetracyclines

(D) institute paregoric syrup

(E) offer skim milk fortified with vitamin D   *(Ref. 66)*

39. In a patient with transient synovitis of the hip, which of the following laboratory results is most likely diagnostic?

(A) leukocytosis

(B) hemolytic anemia

(C) hypoglycemia

(D) positive rheumatoid factor

(E) none of the above   *(Ref. 66)*

40. A family physician's school-aged daughter has had pinworm infection for the first time in her life since admission to school 1 month ago. The most likely source of her pinworm infestation is

(A) the family physician's patients

(B) the girl's schoolmates

(C) the girl's mother

(D) family relatives

(E) neighbors   *(Ref. 66)*

41. At 15 months of age, a male infant is noted to have an open anterior fontanel during a routine visit to your office. You would

(A) order a skull x-ray

(B) order T3 and T4

(C) administer a measles–mumps–rubella (MMR) vaccine

(D) administer corticosteroids

(E) order a chromosomal study   *(Ref. 66)*

42. An 8-day-old infant is seen for red eyes with a yellowish discharge. The palpebral conjunctivae are injected, and no other systemic signs are noted. The most likely diagnosis is

(A) gonococcal conjunctivitis

(B) chemical conjunctivitis

(C) syphilitic conjunctivitis

(D) chlamydial conjunctivitis

(E) allergic conjunctivitis   *(Ref. 2)*

43. A lower urinary tract obstruction in a new-born male is most likely caused by

    (A) hydrocele
    (B) renal artery stenosis
    (C) posterior urethral valves
    (D) cryptorchism
    (E) choriocarcinoma   *(Ref. 15)*

44. A full-time working mother brings her 4-week-old baby for the first office visit. The birth weight was 7 lb 4 oz and the weight in the office is 8 lb 8 oz. She is bottle feeding the baby and is worried about adequate nutrition and weight gain. You would

    (A) reassure her
    (B) order complete blood count (CBC) for the baby
    (C) order CBC for the mother
    (D) advise breast feeding
    (E) advise the use of soybean milk   *(Ref. 66)*

45. A newborn baby presents with jaundice, hepatomegaly, and seizure. The eye ground reveals retinal hemorrhages, and skull x-rays show multiple punctate calcifications. The most likely diagnosis is

    (A) cysticercosis
    (B) cytomegalic inclusion disease
    (C) toxoplasmosis
    (D) Wilson's disease
    (E) biliary obstruction   *(Ref. 66)*

46. A 5-year-old boy was found to have group A beta-hemolytic streptococcal pharyngitis 3 days ago. His 7-year-old sister is complaining of fever and sore throat. The throat is infected, but other parts of physical examination are essentially normal. You would now

    (A) reassure the mother that no treatments are necessary
    (B) order white blood count (WBC)
    (C) order erythrocyte sedimentation rate (ESR)
    (D) prescribe oral tetracyclines
    (E) order throat culture   *(Ref. 3)*

47. A 28-year-old school teacher has brought her 3-year-old boy to your office. She states that her father-in-law stayed with them for 3 weeks last month, and she has just learned that he has had active tuberculosis. The boy is asymptomatic, and the physical examinations are essentially normal. The tuberculin test is negative. Now you would

    (A) start isoniazid (INH) and rifampin combination therapy for 18 months
    (B) reassure the mother that no medications are necessary at this point
    (C) give a booster of the rubeola vaccine
    (D) start INH for 3 months and reevaluate the situation
    (E) give influenza immunization for preventive protection   *(Ref. 66)*

48. By what age does a child learn to ride a tricycle and to count?

    (A) 4 months
    (B) 30 months
    (C) 12 months
    (D) 24 months
    (E) 36 months   *(Ref. 66)*

49. By what age does a child learn to speak a few words?

    (A) 3 months
    (B) 6 months
    (C) 12 months
    (D) 24 months
    (E) 36 months   *(Ref. 66)*

50. By what age does a child use three or four blocks to build a tower?

    (A) 6 months
    (B) 12 months
    (C) 18 months
    (D) 24 months
    (E) 36 months   *(Ref. 66)*

51. A male newborn infant is found to have respiratory distress. He drools saliva exces-

sively, becomes cyanotic, and often chokes and regurgitates. The most likely diagnosis is

(A) esophageal atresia
(B) respiratory distress syndrome
(C) hypertrophic pyloric stenosis
(D) aortic vascular rings
(E) aspiration pneumonia   *(Ref. 66)*

52. A full-term infant, born after an uncomplicated pregnancy and delivery, required resuscitation and continued to have labored respiration. Heart sounds were best heard to the right of the midsternal line. No breath sounds were heard in the left chest. The most likely diagnosis is

(A) dextrocardia
(B) diaphragmatic hernia
(C) atelectasis
(D) hyaline membrane disease
(E) transposition of the great vessels
        (Ref. 66)

53. The varicella vaccine is recommended at the age of

(A) 1 month
(B) 2 months
(C) 6 months
(D) 9 months
(E) 18 months   *(Ref. 66)*

54. By what age does an infant smile?

(A) at birth
(B) by 1 month of age
(C) by 2 months of age
(D) by 6 months of age
(E) by 12 months of age   *(Ref. 66)*

55. A continuous "machinery" murmur at the upper left sternal border is a sign of

(A) aortic insufficiency
(B) aortic stenosis
(C) mitral stenosis
(D) patent ductus arteriosus (PDA)
(E) mitral insufficiency   *(Ref. 66)*

56. A wide fixed split of the pulmonary second sound is a sign of

(A) atrial septal defect (ASD)
(B) PDA
(C) idiopathic hypertrophic subaortic stenosis (IHSS)
(D) mitral valve prolapse (MVP)
(E) ventricular septal defect (VSD)   *(Ref. 66)*

57. A boot-shaped heart on roentgenogram is most likely associated with

(A) peripheral pulmonary arterial stenosis
(B) hypoplastic left ventricle
(C) tetralogy of Fallot
(D) transposition of the great vessels
(E) tricuspid atresia   *(Ref. 66)*

58. In hereditary spherocytosis

(A) the spherocytes are much larger than the regular erythrocytes
(B) the disease is transmitted by a sex-linked recessive trait
(C) the red cell membrane is decreased in osmotic fragility
(D) the anemia is caused by vitamin B_{12} deficiency
(E) hyperbilirubinemia may arise in the neonatal period   *(Ref. 66)*

59. A 4-month-old infant fed by goat milk may develop

(A) botulism
(B) iron deficiency anemia
(C) sickle cell anemia
(D) folic acid deficiency
(E) vitamin C deficiency   *(Ref. 66)*

60. Congenital hip dysplasia is often associated with

(A) plancenta previa
(B) PDA
(C) cleft lip
(D) clubfoot
(E) polydactly   *(Ref. 80)*

61. A 12-year-old boy suffers from recurrent swollen lips and occasional difficulty in breathing. The family history reveals that his father had a similar problem. The cause of the symptoms is

    (A) excessive cholinesterase inhibitor
    (B) deficiency of C-1 esterase inhibitor
    (C) angiotensin-converting enzyme (ACE) inhibitor deficiency
    (D) hepatic hydroxymethylglutaryl coenzyme A (HMG CoA) reductase inhibitor deficiency
    (E) immunoglobulin A (IgA) deficiency
    (Ref. 27)

62. Kayser–Fleischer ring is a sign of

    (A) Guillain–Barré syndrome
    (B) von Recklinghausen's disease
    (C) Kawasaki's disease
    (D) Wilson's disease
    (E) Lowe syndrome
    (Ref. 66)

63. Which of the following diseases has an incubation period of 7 to 10 days?

    (A) scarlet fever
    (B) diphtheria
    (C) skin cancer
    (D) measles
    (E) chickenpox
    (Ref. 66)

64. A normal 12-month-old male infant is seen for routine well-child care. All of his immunizations are up to date, and the mother reports that they live in a community where the fluoride content in the water supply is less than 0.3 ppm. You will order

    (A) Poly-Vi-Flor 0.25 mg 1 cc PO qd
    (B) Vi-Daylin F 1.0 mg chewable PO 1 tablet qd
    (C) Pediaflor 0.5 mg 1 cc PO qd
    (D) Tri-Vi-Flor 1.0 mg chewable PO 1 tablet qd
    (E) fluoride-containing toothpaste tid
    (Ref. 66)

65. A 10-month-old boy developed a 3-day fever of 102°F. An erythematous maculopapular

rash on the trunk appeared at the time of defervescence. The most likely diagnosis is

    (A) roseola infantum
    (B) rubella
    (C) rubeola
    (D) erythema infectiosum
    (E) echovirus infection
    (Ref. 27)

66. Otitis media with effusion is associated with

    (A) breast feeding
    (B) nutritional anemia
    (C) care at home
    (D) passive smoking
    (E) tropical weather
    (Ref. 66)

67. Screening for lead poisoning is best performed for children living at an old building in the inner city by

    (A) hemoglobin level
    (B) urine protoporphyrin level
    (C) ESR
    (D) urine lead level
    (E) blood lead level
    (Ref. 5)

68. A normal 2-month-old female infant is seen for her well-child care. She has never received any immunizations. You will order all of the following EXCEPT

    (A) diphtheria–pertussis–tetanus (DPT) (first shot)
    (B) urinalysis
    (C) hepatitis B (first shot)
    (D) *Haemophilus* vaccine (first shot)
    (E) oral polio vaccine (first dose)
    (Ref. 66)

69. Head circumference does not need to be measured routinely after the age of

    (A) 3 months
    (B) 12 months
    (C) 24 months
    (D) 36 months
    (E) 48 months
    (Ref. 66)

70. Slipped capital femoral epiphysis is characterized by

(A) pain referred from groin to anteromedial thigh and knee

(B) pain referred from low back to anteromedial thigh and knee

(C) pain limited to the entire thigh

(D) pain developed only when the hip is in the position of lateral rotation

(E) elevated ESR of 120 mm/hr or more

(Ref. 66)

71. A 7-year-old boy's intelligence quotient (IQ) test result was 70. He is classified as having

(A) profound mental retardation

(B) severe mental retardation

(C) moderate mental retardation

(D) mild mental retardation

(E) borderline mental retardation   (Ref. 66)

72. Twirling is a sign of

(A) infantile autism

(B) lead poisoning

(C) encopresis

(D) enuresis

(E) lymphosarcoma   (Ref. 66)

73. Clinical disease can be caused by the administration of a(an)

(A) Haemophilus vaccine

(B) influenza vaccine

(C) Sabin vaccine

(D) hepatitis vaccine

(E) DPT vaccine   (Ref. 66)

74. Spontaneous hemarthrosis is a sign of

(A) idiopathic thrombocytopenic purpura (ITP)

(B) classic hemophilia

(C) acute lymphocytic leukemia

(D) rheumatoid arthritis

(E) multiple myeloma   (Ref. 66)

75. Contraindications for further DPT immunizations include

(A) low-grade fever of less than 104°F

(B) anorexia

(C) redness of the injection sites

(D) high-pitched unusual cry

(E) nausea   (Ref. 66)

DIRECTIONS (Questions 76 through 167): Each question consists of an introduction followed by some statements. Mark T (true) or F (false) after each statement.

76. A mother brings her 1-year-old boy to your office for a regular checkup. Physical examinations are essentially normal. You will now

(A) prescribe fluoride supplementation of 10 mg/d

(B) administer MMR vaccine if not in an endemic area

(C) administer polyvalent pneumococcal (Pneumovax) vaccine

(D) administer purified protein derivative (PPD) 5 TU (0.1 mL) intradermally

(E) administer Haemophilus B vaccine if it has never been given   (Ref. 66)

77. Treatments for a 4-year-old girl with acute otitis media include

(A) ampicillin 125 mg 1 tablet PO qd for 10 days

(B) amoxicillin 250 mg 1 tablet PO qd for 10 days

(C) corticosteroid otic solution qid instilled into both ear canals for 10 days

(D) doxycycline 50 mg 1 tablet PO bid for 10 days

(E) aqueous procaine penicillin, 4.8 million IM stat   (Ref. 66)

78. Which of the following clinical presentations is characteristic for Legg–Calvé–Perthes disease?

    (A) high fever
    (B) ESR of 120 mm/hr
    (C) decreased uptake of technetium bone scan in the affected hip
    (D) WBC of 35,000/mm^3
    (E) WBC of 100,000/mm^3 in the synovial fluid of the affected hip   (Ref. 66)

79. Work-ups for a child with acute otitis media include

    (A) WBC
    (B) WBC and differential counts
    (C) tympanocentesis for culture/sensitivity of the causative organism
    (D) CBC
    (E) x-rays of the middle ear   (Ref. 66)

80. Clinical presentations of the Pickwickian syndrome include

    (A) polycythemia
    (B) somnolence
    (C) hyperventilation
    (D) cardiac failure
    (E) obesity   (Ref. 66)

81. Down syndrome is associated with

    (A) teenage mothers
    (B) a hemophiliac family
    (C) an abnormal Y chromosome in the father
    (D) a Philadelphia chromosome in the mother
    (E) repeated spontaneous abortions in the mother   (Ref. 66)

82. In osteomyelitis of the hip, the presenting manifestations often include

    (A) fever
    (B) local pain
    (C) local swelling
    (D) limited movement
    (E) leukocytosis   (Ref. 66)

83. Clinical characteristics of Prader–Willi syndrome include

    (A) hypogonadism
    (B) high intelligence
    (C) strabismus
    (D) obesity
    (E) Y-chromosome defects   (Ref. 66)

84. The wife of one of your family physician colleagues called you up at 6:00 A.M. at your home in a state of panic. She stated that she found many small wiggling worms at her 8-year-old boy's perianal area at 3:00 A.M. Since then, she just can't sleep any longer. You will

    (A) reassure her that this is a common phenomenon in school children and does not need medical attention
    (B) prescribe a minor tranquilizer such as lorazepam (Ativan) to help her sleep
    (C) instruct her to collect worms and make an appointment at the office as soon as possible to bring the boy for care
    (D) ask her to thoroughly bathe the boy three times a day for 2 weeks, then call you back for results
    (E) recommend killing all worms and boiling all bedsheets and clothes the boy used   (Ref. 66)

85. Which of the following individuals are at high risk of developing lead poisoning?

    (A) painters
    (B) individuals who drink moonshine whiskey made in car radiators
    (C) children living in old buildings
    (D) plumbers
    (E) medical technologists   (Ref. 66)

86. An adolescent female patient asks you about the most reliable method to prevent human immunodeficiency virus (HIV). You instruct her to

    (A) use a condom
    (B) take oral contraceptives

(C) practice abstinence

(D) select a partner carefully

(E) receive an HIV test regularly *(Ref. 3)*

87. In osteoid osteoma

(A) pain is improved at night

(B) the ESR is characteristically elevated beyond 120 mm/hr

(C) technetium bone scan reveals decreased uptake

(D) the roentgenographic appearance shows a radiolucent nidus surrounded by sclerotic bone

(E) the treatment choice is steroid injection of the painful lesion *(Ref. 66)*

88. *Yersinia* infections

(A) usually involve the terminal ileum

(B) cause watery stools containing blood and pus

(C) often have symptoms of fever, vomiting, and abdominal pain

(D) may produce arthritis

(E) may produce thyroiditis *(Ref. 66)*

89. Contraindications to live measles vaccines include

(A) allergy to penicillin

(B) allergy to eggs

(C) pregnancy

(D) diabetes mellitus

(E) steroid therapy *(Ref. 66)*

90. Which of the following statements are true concerning rubeola?

(A) Rubeola is completely eradicated in the United States.

(B) Modified measles is caused by passive immunity with immune globulin and subsequent exposure to natural disease.

(C) Immune globulin therapy is recommended for children less than 1 year of age who are at risk.

(D) Live, attenuated measles vaccine is recommended for healthy infants at age 2 months.

(E) Atypical measles may be confused with Rocky Mountain spotted fever.

(Ref. 66)

91. Serious sequelae of pertussis vaccination include

(A) hydrocephalus

(B) encephalopathy

(C) chronic hepatitis

(D) renal insufficiency

(E) pulmonary fibrosis *(Ref. 66)*

92. Absolute contraindications to further pertussis vaccination include

(A) cerebral palsy

(B) fretfulness

(C) severe reactions in a sibling

(D) family history of seizures

(E) persistent, high-pitched cry *(Ref. 66)*

93. Transient tachypnea of the newborn (TTN) is manifested by

(A) tachypnea

(B) expiratory grunting

(C) cyanosis

(D) wheezing rales

(E) temperature of 104°F or more *(Ref. 66)*

94. Regarding the eruptions in smallpox and varicella

(A) in smallpox, all eruptions appear in the same stage

(B) in varicella, eruptions appear in various stages

(C) in smallpox, skin lesions primarily involve the trunk

(D) in varicella, skin lesions primarily involve the extremities

(E) Kaposi's varicelliform eruptions are the hallmark of varicella *(Ref. 66)*

95. Cretinism may show signs of

    (A) high intelligence
    (B) dry skin
    (C) thick hair
    (D) coarse hair
    (E) harsh voice   (Ref. 66)

96. Children who are at risk for developing depression include those who

    (A) are disfigured in some way
    (B) have a chronic disease
    (C) have a physically ill parent
    (D) have a depressed parent
    (E) have a positive family history   (Ref. 66)

97. The problems of urban schoolchildren include

    (A) failing hearing tests
    (B) inadequate immunizations
    (C) failing vision tests
    (D) dental caries
    (E) glasses not updated   (Ref. 5)

98. The health problems of urban schoolchildren are taken care of by

    (A) primary-care physicians
    (B) hospital clinics
    (C) neighborhood health centers
    (D) emergency rooms
    (E) health maintenance organizations
        (HMOs)   (Ref. 5)

99. The lead level in urban children

    (A) is higher than that of suburban children
    (B) is higher than that of rural children
    (C) may lead to behavioral problems and low intelligence scores even in subclinical levels
    (D) may cause stressful situations for the family involving housing and landlord–tenant problems
    (E) is increased if they reside in old buildings built in the 1930s   (Ref. 5)

100. Clinical features that should arouse suspicion of the battered-child syndrome are

    (A) a 5-month-old with a fractured femur caused by getting his leg caught in the crib sides
    (B) a 10-month-old with height and weight less than the third percentile who is unable to crawl or sit and lies in bed motionless with an intense gaze
    (C) a 5-month-old with a burn of the perineum who was placed in a bathtub of water that was too hot
    (D) a 6-month-old with an acute subdural hematoma found on investigation for repeated vomiting to have no history of head trauma
    (E) many bruises (faded and fresh) all over the body of a 2-month-old boy, without adequate explanations   (Ref. 66)

101. Effective punishment includes

    (A) preventing avoidance of and escape from the punisher
    (B) reducing the need for subsequent punishment
    (C) not providing a model of aggressive behavior
    (D) avoidance of producing in the child a hateful attitude toward the punisher
    (E) a clear explanation of the reason for punishment   (Ref. 66)

102. In children, a good way to modify behavior is to

    (A) specify signals to the children so that they understand what is expected of them
    (B) ignore disruptive behaviors
    (C) praise children for improvement in behavior
    (D) award privileges to those showing good behavior
    (E) increase the difficulty of award abruptly without clear explanation   (Ref. 66)

103. The causes of neonatal convulsions include

    (A) anoxia
    (B) addicted mother

(C) maple syrup urine disease

(D) severe infections

(E) hypoglycemia   *(Ref. 66)*

104. A 10-year-old boy has had a bee sting. He may develop

(A) swelling

(B) itching

(C) burning

(D) angioedema

(E) erythema   *(Ref. 66)*

105. At 40 weeks of age, the infant

(A) sits erect for sustained periods

(B) pulls himself to a standing position

(C) grasps objects with his thumb and fore-finger

(D) responds to his name, waves bye-bye

(E) runs two blocks   *(Ref. 66)*

106. Causes of jaundice during the first week of life include

(A) enclosed hemorrhage

(B) rubella syndrome

(C) transient familial neonatal hyperbilirubinemia

(D) Crigler–Najjar syndrome

(E) physiologic jaundice   *(Ref. 66)*

107. Aseptic meningitis means the etiologic agent is possibly

(A) viral

(B) fungal

(C) meningococcal

(D) *Haemophilus influenzae*

(E) tuberculosis   *(Ref. 66)*

108. Iron deficiency anemia in infancy may be due to

(A) low birth weight

(B) acute hemorrhage

(C) early clamping of cord

(D) inadequate diet

(E) blood loss   *(Ref. 66)*

109. Depression in children is characterized by

(A) disturbances of sleep

(B) suicidal ideas

(C) psychomotor retardation

(D) episodes of anxiety

(E) increase of appetite   *(Ref. 66)*

110. Petit mal (absence seizure) usually begins in childhood. It may be characterized by

(A) impairment of consciousness with mild clonic movements

(B) either increased or decreased postural tone

(C) 5-second spike on electroencephalogram (EEG)

(D) automatic movements

(E) autonomic phenomena   *(Ref. 66)*

111. A differential diagnosis of wheezing in children may include

(A) cystic fibrosis

(B) asthma

(C) foreign-body aspiration

(D) atelectasis

(E) acute gastroenteritis   *(Ref. 66)*

112. The common causes of vomiting in children include

(A) URI

(B) gastroenteritis

(C) genitourinary (GU) infection

(D) intestinal obstruction

(E) otitis media   *(Ref. 66)*

113. *Mycoplasma pneumoniae* (Eaton agent) infections may be manifested by

(A) cervical adenitis

(B) lung infiltrates on x-ray chest

(C) clinical responsiveness to erythromycin therapy

(D) increased cold agglutinin titer

(E) maculopapular rashes   *(Ref. 66)*

114. Hand–Schuller–Christian's disease is characterized by

    (A) diabetes mellitus
    (B) exophthalmos
    (C) diabetes insipidus
    (D) skull defects
    (E) maculopapular skin rash   *(Ref. 68)*

115. Which of the following is/are true of Niemann–Pick disease?

    (A) hepatosplenomegaly
    (B) severe psychomotor retardation
    (C) early death
    (D) accumulation of ganglioside
    (E) seizures   *(Ref. 66)*

116. A staph epidemic occurs in a newborn nursery. Management consists of

    (A) admitting all new babies to newly established nurseries staffed by separate uninfected personnel
    (B) admitting new infants to regular nurseries only after all others are discharged
    (C) hexachlorophene bath for new admissions
    (D) aseptic technique to handle the baby admitted
    (E) kanamycin prophylaxis for infants
    (Ref. 66)

117. Croup is suspected by

    (A) low hematocrit value of 20
    (B) high hemoglobin value of 17
    (C) hillar lymphadenopathy on chest x-rays
    (D) barking cough
    (E) appearance of erythema nodosum in the legs
    (Ref. 66)

118. The differential diagnosis of croup includes

    (A) epiglottitis
    (B) peritonsillar abscess
    (C) Ludwig's angina
    (D) bacterial tracheitis
    (E) foreign-body aspiration   *(Ref. 66)*

119. Erythema infectiosum is caused by

    (A) adenovirus A18
    (B) enterovirus C16
    (C) parovirus B19
    (D) Lassa virus B19
    (E) *Helicobacter pylori*   *(Ref. 27)*

120. Clinical manifestations of rickets include

    (A) increased linear growth of the long bones
    (B) delayed dental eruptions
    (C) leg bowing
    (D) enlarged frontal bone
    (E) "rachitic rosary" of the ribs   *(Ref. 66)*

121. The childhood (1 to 14 years) mortality rate

    (A) shows a clearly increasing trend
    (B) dropped below one half of that in the 1950s
    (C) shows a fairly constant pattern since the 1950s
    (D) was 90/100,000 in 1950 and doubled in 1990
    (E) was 90/100,000 in 1950 and increased 10 times in the 1980s due to acquired immune deficiency syndrome (AIDS) epidemic   *(Ref. 66)*

122. The five leading causes of infant deaths in 1993 were

    (A) congenital anomalies
    (B) respiratory distress syndrome
    (C) diabetes mellitus
    (D) retinoblastoma
    (E) Tylenol poisoning   *(Ref. 66)*

123. The five leading causes of childhood deaths in 1993 were

    (A) lupus erythematosus
    (B) AIDS
    (C) homicides
    (D) accidents
    (E) cancers   *(Ref. 66)*

124. With regard to neuroblastoma

    (A) it accounts for 8% of tumors in children
    (B) it is responsible for 11% of cancer deaths in children
    (C) the new cases are approximately 500 per year
    (D) it is more likely to occur in children older than 14 years of age
    (E) 75% occurs in patients between 4 and 14 years of age   *(Ref. 66)*

125. Clinical features of neuroblastoma include

    (A) abdominal pain
    (B) abdominal mass
    (C) weight gain
    (D) increased vanillylmandelic acid (VMA) in urine
    (E) decreased homovanillic (HVA) in urine   *(Ref. 66)*

126. Concerning AIDS

    (A) 1% of the total deaths are of children less than 12 years of age
    (B) 90% of patients are between 13 and 19 years of age
    (C) 1% of patients are between 20 and 29 years of age
    (D) many young adults contracted AIDS as adolescents
    (E) adolescents are at high risk of contracting HIV–AIDS   *(Ref. 68)*

127. Which of the following statements is/are true for adolescents (13 to 19 years)?

    (A) There are 3 million adolescents.
    (B) Adolescents are only one half of the number of the elderly (beyond 65 years).
    (C) The age-specific death rate is around 1%.
    (D) There are more females than males.
    (E) They are an "overserved" group in health care.   *(Ref. 69)*

128. Adolescents are an underserved population because they lack

    (A) transportation
    (B) money

    (C) time
    (D) initiative
    (E) encouragement   *(Ref. 3)*

129. Concerning adolescents' health care, which of the following statements are true?

    (A) ninety five percent of adolescents have regular physician contacts.
    (B) ninety nine percent of adolescents are seen regularly by pediatricians.
    (C) one percent of adolescents are seen regularly by family physicians.
    (D) The typical pediatrician–adolescent encounter lasts 120 minutes.
    (E) Anticipatory guidance lasts for 115 minutes of a 120-minute encounter.   *(Ref. 3)*

130. Most adolescents like to discuss which of the following topics with their physicians?

    (A) diabetes mellitus
    (B) hypertension
    (C) sexually transmitted diseases (STDs)
    (D) drug abuse
    (E) rheumatoid arthritis   *(Ref. 71)*

131. To provide adolescent care, information on which of the following issues will be collected?

    (A) organic problems
    (B) home environment
    (C) family dynamics
    (D) peer activities
    (E) school achievements   *(Ref. 70)*

132. Often, it may be difficult to elicit medical history from an adolescent. The physician should

    (A) abandon the adolescent
    (B) ask for help from the parent
    (C) respect the adolescent's attitude
    (D) encourage the adolescent to express his or her feelings
    (E) be angry at the adolescent   *(Ref. 70)*

133. Which of the following are possible barriers for physicians to care for adolescents?

    (A) dislike adolescents
    (B) minor status
    (C) fear of adolescents
    (D) confidentiality issues
    (E) lack of insurance coverage   (Ref. 70)

134. Transient synovitis of the hip is caused by

    (A) trauma
    (B) tuberculosis
    (C) gonorrhea
    (D) chlamydia
    (E) none of the above   (Ref. 66)

135. Neonatal meningitis is likely to be caused by

    (A) *Streptococcus agalactiae*
    (B) gram-negative enterococci
    (C) *Listeria monocytogenes*
    (D) group A streptococci
    (E) *Pseudomonas aeruginosa*   (Ref. 66)

136. During the first few years of life, the common microorganisms responsible for bacterial meningitis are

    (A) *S. agalactiae*
    (B) *Streptococcus pneumoniae*
    (C) *Neisseria meningitidis*
    (D) *Neisseria gonorrhoeae*
    (E) *H. influenzae* type B   (Ref. 66)

137. Wilms' tumor is associated with

    (A) aniridia
    (B) sharp visual acuity
    (C) hemihypertrophy
    (D) macrocephaly
    (E) high intelligence   (Ref. 66)

138. A 9-year-old boy is brought to the family practice center by his mother for evaluation of a limp and left hip pain of 2 days' duration. Prior to the development of left hip pain, the patient had flu-like symptoms for 2 weeks. The patient denies any known injury to the left hip. There is local tenderness over the left hip joint anteriorly. The left hip motion reveals limited internal rotation and abduction. Temperature is normal. ESR, CBC, and x-rays of the left hip are all within normal limits. The most likely diagnosis is

    (A) osteoarthritis
    (B) gonococcal arthritis
    (C) osteomyelitis
    (D) transient synovitis
    (E) slipped capital femoral epiphysis
                                          (Ref. 66)

139. Hypoplastic left heart syndrome is characterized by

    (A) dyspnea
    (B) hepatomegaly
    (C) grayish-blue color of skin
    (D) heart failure
    (E) strong peripheral pulse   (Ref. 66)

140. Regarding hepatitis B vaccination schedules

    (A) for infants of hepatitis B surface antigen (HBsAg)-negative mothers—one shot only
    (B) for infants of HBsAg-positive mothers—five shots are the minimum
    (C) for infants whose mothers' HBsAg status is unknown—three shots are needed
    (D) for infants of hepatitis B surface antibody (HBsAb)-positive mothers—no vaccinations are recommended
    (E) for infants of HBsAg-positive and HIV-positive mothers—a monthly shot × 12 is required   (Ref. 66)

141. Which of the following groups are recommended for hepatitis B vaccination?

    (A) premature infants
    (B) infants born to HBsAg-positive mothers
    (C) infants born to HBsAg-negative mothers
    (D) infants born to mothers whose HBsAg status is unknown
    (E) infants with sickle cell anemias   (Ref. 66)

142. Which of the following statements is/are true for hepatitis B virus (HBV) carriers?

    (A) The risk of becoming a carrier is lowest during the neonatal period.
    (B) ninety five percent of adolescents who are infected with HBV will become carriers.
    (C) Women who are HIV carriers may pass the virus to their newborn infants.
    (D) A person with a positive HBsAg test is potentially infectious to household members and sexual contacts.
    (E) HBV carriers are 100 times greater at risk to develop hepatoma.   (Ref. 66)

143. The advantage of vaccinating infants against HBV is

    (A) a vaccine delivery system is already in existence
    (B) vaccination is provided prior to HBV exposure
    (C) to prevent HBV carriers
    (D) to prevent HBV occurrences
    (E) to prevent cirrhosis and hepatoma occurrences   (Ref. 66)

144. Which of the following statements is/are true regarding allergic rhinitis?

    (A) It accounts for 95% of physician visits.
    (B) Estimates of prevalence range between 5 and 22% of the population.
    (C) Incidence is highest between 15 and 25 years of age.
    (D) The first development is usually at 5 to 10 years of age.
    (E) Symptoms are most severe during puberty.   (Ref. 66)

145. Newborn circumcision is not recommended in the infant with

    (A) urinary tract infection (UTI)
    (B) balanitis
    (C) bleeding disorders
    (D) posthitis
    (E) paraphimosis   (Ref. 15)

146. The ethnicity of sickle cell patients includes

    (A) African Americans
    (B) those of Mediterranean ancestry
    (C) those of Caribbean origin
    (D) Arabs
    (E) those of East Indian ancestry   (Ref. 66)

147. Adolescent anabolic–androgenic steroid use may

    (A) produce premature epiphyseal closure
    (B) promote further growth
    (C) increase testicular size
    (D) produce male pattern baldness
    (E) increase femininity in female adolescents   (Ref. 3)

148. The sequelae of bacterial meningitis is

    (A) hearing impairment
    (B) hydrocephalus
    (C) ataxia
    (D) learning disability
    (E) seizure disorders   (Ref. 66)

149. The group A beta-hemolytic streptococcus (GABHS) pyogens

    (A) may account for 99% of sore throats in children
    (B) are treated with metronidazole (Flagyl) for 100% effectiveness
    (C) are treated with penicillin traditionally, but penicillin is only effective for less than 1% of patients now
    (D) produce pharyngitis indistinguishable from that of viral origin
    (E) may produce rheumatic fever as a complication   (Ref. 66)

150. A 6-month-old baby is brought in for a well-baby visit. There are marked erythematous, papulous rashes at the perineum. The most likely diagnosis is

    (A) milk allergy
    (B) diaper dermatitis
    (C) atopic dermatitis
    (D) tinea cruris
    (E) perineal impetigo   (Ref. 55)

151. GABHS pharyngitis is manifested by

   (A) fever
   (B) tonsillar inflammation with white exudates
   (C) tender, swollen cervical nodes
   (D) palatal petechiae
   (E) headache   (Ref. 66)

152. Hemorrhagic disease of the newborn may be

   (A) evident on the second or third day
   (B) melena
   (C) bleeding from the navel
   (D) hematuria
   (E) hypovolemic shock   (Ref. 66)

153. In congenital rubella

   (A) hearing loss is conductive in nature
   (B) intelligence is high
   (C) interstitial pneumonia may present with cough, tachypnea, and respiratory distress
   (D) low birth weight is common
   (E) cataracts are common   (Ref. 66)

154. A child has had a common cold syndrome. Physically, he was normal. Strep screening was negative. The mother requests antibiotic therapy. You would now

   (A) prescribe penicillin for 10 days
   (B) prescribe penicillin for 5 days
   (C) reassure the mother that no antibiotic therapy is required
   (D) prescribe ampicillin for 10 days
   (E) advise the use of antibiotic throat spray
                                          (Ref. 66)

155. Which of the following statements is/are true for the common cold syndromes?

   (A) Among children aged 1 to 5 years, the incidence ranges from 6 to 13 times yearly.
   (B) Older children suffer four colds a year.
   (C) More than $500 million are spent for over-the counter (OTC) cold remedies.
   (D) There are 800 brands of cold remedies available without prescriptions.
   (E) It accounts for 100 million physician visits a year.   (Ref. 66)

156. A teenage girl plans to attend a sun bathing contest at the beach. You will tell her about which of the following harmful effects of the sun?

   (A) skin cancer
   (B) wrinkling
   (C) blotchy color
   (D) coarseness
   (E) tendency to bruise easily   (Ref. 66)

157. Which of the following statements is/are true concerning adolescent (13 to 19 years) sexuality?

   (A) Forty percent are sexually active.
   (B) Sixty percent of sexually active girls do not regularly use contraceptives.
   (C) Approximately 50% of adolescents do not use contraceptives the first time they have intercourse.
   (D) Half of premarital pregnancies occur within the first 6 months after sexual initiation.
   (E) Approximately 2.5 million adolescents have had an STD.   (Ref. 69)

158. The incidence of adolescent high school seniors' substance abuse is as follows:

   (A) Twenty percent smoke cigarettes on a daily basis.
   (B) Twenty percent used marijuana in the preceding month.
   (C) Thirty three percent use alcohol more than once a month.
   (D) Fifteen percent have tried cocaine.
   (E) White adolescents are more likely than black or Hispanic adolescents to use alcohol, tobacco, and most other drugs.
                                          (Ref. 69)

159. Which of the following is true with regard to adolescent violence?

(A) Violence and injury account for 75% of adolescent deaths.

(B) Thirty percent of adolescent deaths are from motor vehicle accidents.

(C) Fifty percent of adolescent motor vehicle accident deaths are alcohol related.

(D) Homicide is the leading cause of death among blacks 15 to 19 years of age.

(E) Adolescents experience more abuse and neglect than younger children do.

(Ref. 69)

160. The recommendation for the MMR vaccine is

(A) first dose given at age 15 months

(B) second dose given at age 4 to 6 years

(C) alternatively, second dose can be given at 12 years of age, or at middle school entry

(D) should be given to all pregnant women

(E) children with HIV are contraindicated

(Ref. 66)

161. The recommendations for hepatitis B vaccines for infants of HBsAg-negative mothers are

(A) first shot at birth

(B) second shot at 1 to 2 months of age

(C) third shot at 6 to 18 months of age

(D) alternative schedule: first shot at 1 to 2 months, second shot at 4 months, and third shot at 6 to 18 months

(E) booster at 4 to 6 years for both regular and alternative schedules *(Ref. 66)*

162. The recommendations for hepatitis B vaccines for infants of HBsAg-positive mothers are

(A) first dose within 12 hours of birth

(B) hepatitis B immune globulin (HBIG) within 12 hours of birth

(C) second dose at 1 month of age

(D) third dose at 6 months of age

(E) a booster at 18 months of age

(Ref. 66)

163. The recommendations for *H. influenzae* type B (HIB) vaccines are

(A) HIB vaccine should be given to all infants

(B) HIB titer is given at 2 months (#1), 4 months (#2), 6 months (#3), and 15 months (#4) of age

(C) HIB titer can be given simultaneously with DPT (#1, #2, #3, #4), oral polio vaccine (OPV) (#1, #2, #3), hepatitis B (#2, #3), and MMR (#1)

(D) For children between 15 months and 60 months of age, one dose only is necessary

(E) After 5 years of age, no HIB vaccines are necessary. *(Ref. 66)*

164. The current primary immunization schedule is

(A) at birth—Hep B #1, if mother is carrier + HBIG

(B) 2 months—DPT #1, OPV #1, HIB #1, Hep B #2

(C) 4 months—DPT #2, OPV #2, HIB #2

(D) 6 months—DPT #3, HIB #3, Hep B #3

(E) 15 months—DPT #4, HIB #4, OPV #3, MMR #1 *(Ref. 66)*

165. The immunization schedule for children at age 15 months to 7 years is

(A) 1st visit—DPT #1, OPV #1, MMR #1, HIB

(B) 2 months later—DPT #2, OPV #2

(C) 2 months later—DPT #3

(D) 6 to 12 months later—acellular diphtheria–pertussis–tetanus toxoids (DPaT) #4, OPV #3

(E) 4 to 6 years old—DPTa #5, OPV #4, MMR #2 *(Ref. 66)*

166. The immunization schedule of children beyond 7 years of age is

(A) 1st visit—tetanus–diphtheria (TD) #1, OPV #1, MMR #1

(B) 6 to 8 weeks later—TD #2, OPV #2, MMR #2

(C) 6 to 12 months later—TD #3, OPV #3

(D) 10 years later—TD

(E) hepatitis vaccine (3 doses) is given to

high-risk adolescents   *(Ref. 66)*

167. Spina bifida may be associated with

    (A) meningocele
    (B) muscle paralysis
    (C) incontinence
    (D) hydrocephalus
    (E) UTI   *(Ref. 66)*

DIRECTIONS (Questions 168 through 187): The following clinical set problem consists of clinical information presented in the format of questions or incomplete statements followed by a group of numbered options.

Indicate T if the option is true;
Indicate F if the option is false.

A 4-year-old boy was brought to a family practice center located at the underserved inner city by his mother. Both the mother and the boy are recent immigrants from Mexico and speak only a little English. The boy's aunt presented his complaints as sore throat and loss of appetite. The aunt also indicated that the boy had been treated for anemia back home and requested that you give him strong iron and vitamin shots. The physical examination revealed an infected pharynx and enlarged red tonsils. The remaining examinations were unremarkable. You would now

168. prescribe vitamin E 100 IU 1 tablet tid for 1 month

169. give him a shot of 0.5 mL (0.5 mg) vitamin B_{12} (cyanocobalamin)

170. administer 0.5 mL (25 mg) of ferrous gluconate injection

171. administer IM penicillin G 1 million units

172. take a throat culture

173. prescribe erythromycin 250 mg bid for 5 days

174. order hemoglobin, hematocrit, and red blood cell (RBC) count

175. prescribe ampicillin 250 mg qid for 10 days

176. prescribe ampicillin 250 mg in 5 mL syrup qid for 10 days

One week later, the boy returned to the family practice center with his aunt. The aunt reported that the sore throat has resolved, but the boy has had vague epigastric discomfort for almost a year without improvement. Physical examinations were essentially normal. You would now

177. order upper gastrointestinal (GI) series

178. order gastroendoscopy

179. order stool examination for parasitic ova

180. order gastric juice analysis

181. prescribe cimetidine (Tagamet) 200 mg tid for 1 week

Ascariasis is suspected to be the diagnosis. Which of the following statements aid in identification of the eggs?

182. yellowish oval shape with pluglike ends; measuring $50 \times 23 \mu$

183. asymmetric, flattened on one side; measuring $30 \times 60 \mu$

184. Outer mamillated coverings, measuring $40 \times 60 \mu$

Which of the following medications are effective for ascariasis?

185. piperazine (Antepar)

186. pyrantel pamoate (Antiminth)

187. chloroquine (Aralen)   *(Ref. 66)*

Answers and Explanations

1. **(A)** Because of a deficiency of pancreatic enzyme, pebble-like hard masses of tenacious meconium block the terminal ileum; the bowel proximal to this area is greatly dilated and filled with pasty meconium. Volvulus and gangrene of the dilated loops may occur with perforation. Sweat electrolyte levels are elevated and a chloride level above 60 mEq/L is significant. The gamma globulin is also elevated.

2. **(A)** The cause is unknown, but a deficiency of surfactin and hypoperfusion may be associated. This condition is a major cause of death in the newborn period, with high incidence among premature babies.

3. **(A)** The Barr body is a rounded chromatin mass located near or at the inner surface of nuclear membrane. The number of the chromatin bodies in a cell is one less than the number of X chromosomes in that cell. The sex chromosome type in Turner syndrome is XO, so that the Barr body is 0.

4. **(A)** In boys, the first sign of puberty is testicular enlargement, followed by enlargement of the penis and scrotum (thinning and pigmentation), and appearance of pubic hair (first straight, then curly) and axillary hair.

5. **(C)** Constitutional growth delay is usually familial and is genetically determined. The adolescent is often very much concerned with the shortness of height, but it is normal and the bone age is equal to or only slightly behind the chronologic age.

6. **(D)** Synthesis of red cell G6PD is determined by genes borne on the X chromosome. Thus, G6PD deficiency is an X-linked recessive disease like hemophilia. Since the father's X chromosome carries the pathological trait of G6PD deficiency, all the daughters will become carriers of G6PD deficiency (each daughter has one X chromosome from the father and another X from the mother), and none of the sons will have G6PD deficiency traits (the Y of each son comes from the father and the X of each son comes from the mother). Since the sister of the mother has hemophilia, the sister's two Xs are both affected; one of the affected Xs is derived from the grandmother. The grandfather is a hemophiliac, but the mother is not affected. She carries one affected X for hemophilia (received from the grandfather) and one normal X (received from the grandmother). The father carries normal XY for hemophilia. Thus, half of the daughters will be carriers of hemophilia (one affected X from the mother and one normal X from the father), half of the daughters will be normal (one normal X from the mother and one normal X from the father), half of the sons will be normal (one normal X from the mother and one normal Y from the father) and half of the sons will be carriers of hemophilia (one affected X from the mother and one normal Y from the father).

7. **(D)** Congenital porphyria is characterized by the excretion of urine that is burgundy-red as passed or becomes so upon exposure to light; this begins at birth or shortly thereafter.

8. **(D)** Evaporated milk provides 40 calories/oz; thus, it provides 40 calories/oz × 6 oz = 240 cal. Sugar provides 120 calories/oz; thus, it provides 120 calories/oz × $^3/_4$ oz = 90 calories.

Total calories: 240 calories + 90 calories
= 330 calories

Total fluid: 6 oz + 14 oz + $^3/_4$ oz = 20.75 oz
calories/oz = 330 calories/20.75 oz
= 16 calories

9. **(C)** Symptoms of hypervitaminosis A can occur after a period of several weeks of 10 times the prophylactic dosage (1500 to 5000 IU). Bone pain, loss of hair, cheilosis, and benign intracranial hypertension (pseudotumor cerebri) may be noted as well.

10. **(C)** At birth, 7½ lb is the average weight; the weight is usually doubled by the fifth month and tripled by 12 months (22 lb). The birth weight is quadrupled (30 lb) at 2½ years of age. At 10 years of age, the weight is 10 times that at birth (75 lb).

11. **(B)** The infant will be able to sit steadily by the age of 28 weeks.

12. **(B)** Alkaptonuria is due to the absence in the liver of the enzyme homogentisic acid oxidase. The accumulation of homogentisic acid causes the dark-brown staining of urine-moistened diapers.

13. **(D)** The symptoms of rheumatic fever usually do not develop until some time after the manifestations of the preceding streptococcal infection have disappeared. This latent period lasts from 1 to 5 weeks, and in chorea this may be 2 to 6 months. The presenting manifestation of acute rheumatic fever is commonly arthritis or choreiform movements in school-aged children and carditis in very young children.

14. **(A)** Blue-diaper syndrome is a familial disorder of Hartnup's disease characterized by hypercalcemia, nephrocalcinosis, and indicanuria.

15. **(E)** Common causes of in-toeing in children include metatarsus adductus, medial thigh torsion, and medial femoral torsion (excessive femoral anteversion). Normally, the internal rotation and lateral rotation of the hip is 45° each; in excessive femoral anteversion, the internal rotation is increased and the lateral rotation is decreased. Observation with comprehensive total health care is needed because many show spontaneous resolution. Surgery may be needed at age 8 to 10 years if the condition persists.

16. **(C)** Umbilical hernias are more frequent in females and are more common in African Americans. The majority of umbilical hernias less than 2 cm in size close spontaneously by 5 to 6 years of age. Umbilical hernias are not likely to cause incarceration or strangulation, which requires surgery.

17. **(B)** Abetalipoproteinemia is an autosomal recessive disease characterized by steatorrhea, ataxia, acanthocytosis, and retinitis pigmentosa.

18. **(B)** Amblyopia, also called lazy eye, is a condition in which the eyes are anatomically normal but they perform subnormal visual acuity. The most common cause is strabismus, which should be screened early within four months of age for correction. Anisometropia needs patching of the good eye for correction.

19. **(A)** Four pathophysiologic groups of neonatal infants are at high risk of developing hypoglycemia: (1) infants of diabetic mothers and infants with severe erythroblastosis fetalis; (2) low-birth-weight infants (particularly infants of toxemic mothers); (3) very immature or severely ill infants; and (4) infants with galactosemia, glycogen storage disease, maple syrup urine disease, leucine sensitivity, insulinomas, or Beckwith syndrome. Onset is from a few hours to a week after birth. Symptoms include jitteriness or tremors, cyanosis, apathy, convulsions, tachypnea, weak or high-pitched cry, limpness, difficulty in feeding, eye rolling, sudden pallor, sweating, and hypothermia. If the symptoms per-

sist with the administration of sufficient glucose, other causes must be considered (including infections such as meningitis).

20. **(D)** The meningitic form presents symptoms and signs of meningitis plus those of septicemia (purpura). Endotoxic shock with disseminated intravascular coagulation (DIC) leading to adrenal hemorrhage and circulatory collapse (Waterhouse–Friderichsen syndrome) occurs frequently with meningococcemia (hypotension; widespread purpura; rapid, thready pulse; and coma). The treatment of shock includes hydrocortisone, isoproterenol, antibiotics, and adequate blood-volume replacement.

21. **(C)** See table at bottom of page.

22. **(C)** There is frequently a family history of febrile convulsions. A normal electroencephalogram is obtained about 1 week after the seizure and prognosis is good. Convulsions usually disappear by the age of 3 years.

23. **(C)** Duchenne–Becker muscular dystrophy is characterized by pseudohypertrophy of the calf, deltoid, brachioradialis, and tongue muscles.

24. **(A)** Bedtime crying is easily cured from the start by following a consistent bedtime routine, putting the child to bed, and leaving her. If she cries on being left, it should be ignored. The young child will quickly learn not to cry at bedtime.

25. **(D)** Pediatricians and family physicians have the responsibility of the total health needs of children, including the quality of the child's life in providing comprehensive and continuous care.

26. **(D)** The parents of delinquent children usually communicate their permissiveness to the children, though mostly through unconsciously driven behavior. Approval of the delinquent behavior of the children is often expressed in nonverbal forms, and parental disciplinary behavior usually lacks consistency.

27. **(A)** Screaming is a normal reaction for a child who becomes angry, usually because of frustration at failing to gain his desires, antagonism between himself and his parents, or jealousy between siblings. The behavioral syndrome that includes screaming, breath holding, kicking, and throwing himself on the floor is called a temper tantrum. Most preschool children have tantrums; they are considered pathologic only when frequent and severe.

28. **(D)** Kawasaki's disease is a disease of unknown etiology affecting children under 5 years of age in Japan, the United States, Europe, and Australia. The clinical features include a prolonged or intermittent fever, sterile conjunctivitis, and diffuse reddening of the oral and pharyngeal mucosa with redness and fissuring of the lips. Later in the course of the fever there is redness and induration of the palms, soles, fingers, and toes, followed by desquamation. There is also a polymorphous exanthema of the trunk and limbs with a nonpurulent cervical lymphadenopathy. The frequently associated findings include (1) coronary aneurysm (20% to 36%); (2) carditis, especially myocarditis and pericarditis (70%): appearance of Q waves, prolongation of PR and QT, ST-T wave changes in electrocardiogram (ECG); (3) diarrhea; (4) arthralgia or arthritis; (5) proteinuria and increase of leukocytes in urine sediment;

		0	1	2
A, R	Appearance (color)	Blue, pale	Body pink, extremities blue	Completely pink
P	Pulse	Absent	Below 100	Over 100
G	Grimace (reflex irritability)	No response	Grimace	Cough, sneeze, or vigorous cry
A	Activity (muscle tone)	Flaccid	Some flexion of extremities	Well-flexed, active motion

(6) changes in blood tests: leukocytosis with shift to the left; slight decrease in erythrocyte and hemoglobin levels; increased ESR, lactic dehydrogenase (LDH), creatine phosphokinase (CPK), and immunoglobulin E (IgE), positive C-reactive protein (CRP); increased alpha-2-globulin; and negative antistreptolysin-O (ASLO) titer with thrombocytosis and negative febrile agglutinins; (7) changes occasionally observed: aseptic meningitis, mild jaundice or slight increase of serum glutamic oxaloacetic transaminase (SGOT), hydrops of gallbladder; (8) aneurysms of brachial, vertebral, celiac, and mesenteric arteries; (9) renal and iliofemoral arteries; (10) mitral insufficiency; and (11) anterior uveitis.

29. **(D)** This is a typical example of regression. A toilet-trained, first-born child may temporarily lose bladder and bowel control in response to the arrival of a second child in the family. Regression is the return to an earlier level of emotional adjustment (eg, not toilet-trained) at which gratification was assured.

30. **(C)** Normal adolescence is characterized by a multitude of personality changes. The turmoil involves the adolescent's attempts to establish himself as an independent individual. His efforts are often of a rebellious and radical nature. The adolescent boy may show rebellion, defiance, and antisocial feelings.

31. **(D)** The pathognomonic sign of rabies is to find the neuronal cytoplasm of the Negri body (inclusion body) in the skunk's brain or salivary gland. Examination of these tissues by the fluorescent antibody test is a rapid, reliable means of diagnosis. However, it is sometimes difficult to obtain the biting skunk for observation and examination.

32. **(B)** Congenital dislocation of the hip is a common cause of childhood limp. Usually, there is a positive family history. The mother may note that the infant's hip is stiff when the diaper is changed. Risk factors include female sex, first born, breech presentation, and other associated musculoskeletal abnormalities.

33. **(E)** The slipped capital femoral epiphysis is more common in blacks than in whites, and more common in men than in women. It occurs most commonly in adolescents at puberty, males from 10 to 17 years, and females from 8 to 15 years. It occurs more commonly in obese adolescents and less frequently in very tall individuals.

34. **(D)** Imipramine 25 to 50 mg/d is used for children over 6 years of age who are suffering from enuresis. Side reactions include hypotension, hypertension, tachycardia, restlessness, nightmares, dry mouth, and, rarely, blood dyscrasia. Continuous follow-up with support and understanding is necessary.

35. **(C)** Most full-term infants gain their birth weights by the age of 10 to 14 days.

36. **(C)** A hydrocele is frequently seen at birth; it usually resolves within a few months. Follow-up observation of the baby is recommended. Reassurance is offered to alleviate parental concerns.

37. **(A)** Recurrent abdominal pain in a child is usually caused by emotional stress. Abdominal epilepsy is a rare condition. The incidence of positive organic disorders in recurrent abdominal pain in children is about 7%. Although an IVP study is not required immediately, a urinalysis should be performed to rule out disease in the urinary tract. The family and personal history, together with the clinical examination and minimal investigation, will provide important evidence that there is no demonstrable organic disease and that there is an emotional disorder to account for the symptoms. These patients are usually tense, fussy, timid, anxious, and overconscientious. These children may also show emotional disturbances such as fears, sleep disorders, and school difficulties.

38. **(B)** Simple diarrhea in the child is best treated by supportive measures. Formula and solid foods are temporarily withheld to reduce the solute load reaching the diseased bowel and to diminish fecal water loss. Oral fluids, including warm dilute sugar solution,

soft drinks exhausted of carbonation, and solutions of flavored gelatin mixes, are given frequently. More advanced cases may require intravenous fluid replacement.

39. **(E)** In a typical patient with transient synovitis of the hip, laboratory tests are usually normal. However, ESR may be elevated in some patients, but the alpha-2-globulin is rarely greater than 1.0 mg/dL.

40. **(B)** All options are possible, because pinworms are nondiscriminative for socioeconomic classes. However, the most likely source of infection is from the girl's schoolmates. Thus, the control of pinworm infestations is difficult; all schoolchildren need to practice hygienic behaviors.

41. **(C)** In a normal infant, the anterior fontanel closes between 9 and 18 months of age, and an open anterior fontanel occurring at 15 months of age is within the limits of the normal developmental stage; no work-ups are necessary at this time. MMR primary immunization is recommended at 15 months of age. Persistent open fontanel may be caused by chromosomal abnormalities (Down syndrome, trisomy 13 or 18), hypothyroidism, malnutrition, rubella syndrome, and skeletal disorders.

42. **(D)** Gonococcal and chemical (resulting from silver nitrate use for newborns) conjunctivitis usually occur in the early postnatal days. Chlamydial conjunctivitis is characterized by late onset at 7 to 14 days of age. Red eyes, purulent discharges, and palpebral conjunctival infections are consistent with infection by *Chlamydia trachomatis*. A Gram stain of the conjunctival exudate shows polymorphonuclear and mononuclear cells; a Giemsa stain of epithelial cell scrapings reveals intracellular inclusions. When in doubt, positive culture establishes the diagnosis. Fifty percent may be complicated by pneumonia, particularly in older babies aged 3 to 16 weeks.

43. **(C)** The most common cause of lower urinary tract obstruction is the posterior urethral valves. In male newborns, these valves are formed by the mucosal folds to obstruct the lower urinary tract at the prostatic level. The male newborn presents with a dribbling urinary stream. A suprapubic mass is frequently noted.

44. **(A)**

$$7 \text{ lb } 4 \text{ oz} = 7.25 \text{ lb}$$
$$= 3.3 \text{ kg } (1 \text{ lb} = 0.45 \text{ kg})$$
$$8 \text{ lb } 8 \text{ oz} = 3.8 \text{ kg}$$
$$3.8 \text{ kg} - 3.3 \text{ kg} = 0.5 \text{ kg} = 500 \text{ g}$$
$$4 \text{ weeks} = 28 \text{ days } (1 \text{ week} = 7 \text{ days})$$

The baby is presumed to regain her prior weight at 10 days of age, so that during the past 18 days (28 days − 10 days = 18 days) the baby has gained 28 g/d (500 g/18 d = 28 g/d). The average baby gains 25 g/d over this period, and anything over 20 g/d is normal. Although the mother's desire for breast feeding should be encouraged, it may not be practical for a full-time working mother to breast feed her baby during working hours.

45. **(B)** Cytomegalic inclusion disease usually presents with jaundice, hepatosplenomegaly, prematurity, microcephaly, chorditis, necrotizing retinitis, retinal hemorrhages, microphthalmia, cataract, optic atrophy, and optic disk malformation. Interferon inducers (poly I:C) and arabinoside (Vidarabine) may be useful.

46. **(E)** Distinguishing between viral pharyngitis and streptococcal pharyngitis is often not easy. Close contact with the sick sibling makes the patient at increased risk for streptococcal infection. Throat culture should be performed to confirm the diagnosis.

47. **(D)** INH single-drug therapy should be instituted for the close contacts (such as household contacts) of patients with an active case of tuberculosis, even though the contacts' tuberculin skin tests are negative; early treatment prior to the hematogenous dissemination will promptly eradicate the tubercle bacilli before hypersensitivity develops. INH should continue for 3 months if the tuber-

culin test remains negative and no evidence of disease is present. If there is positive conversion of the tuberculin test, INH (10 to 20 mg/kg) should be continued for a total of 12 months of chemoprophylaxis. In a tuberculin-positive child who receives a rubeola vaccine or who has had rubeola, pertussis, or influenza, 1 month of INH chemoprophylaxis is required. The initial therapy for tuberculosis is INH and rifampin (10 mg/kg) for 12 months.

48. **(E)** A child can ride a tricycle at 3 years. The child is able to state the age and the sex (boy or girl). The child can ascend stairs by age 3 and descend by age 4. By 3 years, most children can stand on one foot for a short period of time, and by 5 years, they can hop on one foot.

49. **(C)** A child learns to speak communicatively (eg, mama, dada) by age 1. In addition, a child may know the names of a few objects.

50. **(C)** A child can put a 1-inch cube on top of another, and can build a tower of three or four blocks by 18 months. At 24 months, the child can build six cubes.

51. **(A)** The diagnosis of esophageal atresia should be considered in any newborn infant with respiratory distress, excessive salivation, or cyanosis. Inability to pass a small, relatively rigid rubber catheter through the esophagus into the stomach usually establishes the diagnosis. One to three milliliters of water-soluble contrast medium is introduced into the tube and an x-ray is taken with the infant in the upright position. This will define the level of the blind proximal pouch, and the presence of air in the stomach and gastrointestinal tract will confirm communication between the distal esophagus and the trachea. Direct anastomosis is the treatment of choice.

52. **(B)** Usually, an infant with diaphragmatic hernia (foramen of Bochdalek) presents in a state of acute respiratory distress with cyanosis and markedly increased respiratory rate and effort. The affected hemithorax is usually dull to percussion, and there is evidence of shift of mediastinal structures to the opposite side. The diagnosis is almost always apparent on standard roentgenogram of the thorax, which often clearly demonstrates gas-filled intestines. Immediate surgical repair is indicated.

53. **(E)** The varicella vaccine is recommended for all children 1 to 12 years old without a past history of clinical varicella. Children with immunodeficiency are not recommended for immunization.

54. **(C)** A child smiles (on social contact) by 2 months of age.

55. **(D)** In PDA, the physical signs may show hyperactive left ventricular impulses, bounding pulses, wide pulse pressure, third heart sound, and the continuous murmur. Indomethacin is useful in premature babies.

56. **(A)** ASD causes constant splitting of pulmonary second sound, clubbing, and cyanosis. This is a congenital disease, but the symptoms may not develop until 30 or 40 years later. The symptoms include fatigue, palpitation, and dyspnea on exertion. Pulmonary embolism or paradoxic embolism (stroke) may occur.

57. **(C)** Tetralogy of Fallot includes pulmonary stenosis, VSD, hypertrophic right ventricle, and dextroposition of the aorta. Roentgenogram reveals a normal-sized, boot-shaped heart with decrease of pulmonary markings.

58. **(E)** Hereditary spherocytosis is transmitted by dominant inheritance and causes familial hemolytic anemia and acholuric jaundice with splenomegaly. The spherocytic red cell is smaller than the normal erythrocyte and lacks the central pallor of the biconcave disk; the osmotic fragility is increased.

59. **(D)** Folic acid deficiency, possibly due to feeding of goat's milk, usually causes megaloblastic anemia to develop at 4 to 7 months of age, with hypersegmented neutrophils.

60. **(D)** Congenital hip dysplasia is associated with breech delivery. It is more common in girls and may also be associated with pes equinovarus (clubfoot) and arthrogryposis. Physical examination shows loss of abduction of the thigh and a hip click.

61. **(B)** The clinical syndrome is the hereditary angioedema resulting from the deficiency of C-1 esterase inhibitor, which produces excessive vasoactive mediators, causing swelling of the skin, extremities, and respiratory and GI tracts. The patient may complain of abdominal pain, nausea, and vomiting. Danazol (300 to 800 mg/d) and stanozolol (2 mg tid) are used for prophylaxis.

62. **(D)** Wilson's disease (hepatolenticular degeneration) is characterized by Kayser–Fleischer ring, a greenish-yellow ring near the margin of the iris; liver cirrhosis; and mental retardation. The disease is usually clinically detectable after 5 years.

63. **(D)**

Incubation Period (Days)	Illness
10–21	Chickenpox
7–14	Measles
7–14	Poliomyelitis
2–6	Diphtheria
2–5	Scarlet fever

64. **(A)**

Age
Birth–6 months
6 months–3 years
3 years–6 years
6 years–16 years

Fluoride Content of Water Supply		
<0.3 ppm	0.3 to 0.6 pp	>0.6 ppm
0	0	0
0.25 mg	0	0
0.05 mg	0.25 mg	0
1.00 mg	0.50 mg	0

65. **(A)** Roseola infantum (exanthem subitum) is caused by herpesvirus type 6. It usually shows suboccipital lymphadenopathy and leukopenia (with relative lymphocytosis); the treatment is symptomatic.

66. **(D)** Passive smoking (eg, parental smoking in the presence of the child) is found to be associated with an increased risk of otitis media with effusion. The mother should be counseled about the benefit of decreasing the child's exposure to smoking.

67. **(B)** All children between the ages of 1 and 4 years who live in or visit poorly kept buildings built before 1950, or who are exposed to industrial pollution containing lead fumes, should be screened.

68. **(B)** Laboratory tests are not necessary for every well-baby visit unless the history and physical indicate the need.

69. **(D)** Head circumference is particularly useful in identifying hydrocephalus. After 3 years of age, the head circumference does not need to be measured routinely during the regular well-child check.

70. **(A)** In slipped capital femoral epiphysis, the femoral head is displaced posteriorly and inferiorly to the femoral neck; consequently, the femoral neck rotates laterally and slides upward. This is shown by roentgenography. Almost all patients complain of pain referred from the groin to the anteromedial aspect of the thigh and knee. There is usually no fever, and ESR is within normal limits.

71. **(E)** The levels of mental retardation are classified as follows: borderline (IQ 68 to 85); mild (IQ 52 to 67); moderate (IQ 36 to 51); severe (IQ 20 to 35); and profound (IQ <20).

72. **(A)** Infantile autism is characterized by lack of communicative skills and interpersonal sensitivities, an obsessive need for sameness, and twirling.

73. **(C)** On rare occasions, paralytic diseases can be developed in susceptible recipients and their close contacts of the live polio vaccines.

74. **(B)** Classic hemophilia is an X-linked disease due to deficiency of factor VIII in the plasma. The hallmark is hemarthrosis; the partial prothrombin time (PTT) is greatly prolonged.

75. **(D)** Adverse reactions of DPT immunizations include fever, anorexia, pain, drowsiness, swelling and redness at the injection sites, and vomiting. Patients with the following adverse reactions are not recommended for subsequent DPT immunizations: seizures; collapse with shocklike state; encephalopathy; high fever (more than 104.9°F); persistent cry (3 to 21 hours); and high-pitched, unusual cry.

76. **(A)-F, (B)-F, (C)-F, (D)-T, (E)-T.** Pneumococcal vaccines are given to high-risk individuals over 2 years of age. HIB is recommended for children 2 months to 5 years of age against *H. influenzae* type B. Fluoride supplementation is recommended for the community in which the water fluoride level is less than 0.7 ppm. For children younger than 3 years of age, fluoride supplementation is 0.5 mg/d; for children older than 3 years, it is 1 mg/d.

77. **(A)-F, (B)-F, (C)-F, (D)-F, (E)-F.** The recommended treatments for a 4-year-old child are ampicillin, 250 mg, 1 teaspoonful qid for 10 days or amoxicillin, 250 mg, 1 teaspoonful tid for 10 days; erythromycin or trimethoprim and sulfamethoxazole are alternative drugs.

78. **(A)-F, (B)-F, (C)-T, (D)-F, (E)-F.** Legg–Calvé–Perthes disease (coxa plana) is an avascular necrosis of the femoral head. There is no fever, and WBCs, ESR, and synovial fluid analyses are normal. In the early stage, roentgenogram is normal, but the technetium bone scan reveals decreased uptake in the femoral head.

79. **(A)-F, (B)-F, (C)-F, (D)-F, (E)-F.** Work-ups for a child with acute otitis media include a careful and detailed history and physical examination. When there is no response toward treatments, tympanocentesis is needed for culture and sensitivity of the causative organism.

80. **(A)-T, (B)-T, (C)-F, (D)-T, (E)-T.** Pickwickian syndrome is characterized by extreme obesity, hypoventilation, somnolence, hypoxemia, cyanosis, and right-sided cardiac failure resulting from pulmonary hypertension. Weight reduction is an important treatment regimen.

81. **(A)-F, (B)-F, (C)-F, (D)-F, (E)-T.** Advanced maternal age increases the risk of Down syndrome in the offspring, particularly when the pregnant women have had previous multiple spontaneous abortions and excessive radiation exposures. When the mother's age is 35 years, the incidence of Down syndrome is 1:365; at age 39, it is 1:139; at age 45, it is 1:32. The incidence of another Down baby for a mother who has a Down baby previously is 1% to 2%.

82. **(A)-T, (B)-T, (C)-T, (D)-T, (E)-T.** In osteomyelitis of the hip, the child is usually febrile; the affected hip is swollen, painful, and limited in movement. There is leukocytosis, and ESR is elevated. Blood culture may be positive. Roentgenogram is characterized by lytic lesions, soft-tissue swelling, periosteal reaction, cortical irregularity, demineralization, and sequestrum formation; but it may be normal in the early stage, while bone scan will show increased uptake.

83. **(A)-T, (B)-F, (C)-T, (D)-T, (E)-F.** Prader–Willi syndrome is characterized by obesity, mental retardation, hypotonia, binge eating, strabismus, small hands and feet, and hypogonadism. It is associated with a small deletion on the long arm of chromosome 15.

84. **(A)-F, (B)-F, (C)-T, (D)-F, (E)-F.** The case presented is most likely due to pinworm infection (*Enterobius vermicularis*). Although the diagnosis can be made by the identification of the sharply pointed tail of the adult female gravid worms (thus the name of pinworms)

with a length of 1 cm, it is advisable to instruct the mother to preserve the worms in 75% ethyl alcohol and bring them to the office for microscopic examinations. Once the boy's problem is resolved, the mother will be able to sleep and the minor tranquilizer will not be necessary. Frequent bathing may offer symptomatic relief, and boiling of bed sheets and clothes may reduce transmission of infections. However, practical and useful therapeutic plans are established through thorough evaluation of data gathered from history, physicals, and laboratory results in a formal, professional office setting.

85. **(A)-T, (B)-T, (C)-T, (D)-T, (E)-F.** Occupational exposures include painters, plumbers, solderers, individuals working at lead-smelting plants, and individuals working at plants producing batteries, brass, ceramics, enamel, glass, insecticides, lubricants, and matches.

86. **(A)-F, (B)-F, (C)-T, (D)-F, (E)-F.** Abstinence is reliable, but not necessarily practical. The use of rubber condoms may inhibit spread of HIV. Regular, periodic HIV tests are also helpful in detecting HIV early.

87. **(A)-F, (B)-F, (C)-F, (D)-T, (E)-F.** Osteoid osteoma is a small, benign, painful bone lesion with normal ESR. The pain increases at night and is relieved by NSAIDs. There is local tenderness, and the affected limb may show atrophy, mostly located in the femur or tibia. Technetium bone scan increases uptake, and the treatment is surgical excision.

88. **(A)-T, (B)-T, (C)-T, (D)-T, (E)-T.** *Yersinia* infections are common. In children, infection occurs by the ingestion of contaminated foods, primarily milk products and tofu. The symptoms and signs may mimic acute appendicitis.

89. **(A)-F, (B)-T, (C)-T, (D)-F, (E)-T.** Contraindications include allergy to eggs, allergy to neomycin, pregnancy, immunodeficiency, systemic malignancy, and therapy with steroids or antineoplastic agents.

90. **(A)-F, (B)-T, (C)-T, (D)-F, (E)-T.** Atypical measles occurs in the recipients of killed measles vaccine after exposure to natural disease. Live, attenuated vaccine is recommended for children at the age of 15 months in nonendemic areas. Children at the age of 6 months may be vaccinated during epidemics. Children vaccinated before 1 year of age are to be revaccinated at 15 months of age.

91. **(A)-F, (B)-T, (C)-F, (D)-F, (E)-F.** Serious sequelae of pertussis vaccination that may last more than 1 year include (1) encephalopathy; (2) complex febrile seizures that are more than 10 minutes in duration, are repetitive over 24 hours, or are focal in nature; (3) afebrile seizures that are less than 30 minutes in duration. Serious sequelae unlikely to last 1 year include (1) simple febrile seizures; (2) anaphylaxis; and (3) shocklike episode with vascular collapse, hypotonicity, and unresponsiveness for more than 10 minutes.

92. **(A)-F, (B)-F, (C)-F, (D)-F, (E)-T.** Absolute contraindications to further pertussis vaccination include high fever (higher than 104.9°F), seizures, collapse with shocklike state, encephalopathy, and persistent and unusual high-pitched cry.

93. **(A)-T, (B)-T, (C)-T, (D)-F, (E)-F.** TTN is characterized by rapid improvement in 2 to 4 hours. Chest x-rays usually show prominent pulmonary vascular markings and occasionally cannot be differentiated from hyaline membrane disease. However, in 2 to 4 hours, the chest x-rays will clear up and physically the baby is in a good health status. The temperature is usually normal or even subnormal (hypothermia).

94. **(A)-T, (B)-T, (C)-F, (D)-F, (E)-F.** Kaposi's varicelliform eruptions are caused by herpes simplex. The distribution of eruptions in smallpox is centrifugal with the same stage of eruptions, while the distribution of eruptions in chickenpox is centripetal, with different stages (macules, papules, vesicles, and crusts) all simultaneously present.

95. **(A)-F, (B)-T, (C)-T, (D)-T, (E)-T.** Cretinism may show signs of mental retardation; dry, baggy skin; scanty, coarse hair; thick tongue;

umbilical hernia; coarse, harsh voice; short, pudgy extremities; and delayed dentition.

96. **(A)-T, (B)-T, (C)-T, (D)-T, (E)-T.** Precipitating factors include a positive family history; illnesses requiring hospitalization; loss of a parent through separation, divorce, or death; loss of a significant relationship with a friend or a pet; a move of the family from one residence or city to another; experiences that damage self-esteem, including school failure and social exclusion; and concerns of growing responsibilities.

97. **(A)-T, (B)-T, (C)-T, (D)-T, (E)-T.** Studies from New York City and Chicago revealed that 24 to 28% of schoolchildren had incomplete or inadequate immunizations. Many students failed vision tests for the 20/30 score, and there were students whose glasses had not been updated. Many students had untreated dental caries, and many students failed hearing tests. The prevalence of anemia and lead poisoning was low.

98. **(A)-T, (B)-T, (C)-T, (D)-T, (E)-T.** Over 50% of children use a primary-care physician. Twenty-five percent use a hospital clinic, with the remain-der seeking out neighborhood health centers, medical groups, and emergency rooms.

99. **(A)-T, (B)-T, (C)-T, (D)-T, (E)-T.** Lead poisoning in urban children is estimated to be less than 0.1%; however, in those children from lower socioeconomic sections of large cities living in old, poorly kept buildings built before 1950, the lead level is estimated to be 7 to 10%. For these high-risk groups, lead screening is necessary.

100. **(A)-T, (B)-T, (C)-T, (D)-T, (E)-T.** Battered child syndrome is frequently diagnosed by a high index of suspicion. Subdural hematoma with absence of diagnostic evidence is frequently caused by violent shaking. Stories of babies under 6 months old trying to get out of a crib and fracturing the femur are suspicious. The child with failure to thrive due to caloric deprivation usually has a weight and height less than the third percentile. Hot wa-

ter burns on the perineum are usually done by parents for the punishment of enuresis or resistance to toilet training.

101. **(A)-T, (B)-T, (C)-T, (D)-T, (E)-T.** Effective punishment must do at least four things: (1) Prevent avoidance of and escape from the punisher; (2) reduce the need for subsequent punishment; (3) not provide a model of aggressive behavior; and (4) avoid teaching the child a hateful attitude toward the punisher.

102. **(A)-T, (B)-T, (C)-T, (D)-T, (E)-F.** The following three procedures are useful in changing children's behavior: (1) Give clear signals. Make the rules clear so that the children know what is expected of them. Repeat the rules as necessary. (2) Ignore disruptive behaviors. Do not attend to the behaviors you wish to weaken. Get involved with other children showing behaviors you wish to strengthen. Praise a child showing behavior incompatible with disruptive behaviors. (3) Praise the children for improvement in behavior. Acknowledge the children who are behaving well, rather than badly. Tell the children what it is that they are doing that you approve of. Award privileges when the children show good behavior.

103. **(A)-T, (B)-T, (C)-T, (D)-T, (E)-T.** Neonatal convulsions usually point to a disorder of the central nervous system and suggest anoxic brain damage, intracranial hemorrhage, cerebral anomaly, subdural effusion, meningitis, tetany, or, rarely, pyridoxine deficiency, hypoglycemia, hyponatremia, or hypernatremia.

104. **(A)-T, (B)-T, (C)-T, (D)-T, (E)-T.** Stinging with hymenoptera insect allergy is best managed by desensitization therapy. The reactions after subsequent stinging have been markedly reduced in 90% of hyposensitized individuals. Local reaction includes swelling, itching, and burning; the systemic reaction includes generalized urticaria, anaphylactic shock (hypotension, cyanosis, unconsciousness), wheezing, dyspnea, laryngeal edema with hoarseness, abdominal pain, vomiting, and angioedema.

105. **(A)-T, (B)-T, (C)-T, (D)-T, (E)-F.** At 40 weeks, in addition, an infant will be able to creep or crawl.

106. **(A)-T, (B)-T, (C)-T, (D)-T, (E)-T.** The causes of jaundice during the first week of life include physiologic jaundice, cretinism, Crigler–Najjar syndrome, transient familial hyperbilirubinemia, novobiocin, vitamin K, sepsis, hepatitis, toxoplasmosis, cytomegalic inclusion disease, rubella, and galactosemia.

107. **(A)-T, (B)-T, (C)-F, (D)-F, (E)-T.** The causes of aseptic meningitis include bacteria (infections partially treated), parameningeal foci, virus, fungus, tuberculosis, malignancy, and trichinosis.

108. **(A)-T, (B)-F, (C)-T, (D)-T, (E)-T.** Iron deficiency in infancy is rarely due to acute hemorrhage. Sixty percent of body iron concentration at birth is contained in circulating hemoglobin.

109. **(A)-T, (B)-T, (C)-T, (D)-T, (E)-F.** Compared with adults, children are less likely to manifest vegetative signs of depression. However, they frequently develop sleep problems and loss of appetite. In smaller children, depression may lead to failure to thrive.

110. **(A)-T, (B)-T, (C)-F, (D)-T, (E)-T.** Petit mal is characterized by episodes of abrupt, momentary loss of consciousness accompanied by cessation of voluntary activities. While having a petit mal attack, some children may perform semipurposeful motor acts, such as snapping of fingers, patting movements, or walking around in circles (petit mal automatism). When attacks occur in close succession for a prolonged period of time, mental function is continually impaired, and the child remains dazed and confused. Myoclonic jerks may also present, known as petit mal status. The EEG abnormality consists of bursts of generalized bilaterally synchronous three-per-second spikes, and wave complexes appear, usually against a background of normal activity. Bursts lasting longer than 5 seconds are often associated with clinical attacks.

111. **(A)-T, (B)-T, (C)-T, (D)-T, (E)-F.** Wheezing is a musical, high-pitched, continuous expiratory (and sometimes inspiratory) sound, usually associated with a prolonged expiratory phase. It is caused by partial obstruction of the central, medium-sized airway. Wheezing is a common complaint in children, and the list of differential diagnoses includes asthma, cystic fibrosis, bronchiectasis, bronchiolitis, pneumonia, atelectasis, pulmonary tuberculosis, alpha-1-antitrypsin deficiency, foreign-body aspiration, hypersensitivity pneumonitis, and chronic aspiration.

112. **(A)-T, (B)-T, (C)-T, (D)-T, (E)-T.** Children react by vomiting to most insults, especially infections. Frequently, vomiting will precede fever.

113. **(A)-T, (B)-T, (C)-T, (D)-T, (E)-T.** A few patients have no abnormal physical findings, although some have maculopapular or urticarial rash, which usually disappears within 48 hours. Chest x-ray usually shows evidence of pneumonia before physical signs are apparent.

114. **(A)-F, (B)-T, (C)-T, (D)-T, (E)-T.** Cholesterol is deposited in the reticulum cells in the disease. The classic triad consists of punched-out lesions in the skull, bilateral exophthalmos, and diabetes insipidus. There is a variety of skin lesions, including a diffuse papular eruption of vesicular nature in the young patient; a scaly and petechial dermatitis; and a moist, denuded involvement in intertriginous areas.

115. **(A)-T, (B)-T, (C)-T, (D)-F, (E)-T.** Niemann–Pick disease is characterized in the tissues by vacuolated foam cells whose most striking chemical feature is the cytoplasmic accumulation of sphingomyelin (phospholipid).

116. **(A)-T, (B)-T, (C)-T, (D)-T, (E)-F.** The routine administration to an infant in the nursery of full therapeutic doses of an antibiotic effective against the staphylococcal strain from the day of admission through the day of discharge is not a preferable aspect of man-

agement. Erythromycin is usually the drug of choice; kanamycin is too toxic.

117. **(A)-F, (B)-F, (C)-F, (D)-T, (E)-F.** Diagnosis of croup is by characteristic clinical syndrome, including barking or seal-like cough, acute stridor, wheezing, mild respiratory distress, "steeple" sign on the posteroanterior view of the neck x-rays, fever, and normal or elevated WBCs.

118. **(A)-T, (B)-T, (C)-T, (D)-T, (E)-T.** There are no special diagnostic tests available; the diagnosis is by exclusion, using sound clinical judgment. Differential diagnosis is thus very important. It often includes epiglottitis, bacterial tracheitis, Ludwig's angina, peritonsillar abscess, diphtheria, paraquat poisoning, and foreign-body obstruction of the upper airway. These potentially life-threatening conditions must be identified because they require specific interventions.

119. **(A)-F, (B)-F, (C)-T, (D)-F, (E)-F.** Erythema infectiosum is called Fifth disease, characterized by facial erythema as "slapped cheek" rash. Erythema is developed in a fishnet-like pattern on the extremities, trunk, and buttocks. The eruption may recur at the previously affected sites of face and body in 2 to 3 weeks. Women with parvovirus exposure may develop arthritis and pruritus. Pregnant women may have an increased risk of spontaneous abortion.

120. **(A)-F, (B)-T, (C)-T, (D)-T, (E)-T.** Rickets is hypovitaminosis D, which may result in hypocalcemia (tetany, seizures), decreased linear growth in legs with bowing, rachitic rosary (enlargement) of the ribs, pathologic fractures, enlarged frontal bone, and delayed dentition. Breast-fed infants without adequate vitamin D intake are at increased risk.

121. **(A)-F, (B)-T, (C)-F, (D)-F, (E)-F.** In 1950, the childhood mortality (1 to 14 years) was 88/100,000. In 1979, it was 40/100,000 (dropped to one half); in 1985, it was 35/100,000; and in 1989, it was 32/100,000.

122. **(A)-T, (B)-T, (C)-F, (D)-F, (E)-F.** In 1990, the five leading causes of infant deaths (in descending order) were congenital anomalies, sudden infant death syndrome (SIDS), respiratory distress syndrome, disorders related to short gestation and unspecified low birth weight, and newborn affected by maternal complications of pregnancy. The sixth through tenth causes were intrauterine hypoxia and birth asphyxia; infections specific to the perinatal period; accidents and adverse effects; newborn affected by complications of placenta, cord, and membrane; pneumonia; and influenza.

123. **(A)-F, (B)-F, (C)-T, (D)-T, (E)-T.** In 1990, the six leading causes of childhood deaths ranging from 1 to 14 years (in descending order) were accidents and adverse effects, cancer, congenital anomalies, homicide, heart disease, pneumonia, and influenza.

124. **(A)-T, (B)-T, (C)-T, (D)-F, (E)-F.** There are 500 newly diagnosed neuroblastoma cases yearly. It accounts for 8% of all childhood tumors, yet accounts for 11% of total pediatric cancer deaths. Fifty percent occur at ages under 2; 75% occur at ages under 4. It is rare in individuals older than 14.

125. **(A)-T, (B)-T, (C)-F, (D)-T, (E)-F.** Common presentations of neuroblastoma include abdominal pain or mass, fever, weight loss, bone pain, anemia, diarrhea, and hypertension. Other symptoms of metastasis include enlarged liver, unilateral nasal obstruction, periorbital ecchymoses, and heterochromia iridis. Urinary VMA and HVA are increased.

126. **(A)-T, (B)-F, (C)-F, (D)-T, (E)-T.** Between 1982 and 1991, there were 1,724 AIDS deaths of children under 12 years of age (1% of total AIDS deaths). More than two or three adolescents with AIDS were infected through sexual contact with adults. Although only 440 people with AIDS (fewer than 1%) are between 13 and 19 years of age, the prevalence of HIV infection among adolescents is a source of concern. Because it takes an estimated 5 to 10 years for the HIV infection to

result in AIDS, many young adults who have AIDS contracted the virus as adolescents. Approximately 20% of people identified as having AIDS are between 20 and 29 years of age.

127. **(A)-F, (B)-F, (C)-T, (D)-T, (E)-F.** There are approximately 35 million adolescents in the United States, comparable with the number of elderly. The adolescents are relatively healthy, with an age-specific death rate of 1%. There are more females than males (male and female sex ratio is 100 to 134). They are a relatively underserved population.

128. **(A)-T, (B)-T, (C)-T, (D)-T, (E)-T.** For an adolescent to see a family physician, he or she needs parental approval (or consent, or at least encouragement), time away from school (unless evening or weekend hours are available), transportation to visit the office, money to pay for the visit, and enthusiasm to make a suitable appointment.

129. **(A)-F, (B)-F, (C)-F, (D)-F, (E)-F.** Only 12% of adolescents have regular physician contacts. Thirty-five percent were seen by family (general) physicians, and 23% by pediatricians. The average pediatrician visit lasts 8 minutes, with 7 seconds for anticipatory guidance. Less time is spent discussing issues pertinent to their health or well-being.

130. **(A)-F, (B)-F, (C)-T, (D)-T, (E)-F.** The following topics are what adolescents want to discuss with their physicians: nutrition (60% responded by physicians), growth (60%), alcohol use (44%), drug abuse (46%), birth control (33%), and STDs (26%).

131. **(A)-T, (B)-T, (C)-T, (D)-T, (E)-T.** To provide comprehensive and continuous total health care for adolescents, a biopsychosocial model is adopted to collect information on physical health (including traumas), home environment (family dynamics), school achievement (grades, awards, hobbies), work experiences, peer contacts (drug, cigarette, and alcohol habits), and sexual activities (contraceptives, HIV risks).

132. **(A)-F, (B)-F, (C)-T, (D)-T, (E)-F.** Adolescents are egocentric about their own existence and accordingly think the world revolves around them. Adolescents' obstructive behavior in the history-taking is but an attempt to shield themselves from inspection/evaluation by the physician, a self-protective action. Thus, an adolescent may become quiet, obnoxious, or irritating. The physician needs to respect the adolescent, show genuine trust and concern, encourage expression of feelings, and challenge the thought by raising questions. When rapport is established, the interview will become smooth and productive.

133. **(A)-F, (B)-T, (C)-F, (D)-T, (E)-T.** Adolescents are the underserved population. There has been a call by numerous groups, including the American Academy of Pediatrics and the American College of Physicians, to make adolescent medicine a greater component of medical education to address adolescents' special needs. Adolescents do have unique health-care needs, which largely derive from the diversity of cofactors that contribute to physical dysfunction, many with origins in psychologic and social development. With heightened interests from medical professionals, the health needs of adolescents will be met.

134. **(A)-F, (B)-F, (C)-F, (D)-F, (E)-T.** Transient synovitis of the hip is a self-limiting disease with unknown etiology. Often, the patient may elicit URIs of viral origin 1 to 2 weeks prior to the development of the hip synovitis.

135. **(A)-T, (B)-T, (C)-T, (D)-F, (E)-F.** During the first 2 months of life, the causal organisms reflect the maternal environment, most likely occurring in high-risk infants, including prematurity, prolonged rupture of membranes, and invasive fetal monitoring. The clinical syndrome may be dominated by hypotension and pneumonia.

136. **(A)-F, (B)-T, (C)-T, (D)-F, (E)-T.** From 2 months to 12 years, the most common bacterial agents for meningitis are *H. influenzae* type B, *S. pneumoniae,* and *N. meningitidis.*

Any acute febrile illness with temperature beyond 103°F has a high index of suspicion.

137. **(A)-T, (B)-F, (C)-T, (D)-F, (E)-F.** Wilms' tumor is a nephroblastoma with an incidence of 1/10,000 children. It accounts for 15% of all childhood neoplasms. The heritable form is inherited as an autosomal dominance with incomplete penetrance. It is associated with genitourinary anomalies, aniridia (blindness), microencephaly, mental retardation, and hemihypertrophy. Presenting symptoms include an asymptomatic abdominal mass which does not cross the midline. Hematuria, hypertension, and polycythemia may develop. The deletion of band P13 on chromosome 11 may be related to its oncogenesis.

138. **(A)-F, (B)-F, (C)-F, (D)-T, (E)-F.** The presentation is characteristic for transient synovitis ("toxic synovitis"), which should be differentiated from septic arthritis. Occasionally, the transient synovitis may show elevated temperatures and elevated ESR, and it should be differentiated from osteomyelitis, collagen diseases, and septic arthritis. When temperature is normal and ESR is not elevated, the differential diagnosis includes osteoid osteoma, Legg–Calvé–Perthes disease, and slipped capital femoral epiphysis. The slipped capital femoral epiphysis can be differentiated by roentgenograms, and Legg–Calvé–Perthes disease can be determined by bone scans.

139. **(A)-T, (B)-T, (C)-T, (D)-T, (E)-F.** Hypoplastic left heart syndrome is the underdevelopment of the left heart due to atresia of the aortic or mitral orifices and hypoplasia of the ascending aorta. The left ventricle is small and nonfunctional. Heart failure develops in the first few weeks of life manifested by dyspnea, hepatomegaly, weak or absent peripheral pulses, and a grayish-blue–colored skin.

140. **(A)-F, (B)-F, (C)-T, (D)-F, (E)-F.** Regardless of the mother's HBsAg status, all infants should receive three shots.

141. **(A)-T, (B)-T, (C)-T, (D)-T, (E)-T.** All infants are recommended to get vaccinations. Disease caused by HBV and its complications—cirrhosis and liver cancer—is preventable by vaccination. Universal infant immunization against HBV will prevent this serious and deadly disease.

142. **(A)-F, (B)-F, (C)-T, (D)-T, (E)-T.** The risk of becoming a carrier varies inversely with age and is highest in the neonatal period (90%), 25 to 50% for children aged 1 to 5 years, and lowest in adolescents and adults (6 to 10%). A carrier may increase the risk of developing cirrhosis and hepatoma.

143. **(A)-T, (B)-T, (C)-T, (D)-T, (E)-T.** HBV infection produces a typical illness in 5 to 15% of children 1 to 5 years of age. Symptomatic infections occur in 33 to 50% of older children and adults. Vaccination not only prevents hepatitis B; it also prevents carrier's status, which may develop into cirrhosis and hepatoma.

144. **(A)-F, (B)-T, (C)-T, (D)-T, (E)-T.** It is estimated that the prevalence of allergic rhinitis is around 5 to 22% of the total population. There are around 40 million people afflicted with it, and it accounts for 2.5% of physician visits. Immunoglobulin E (IgE) levels are highest and symptoms are most severe during puberty. The highest incidence is between 15 and 25 years; additional peak is at childhood and adolescence.

145. **(A)-F, (B)-F, (C)-T, (D)-F, (E)-F.** Circumcision is indicated in recurrent balanitis, posthitis, and paraphimosis. Most often, it is requested for cultural and religious customs. The incidence of URIs and cancer of the penis is reduced. The complications include hemorrhage, sepsis, excessive removal of foreskin, inadvertent amputation of the distal glands, and the formation of the urethrocutaneous fistulas. Contraindications include bleeding disorders, neonatal illnesses, genital anomaly, and prematurity.

146. **(A)-T, (B)-T, (C)-T, (D)-T, (E)-T.** There are more than 50,000 sickle cell patients, mostly African Americans. One African-American child in every 375 is affected by sickle cell

disease. It is the most prevalent genetic disease. In addition, the following ethnic groups are at a higher risk: those of Mediterranean, Caribbean, South and Central American, and East Indian ancestry, and Arabs. A universal screening of all infants is helpful in early identification of patients.

147. **(A)-T, (B)-F, (C)-T, (D)-T, (E)-F.** Many adolescent athletes believe that anabolic–androgenic steroid use may increase gains in strength and mass without exercise. Many also believe steroid use will increase vitality, maintain youth, promote physical growth, and guarantee sexual performance. Very few realize the side effects of premature epiphyseal closure, limiting further growth, testicular atrophy, male pattern baldness, facial hair in females, breast development in males, and dependence syndrome.

148. **(A)-T, (B)-T, (C)-T, (D)-T, (E)-T.** With prompt treatment by appropriate antibiotics, bacterial meningitis may leave no appreciable sequelae. However, neurologic sequelae may be found in 10 to 20% of the survivors whose treatments were delayed. Common sequelae include seizure disorders, hydrocephalus, mental retardation, hearing loss, hemiparesis, motor deficits, learning disability, and behavior problems. Hearing loss is of the sensorineural type, and bacterial meningitis is the leading cause of acquired deafness in infancy and childhood, accounting for 8 to 10% of cases of deafness in school-aged children.

149. **(A)-F, (B)-F, (C)-F, (D)-T, (E)-T.** Most sore throats (pharyngitis) are of viral origin; GABHS contributes to 10 to 20% (average of 15%). Treatment is penicillin for 10 days to prevent complications of rheumatic fever and glomerulonephritis.

150. **(A)-F, (B)-T, (C)-F, (D)-F, (E)-F.** An artificial intertriginous area is created under a wet diaper, predisposing to candidal infection, characterized by red base and satellite pustules.

151. **(A)-T, (B)-T, (C)-T, (D)-T, (E)-T.** GABHS is diagnosed by throat culture; however, systemic symptoms favor the diagnosis of GABH pharyngitis over viral infection. Common features include fever; inflamed tonsils with white exudate; tender, swollen cervical nodes; palatal petechiae; abdominal pain; headache; lethargy; anorexia; vomiting; malaise; and generalized urticaria. A scarlet fever rash is nearly always diagnostic. Hoarseness, cough, and rhinitis are more typical of viral pharyngitis.

152. **(A)-T, (B)-T, (C)-T, (D)-T, (E)-T.** Hemorrhagic disease of the newborn is due to deficiency of vitamin K-dependent coagulation factors. Prophylactic administration of vitamin K will prevent decline in prothrombin level and will reduce the possibility of hemorrhage.

153. **(A)-F, (B)-F, (C)-T, (D)-T, (E)-T.** Congenital rubella syndrome may include congenital heart diseases (pulmonary artery stenosis [PAS], PDA, VSD), mental retardation, cataract and glaucoma, and sensorineural hearing impairment.

154. **(A)-F, (B)-F, (C)-T, (D)-F, (E)-F.** Most common cold syndromes are due to rhinovirus, and antibiotics are not indicated. Many parents are unaware or fail to understand that viral disease of common cold does not respond to penicillin or ampicillin and thus seek antibiotics for cure. Instead of satisfying the parents' demand for antibiotics, it is better to explain the truth to the parents so that they will know not to seek antibiotics next time.

155. **(A)-T, (B)-T, (C)-T, (D)-T, (E)-T.** During childhood, 50% of physician visits for acute illness are related to common cold syndromes. Most common cold syndromes are benign, self-limited diseases, requiring symptomatic support for the patient and reassurance for the parent. However, the patient/parent/physician encounters are the basis of establishing rapport and the provisions of comprehensive, continuous, and total preventive health care.

156. **(A)-T, (B)-T, (C)-T, (D)-T, (E)-T.** The harmful effects of the sun may not be visible for photoaging until the age of 30s to 50s. Adolescence is the time to take preventive action by avoiding extended direct sun exposure, by wearing protective clothing and headgear, and by using a sun protection product with a sun protective factor (SPF) of at least 15. Adolescence is the time to begin, and one should continue for a lifetime.

157. **(A)-T, (B)-T, (C)-T, (D)-T, (E)-T.** By the time they are 18 years old, 65% of boys and 51% of girls are sexually active. Eleven percent of adolescent girls become pregnant each year, and 4% have an abortion. Adolescents who get pregnant while in high school are more likely to drop out of school, become dependent on welfare, and become single parents. Between 1950 and 1985, the nonmarital birth rate among adolescents younger than 20 years of age increased 300% for whites and 16% for blacks. One in four sexually active adolescents will contract an STD before graduating from high school. STD rates are substantially higher among black than white adolescents.

158. **(A)-T, (B)-T, (C)-T, (D)-T, (E)-T.** Cigarettes, alcohol, and marijuana are the first-line gateway drugs, which lead to other "hard" drugs. Adolescents who currently drink alcohol are 10 times more likely than nondrinkers to use marijuana and 11 times more likely to use cocaine.

159. **(A)-T, (B)-T, (C)-T, (D)-T, (E)-T.** Over the past 20 years, the suicide rate tripled among 10- to 14-year-olds and doubled among 15- to 19-year-olds. Whites are three times more likely than blacks to commit suicide. Abuse and neglect increased 74% during the past decade. Consequences of abuse include depression, insomnia, and other psychologic difficulties during adolescence and adulthood.

160. **(A)-T, (B)-T, (C)-T, (D)-F, (E)-F.** The MMR vaccine can be given at age 12 months during epidemics; MMR should not be given to pregnant women or women who plan to get pregnant in the next 3 months. MMR is needed for all children with positive HIV.

161. **(A)-T, (B)-T, (C)-T, (D)-T, (E)-F.** This is the same as the preexposure schedule: first visit—#1 shot; 1 month later—#2 shot, 6 months after #1 shot—#3 shot. A booster is not recommended.

162. **(A)-T, (B)-T, (C)-T, (D)-T, (E)-F.** This is the postexposure schedule: First visit—HBIG + #1 shot; 1 month later—#2 shot; 6 months from the first visit—#3 shot. A booster shot is not routinely recommended.

163. **(A)-T, (B)-T, (C)-T, (D)-T, (E)-T.** After age 5, HIB vaccines are given to children with chronic lung diseases, asplenia, sickle cell disease, and chemotherapy for Hodgkin's lymphoma.

164. **(A)-T, (B)-T, (C)-T, (D)-T, (E)-T.** DPT #4—acellular P vaccine; 4 to 6 years—DPaT #5 (acellular diphtheria–pertussis–tetanus vaccine), OPV #4, MMR #2; 14 to 16 years—TD.

165. **(A)-T, (B)-T, (C)-T, (D)-T, (E)-T.** At age 15 months, only one dose of HIB is necessary. This is an accelerated immunization program, and the interval between immunization visits can be shortened to 4 to 6 weeks (if necessary) to complete the series as soon as possible.

166. **(A)-T, (B)-T, (C)-T, (D)-T, (E)-T.** HIB vaccines are no longer needed for children beyond the age of 5; Hep vaccines are given in three dosages (first visit, 1 month later, 5 months later) for high-risk adolescents (drug abuse, multiple sexual partners, STDs, multiparity).

167. **(A)-T, (B)-T, (C)-T, (D)-T, (E)-T.** Spina bifida is a multifactorial trait. It occurs in 2 in 1000 live births. There is a higher incidence in patients of Northern European and Egyptians origins and a lower incidence in blacks, Asians, and Ashkenazi Jews. Spina bifida occulta may have no symptoms. Spina bifida manifesta may develop meningocele, hydromeningocele, hydrocephalus, UTI, incon-

tinence, muscle paralysis, clubfeet, dislocated hip, kyphosis, scoliosis, and mental retardation. Prenatal diagnosis with alpha-fetoprotein determination may be helpful.

168. (F)

169. (F)

170. (F)

171. (F)

172. (T)

173. (F)

174. (T)

175. (F)

176. (F)

177. (F)

178. (F)

179. (T)

180. (F)

181. (F)

182. (F)

183. (F)

184. (T)

185. (T)

186. (T)

187. (F)

The most common cause of pharyngotonsillitis is viral in origin and the treatment is symptomatic. Streptococcal sore throat requires a 10-day course of penicillin treatment. The identification of beta *Streptococcus* often needs positive throat culture (this patient's throat culture is negative) in addition to clinical findings. This patient's laboratory results fail to confirm the suspicion of anemia and the initiation of therapy can be delayed at this time. The eggs of *Ascaris lumbricoides* are characterized by bile-stained, mamillated outer shells. A single dose of pyrantel pamoate (11 mg/kg) is effective; a 2-day course of piperazine (75 mg/kg) is also commonly administered.

Also of Interest

New for 1998

CMDT on CD-ROM 1998
Expanded Multimedia Edition
McPhee et al.
1998, ISBN 0-8385-1480-4, A1480-1

The CURRENT Series

CURRENT Medical Diagnosis & Treatment 1998
Thirty-seventh Edition
Tierney et al.
1997, ISBN 0-8385-1524-X, A1524-6

CURRENT Pediatric Diagnosis & Treatment
Thirteenth Edition
Hay et al.
1997, ISBN 0-8385-1400-6, A1400-9

CURRENT Diagnosis & Treatment in Gastroenterology
Grendell et al.
1996, ISBN 0-8385-1448-0, A1448-8

CURRENT Diagnosis & Treatment in Orthopedics
Skinner
1995, ISBN 0-8385-1009-4, A1009-8

CURRENT Diagnosis & Treatment in Cardiology
Crawford
1995, ISBN 0-8385-1444-8, A1444-7

CURRENT Diagnosis & Treatment in Vascular Surgery
Dean et al.
1995, ISBN 0-8385-1351-4, A1351-4

CURRENT Surgical Diagnosis & Treatment
Tenth Edition
Way
1994, ISBN 0-8385-1439-1, A1439-7

CURRENT Obstetric & Gynecologic Diagnosis & Treatment
Eighth Edition
DeCherney & Pernoll
1994, ISBN 0-8385-1447-2, A1447-0

CURRENT Critical Care Diagnosis & Treatment
Bongard & Sue
1994, ISBN 0-8385-1443-X, A1443-9

CURRENT Emergency Diagnosis & Treatment
Fourth Edition
Saunders & Ho
1992, ISBN 0-8385-1347-6, A1347-2

Other Related Titles

Behavioral Medicine in Primary Care
Feldman & Christensen
1997, ISBN 0-8385-0636-4, A0636-9

Evidence-Based Medicine
A Framework for Clinical Practice
Friedland et al.
1998, ISBN 0-8385-2476-1, A2476-8

 To order or for more information, visit your local health science bookstore or call Appleton & Lange toll free at **1-800-423-1359**.